Essentials of Anesthesiology, Critical Care and Resuscitation
for Medical Students

Essentials of Anesthesiology, Critical Care and Resuscitation
for Medical Students

As per the Competency-based Medical Education Curriculum (NMC)

Mukul Chandra Kapoor

Professor, Head and Chief Consultant
Department of Anesthesiology and Critical Care
Amrita School of Medicine and Amrita Institute of Medical Sciences
Faridabad, Haryana, India

Formerly
Director Anesthesia
Max Hospitals
Saket, Delhi, India
and
Professor
Senior Adviser Anesthesiology and Cardiothoracic Anesthesiology
Armed Forces Medical Services
Pune, Maharashtra, India

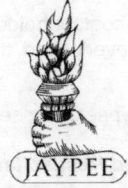

JAYPEE BROTHERS MEDICAL PUBLISHERS
The Health Sciences Publisher
New Delhi | London

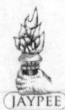 **Jaypee Brothers Medical Publishers (P) Ltd**

Headquarters

Jaypee Brothers Medical Publishers (P) Ltd
EMCA House, 23/23-B
Ansari Road, Daryaganj
New Delhi - 110 002, India
Landline: +91-11-23272143,+91-11-23272703,
+91-11-23282021,+91-11-23245672
Email: jaypee@jaypeebrothers.com

Corporate Office

Jaypee Brothers Medical Publishers (P) Ltd
4838/24, Ansari Road, Daryaganj
New Delhi 110 002, India
Phone: +91-11-43574357
Fax: +91-11-43574314
Email: jaypee@jaypeebrothers.com

Overseas Office

J.P. Medical Ltd
83 Victoria Street, London
SW1H 0HW (UK)
Phone: +44 20 3170 8910
Fax: +44 (0)20 3008 6180
Email: info@jpmedpub.com

Website: www.jaypeebrothers.com
Website: www.jaypeedigital.com

© 2023, Jaypee Brothers Medical Publishers

The views and opinions expressed in this book are solely those of the original contributor(s)/author(s) and do not necessarily represent those of editor(s) and publisher of the book.

All rights reserved. No part of this publication may be reproduced, stored or transmitted in any form or by any means, electronic, mechanical, photocopying, recording or otherwise, without the prior permission in writing of the publishers/editors.

All brand names and product names used in this book are trade names, service marks, trademarks or registered trademarks of their respective owners. The publisher is not associated with any product or vendor mentioned in this book.

Medical knowledge and practice change constantly. This book is designed to provide accurate, authoritative information about the subject matter in question. However, readers are advised to check the most current information available on procedures included and check information from the manufacturer of each product to be administered, to verify the recommended dose, formula, method and duration of administration, adverse effects and contraindications. It is the responsibility of the practitioner to take all appropriate safety precautions. Neither the publisher nor the author(s)/editor(s) assume any liability for any injury and/or damage to persons or property arising from or related to use of material in this book.

This book is sold on the understanding that the publisher is not engaged in providing professional medical services. If such advice or services are required, the services of a competent medical professional should be sought.

Every effort has been made where necessary to contact holders of copyright to obtain permission to reproduce copyright material. If any have been inadvertently overlooked, the publisher will be pleased to make the necessary arrangements at the first opportunity.

Inquiries for bulk sales may be solicited at: jaypee@jaypeebrothers.com

Essentials of Anesthesiology, Critical Care and Resuscitation for Medical Students

First Edition: **2023**

ISBN: 978-93-5465-977-5

Printed at Rajkamal Electric Press, Kundli, Haryana.

"I cannot teach anybody anything. I can only make them think."
—**Socrates**

Dedicated to...

I express my deep gratitude and dedicate this book to my parents, who made me capable and molded me to achieve heights. I also dedicate this book to my family for supporting me in all my academic ventures. I also dedicate it to my students for showing me how to teach better. Last but not least, I dedicate this to the almighty omnipresent, omnipotent, and omniscient Paramatma and Amma, the revered selfless, and compassionate saint who showered her grace on me.

Contributors

Anju Grewal
Professor and Head
Department of Anesthesiology
Dayanand Medical College and Hospital
Ludhiana, Punjab, India

Archana Puri
Senior Consultant
Department of Anesthesiology
Max Super Speciality Hospital
Saket, New Delhi, India

Maj Gen Deepak Kumar Sreevastava
Senior Consultant
Anesthesiology
Armed Forces Medical Services

Deepak Pahwa
Senior Consultant and Assistant Professor
Department of Anesthesiology
Amrita School of Medicine and
Amrita Institute of Medical Sciences
Faridabad, Haryana, India

DV Bhargava
Classified Specialist
(Anesthesiology and Cardiothoracic Anesthesiology)
Armed Forces Medical Services

Indu Bala Maurya
Assistant Professor
Department of Anesthesiology
Kalyan Singh Super Speciality Cancer Institute
Lucknow, Uttar Pradesh, India

Jyotsna Agarwal
Associate Professor
Department of Anesthesiology and Critical Care
Hamdard Institute of Medical Sciences and Research
New Delhi, India

Kiran Mahendru
Assistant Professor
Department of Anesthesiology
Dayanand Medical College and Hospital
Ludhiana, Punjab, India

Mahima Singh
Associate Consultant
Institute of Anesthesiology
Pain and Perioperative Medicine
Sir Ganga Ram Hospital
New Delhi, India

Manish Bharti
Senior Consultant and Intensivist
Department of Critical Care Medicine
School of Medical Sciences and Research
Greater Noida, Uttar Pradesh, India

Manish Jagia
Director
Department of Anesthesia and Critical Care
Moolchand Hospital
New Delhi, India

Meenu Chadha
Head
Department of Anesthesia
Convenient Hospitals Ltd
Indore, Madhya Pradesh, India

Mukul Chandra Kapoor
Professor, Head and Chief Consultant
Department of Anesthesiology and Critical Care
Amrita School of Medicine and
Amrita Institute of Medical Sciences
Faridabad, Haryana, India

Parul Gupta
Consultant Anesthesia
Madhukar Rainbow Children's Hospital
New Delhi, India

Pradeep Pendlaya
Professor
Department of Anesthesiology
ASRAM Medical College
Eluru, Andhra Pradesh, India

Pratibha Jain Shah
Professor and Head
Department of Anesthesiology and Critical Care
Pt Jawahar Lal Nehru Memorial Medical College
Raipur, Chhattisgarh, India

Pratibha Panjiar
Associate Professor
Department of Anesthesiology and Critical Care
Hamdard Institute of Medical Sciences and Research
New Delhi, India

Rakesh Garg
Additional Professor
Department of Onco-Anesthesia and Palliative Medicine
Dr BR Ambedkar Institute Rotary Cancer Hospital
All India Institute of Medical Sciences
New Delhi, India

Rakhee Goyal
Head of Department
Anesthesia and Critical Care
Madhukar Rainbow Children's Hospital
New Delhi, India

Brig Ram Murti Sharma (Retd)
Professor and Head
Department of Critical Care Medicine
School of Medical Sciences and Research
Greater Noida, Uttar Pradesh, India

Contributors

Maj Gen Rashmi Datta (Retd)
Senior Consultant
Professor and Head
Department of Emergency
Medicine
Hamdard Institute of Medical
Sciences and Research and Hakeem
Abdul Hameed Centenary Hospital
New Delhi, India

Richa Jain
Associate Professor
Department of Anesthesiology
Dayanand Medical College and
Hospital
Ludhiana, Punjab, India

Sangeeta Pathak
Director—Transfusion Services
Max Super Speciality Hospital
Saket, New Delhi, India

Shaloo Garg
Senior Consultant and Professor
Department of Anesthesiology
Amrita School of Medicine and
Amrita Institute of Medical Sciences
Faridabad, Haryana, India

Lt Col Siddharth Chaki
Classified Specialist Anesthesiology
Armed Forces Medical Services

Sunil Singh
Consultant and Head
Department of Anesthesiology and
Medical Superintendent
Aarvy Healthcare
Gurugram, Haryana, India

Tushar Chokshi
Consultant Anesthesiology
Sterling Hospital
Ahmedabad, Gujarat, India

Preface

The sciences of Anesthesiology has made tremendous progress in the last century. The specialty matured from being an allied subject to achieving the status of a significant primary specialty. For the last few decades, working knowledge of Anesthesiology has been considered essential for any practicing doctor. Specialization in Anesthesiology is a favored choice with the growth in importance of the subject.

When the Medical Council of India revised the Undergraduate Training of Medical Graduates Curriculum in 2018–19, the syllabus committee decided to enhance the time allocated to Anesthesiology teaching significantly. The earlier teaching program devoted just a few lectures and a short posting to the specialty. The new curriculum ('Competency-based Undergraduate Curriculum for the Indian Medical Graduate' of the Medical Council of India - Vol III) allocates 40 lectures/demonstrations to subjects in the domain of Anesthesiology, Critical Care, and Resuscitation. The syllabus also mandates multiple technical competency-based assessments and Objective Structured Clinical Examination (OSCE) based assessments in these domains.

With a change in the medical education administration from the Medical Council of India (MCI) to the National Medical Council (NMC), significant medical education reforms are in process. A standard Medical Graduates Exit Examination is now mandatory per the NMC Act. All universities are required to follow a common prescribed syllabus and teaching pattern.

Most available Anesthesiology books focus on postgraduate training. With no concise book available, medical graduates struggle to acquire anesthesiology knowledge and depend on MCQs primarily taught in coaching centers. This book is written to cater to the requirements of undergraduate medical students. The book covers all topics prescribed in the new syllabus and also covers Resuscitation, an essential skill for all medical personnel.

The chapters are written by experienced authors who are all established and accomplished teachers. I am highly indebted to them for sparing their valuable time to promote this effort selflessly. I could plunge into this project due to their kind acceptance to advance knowledge in the fields dear to them.

The language of the book is simple yet technical. The knowledge in the book is limited to matters relevant to undergraduates. An attempt has been made to explain the subject in precise and easy-to-understand language. The book also covers all the knowledge needed to answer OSCE on different topics successfully.

Emergency medicine has been given the status of an independent subject. No standard textbook covers most aspects of managing patients in the emergency room. A significant part of this book will also benefit students of emergency medicine. This book will also benefit students trained outside the country. It will help provide the requisite knowledge to clear the Foreign Medical Graduates Examination.

I am very grateful to the whole team of M/s Jaypee Brothers Medical Publishers (P) Ltd, New Delhi, India, who helped and guided me, Shri Jitendar P Vij (Group Chairman), Mr Ankit Vij (Managing Director), Mr MS Mani (Group President), Dr Madhu Choudhary (Director-Educational Publishing), Ms Pooja Bhandari (Production Head), Ms Sunita Katla (Executive

Assistant to Group Chairman and Publishing Manager), Ms Samina Khan (Executive Assistant to Director-Educational Publishing), Dr Sakshi Sanjeevani (Development Editor), Mr Rajesh Sharma (Production Coordinator), Ms Seema Dogra (Cover Visualizer), Mr Rahul Jadli (Proofreader), Mr Dinesh Bhardwaj (Typesetter), Mr Gopal Singh Kirola (Graphic Designer) and their team members, for all their support to work in this project and make it a success. Without their cooperation, I could not have completed this project.

Mukul Chandra Kapoor

Contents

1. **Evolution of Anesthesiology as a Specialty**   1
   - History 1
   - Development of Anesthetic Techniques 5
   - Development of Anesthetic Agents 7
   - Development of Anesthesia Delivery Systems 8

2. **Preoperative Assessment**   10
   - Objective of Preanesthetic Checkup 10
   - General Clinical Assessment 11
   - Preoperative Assessment of Organ Systems 13
   - Preoperative Testing 14
   - Risk Assessment 14
   - Preoperative Optimization 16
   - Preoperative Drug Therapy 18
   - Informed Consent and Counseling 19
   - Premedication 19
   - Review PAC 20

3. **Airway**   22
   - Anatomy of the Upper Airway 22
   - Anatomy of Lower Airway 28
   - Upper Airway Obstruction 28
   - Airway Management 29
   - Airway Assessment 31
   - Laryngoscopy and Intubation 31
   - Managing Difficult Airway 33
   - Emergent Tracheostomy 34

4. **General Anesthesia**   37
   - Process of GA 38

5. **Pharmacology of Anesthetic Agents**   44
   - Intravenous Agents 44
   - Propofol 44
   - Etomidate 45
   - Sodium Thiopental (Penthotal) 46
   - Ketamine 47
   - Midazolam 48
   - Dexmedetomidine 49
   - Inhalation Agents 49
   - Nitrous Oxide 49
   - Isoflurane 51
   - Sevoflurane 51
   - Desflurane 52
   - Opioids 53
   - Morphine 53
   - Fentanyl 55
   - Remifentanil 56

6. **Structure of Neuromuscular Junction and Neuromuscular Transmission in Skeletal Muscles**   58
   - Neuromuscular Junction 58
   - Neuromuscular Transmission 60
   - Neuromuscular Blockers 61
   - Monitoring Neuromuscular Blockade 63
   - Antagonism of Neuromuscular Block 63
   - Residual Neuromuscular Blockade 64

7. Central Neuraxial Blockade   67

- Relevant Spinal Cord Anatomy 67
- Technique of Performing CNB 71
- Types of CNB 71
- Principle of Central Neuraxial Blockade 73
- Physiological Effects of Central Neuraxial Block 74
- Management After CNB 75
- Complications of CNB 76

8. Regional Anesthesia   78

- Regional Anesthesia 78
- Physiology of Pain 79
- Local Anesthetics 79
- Brachial Plexus Block 84
- Lower-extremity Blocks 89

9. Monitoring of a Patient Under Anesthesia   92

- Standards for Monitoring Under Anesthesia 93

10. Ensuring Homeostasis Under Anesthesia   108

- Arterial Blood Pressure Control 108
- Oxygen Carriage 109
- Acid-base Balance and its Relevance 112
- Body Temperature 113
- Intervention to Maintain Homeostasis Based on Monitoring 113

11. Organ Protection During Anesthesia   116

- Central Nervous System Protection 116
- Cardiovascular System Protection 119
- Respiratory System Protection 119
- Kidney Protection 120
- Gastrointestinal Tract and Liver Protection 121
- Others 121

12. Postoperative Care   123

- Post-anesthesia Care Unit 123
- Postoperative Nausea and Vomiting 125
- Mental Care 125
- PACU Recovery Assessment 125
- Crash Cart 126
- Common Complications in the Recovery Room 126

13. Intensive Care   129

- Structure and Function of Intensive Care Unit 129
- Management of an Unconscious Patient 130
- Mechanical Ventilation 131
- Hemodynamic Management and Vasoactive Drug Therapy 133
- Monitoring 135
- Prevention and Treatment of Infections 136
- Nutrition 137
- General Supportive and Nursing Care 138

14. Special Anesthesia Techniques   140

- Total Intravenous Anesthesia 140
- Conduct of TIVA 142
- Equipment used in TIVA/TCI System 143
- Types of Automated Drug Delivery Systems 143
- Drugs used 145

- Monitoring in TIVA 145
- Advantages of TIVA 146
- Disadvantages of TIVA 146
- Anesthesia at Remote Locations 146
- Dissociative Anesthesia 148

15. Daycare Anesthesia — 151

- Set up for Daycare Surgery 151
- Principles of Daycare Anesthesia 152
- Goals of Daycare Anesthesia 153
- Mode of Daycare Anesthesia 153
- Preanesthetic Checkup 153
- General Anesthesia 155
- Total Intravenous Anesthesia 155
- Regional Anesthesia 156
- Monitored Anesthesia Care 156
- Postoperative Management 156
- Other Considerations and Discharge 157
- Procedural Sedation Inside and Outside Operation Room 157

16. Anesthesia for the Elderly — 160

- Changes in the Cardiovascular System 160
- Changes in the Respiratory System 161
- Changes in the Hepatic and Renal System 161
- Changes in the Central Nervous System 161
- Changes in the Endocrine System 162
- Changes in the Musculoskeletal System 162
- Changes in the Pharmacology 162
- Preoperative Evaluation 162
- Laboratory Investigations 163
- Intraoperative Management 163
- Anesthetic Management 163
- Points to Remember 164
- End of Surgery Checklist 164
- Postoperative Care 164
- Rehabilitation 165

17. Intravenous Access and Fluid Therapy — 166

- Intravenous Access 166
- Peripheral Venous Access 166
- Central Venous Access 169
- Fluid Therapy 172
- Common Causes of Preoperative Hypovolemia 172
- Fasting before Anesthesia and Surgery 173
- Preoperative Fluid Intake Reduces the Risk of Pulmonary Aspiration 173
- Enhanced Recovery After Surgery 173
- Intravenous Fluids 173
- Preoperative Fluid Therapy 174

18. Blood and Blood Product Transfusion — 178

- Importance of Blood Transfusion 179
- Sourcing Blood Products 180
- Blood Grouping and Cross-matching 180
- Blood Component Preparation and Preservation 181
- Uses of Blood Components 182

- Quality Control of Blood Production and Storage 182
- Safe Transfusion and Monitoring 183
- Blood Transfusion Reactions 184
- Challenges in Blood Transfusion 184

19. Pain Pathways and Chronic Pain — 186

- Nociception 186
- Pain 186
- Pain Processing 188
- Pain Pathways 188
- Pain Inhibitory Mechanisms 190
- Pain Assessment 191
- Pain Management 192

20. Patient Safety in Operation Theatre — 197

- Patient Identification Safety 197
- Role of Communication in Safety 198
- Safety in Patient Positioning 198
- Safety Under Anesthesia 200
- Infection Control 200
- General Safety Measures 202

21. Resuscitation — 205

- Basic Cardiopulmonary Life Support (BCLS) for an Adult 206
- Early High-quality CPR 208
- Comprehensive Cardiopulmonary Life Support (CCLS) for an Adult 210
- Early Recognition and Management of Precardiac Arrest Condition 211
- Early Comprehensive Life Support and Post-resuscitation Care 215
- Pediatric Cardiopulmonary Resuscitation 215
- Trauma Care 221
- Life-threatening Thoracic Injuries 224

22. Medicolegal Aspects and Investigation of Anesthetic Death — 229

- Medical Ethics 229
- Consent 229
- Standard of Care 230
- Recordkeeping 230
- Mortality Related to Anesthesia 232

23. Career in Anesthesiology — 236

- Evolution of Modern Anesthesiology 236
- Changing Profile of the Anesthesiologist 237
- Extended Role of Anesthesiologists Today 237
- Advances in Drugs and Techniques 237
- Postgraduate Training 237
- Subspecialization in Anesthesiology 238
- Increased Demand for Anesthesiologists 238
- Critical Care 238
- Perioperative Medicine 238
- Perioperative Surgical Home 239
- Safe Surgery 239
- Pride of Place in the Medical Profession 239
- Anesthesiology as a Career 239

24. Ethics in Clinical Anesthesiology — 241

- Ethics in Anesthesia Practice 241
- ASA Ethical Guideline 243

Index — 245

Competency Table

Number	COMPETENCY The student should be able to	Core (Y/N)	Suggested Teaching Learning method	Suggested Assessment method	Chapter	Page number
AS1.1	Describe the evolution of anesthesiology as a modern specialty	N	Lecture	Written/ Viva voce	1	1
AS1.2	Describe the roles of Anesthesiologist in the medical profession (including as a peri-operative physician, in the intensive care and high dependency units, in the management of acute and chronic pain, including labor analgesia, in the resuscitation of acutely ill)	K	Lecture	Written/ Viva voce	1, 23	3, 192, 237
AS1.3	Enumerate and describe the principle of ethics as it relates to anesthesiology	K	Lecture	Written/ Viva voce	24	241
AS1.4	Describe the prospects of anesthesiology as a career	K	Lecture	Written/ Viva voce	23	236
AS2.1	Enumerate the indications, describe the steps and demonstrate in a simulated environment, Basic Life Support in adults, children and neonates	K/S	DOAP session	Skill assessment	21	206
AS2.2	Enumerate the indications, describe the steps and demonstrate in a simulated environment, Advanced Life Support in adults and children	S	DOAP session	Skill assessment	21	210
AS3.1	Describe the principles of preoperative evaluation	K	Lecture, Small group discussion	Written/ Viva voce	2	10
AS3.2	Elicit, present and document an appropriate history including medication history in a patient undergoing surgery as it pertains to a preoperative anesthetic evaluation	S	DOAP session, Bedside clinic	Skill station	2	10

Competency Table

Number	COMPETENCY The student should be able to	Core (Y/N)	Suggested Teaching Learning method	Suggested Assessment method	Chapter	Page number
AS3.3	Demonstrate and document an appropriate clinical examination in a patient undergoing general surgery	S	DOAP session, Bedside clinic	Skill station	2	14
AS3.4	Choose and interpret appropriate testing for patients undergoing surgery	S	DOAP session, Bedside clinic	Skill station	2	14
AS3.5	Determine the readiness for general surgery in a patient based on the preoperative evaluation	S	DOAP session, Bedside clinic	Skill station	2	14
AS3.6	Choose and write a prescription for appropriate premedications for patients undergoing surgery	S	DOAP session, Bedside clinic	Skill station	2	19
AS4.1	Describe and discuss the pharmacology of drugs used in induction and maintenance of general anesthesia (including intravenous and inhalation induction agents, opiate and non-opiate analgesics, depolarizing and non depolarizing muscle relaxants, anticholinesterases)	K	Lecture, Small group discussion	Written/ Viva voce	5	44
AS4.2	Describe the anatomy of the airway and its implications for general anesthesia	K	Lecture, Small group discussion	Written/ Viva voce	3	22
AS4.3	Observe and describe the principles and the practical aspects of induction and maintenance of anesthesia	S	Lecture, Small group discussion, DOAP session	Written/ Viva voce	4	38
AS4.4	Observe and describe the principles and the steps/techniques in maintenance of vital organ functions in patients undergoing surgical procedures	S	Lecture, Small group discussion, DOAP session	Written/ Viva voce	10	108
AS4.5	Observe and describe the principles and the steps/techniques in monitoring patients during anesthesia	S	Lecture, Small group discussion, DOAP session	Written/ Viva voce	9	92

Competency Table

Number	COMPETENCY The student should be able to	Core (Y/N)	Suggested Teaching Learning method	Suggested Assessment method	Chapter	Page number
AS4.6	Observe and describe the principles and the steps/techniques involved in day care anesthesia	S	Lecture, Small group discussion, DOAP session	Written/ Viva voce	15	151
AS4.7	Observe and describe the principles and the steps/techniques involved in anesthesia outside the operating room	S	Lecture, Small group discussion, DOAP session	Written/ Viva voce	15	157
AS5.1	Enumerate the indications for and describe the principles of regional anesthesia (including spinal, epidural and combined)	K	Lecture, Small group discussion	Written/ Viva voce	7	70
AS5.2	Describe the correlative anatomy of the brachial plexus, subarachnoid and epidural spaces	K	Lecture, Small group discussion	Written/ Viva voce	7,8	67,84
AS5.3	Describe the principles and steps/techniques involved in peripheral nerve blocks	S	Lecture, Small group discussion, DOAP session	Written/ Viva voce	8	80
AS5.4	Describe the pharmacology of commonly used drugs and adjuvant agents in regional anesthesia	S	Lecture, Small group discussion, DOAP session	Written/ Viva voce	8	79
AS5.5	Observe and describe the principles and steps/techniques involved in caudal epidural in adults and children	S	Lecture, Small group discussion, DOAP session	Written/ Viva voce	7	73
AS5.6	Observe and describe the principles and steps/techniques involved in common blocks used in surgery (including brachial plexus blocks)	S	Lecture, Small group discussion, DOAP session	Written/ Viva voce	8	84
AS6.1	Describe the principles of monitoring and resuscitation in the recovery room	S	Lecture, Small group discussion, DOAP session	Written/ Viva voce	12	123

Competency Table

Number	COMPETENCY The student should be able to	Core (Y/N)	Suggested Teaching Learning method	Suggested Assessment method	Chapter	Page number
AS6.2	Observe and enumerate the contents of the crash cart and describe the equipment used in the recovery room	S	Lecture, Small group discussion, DOAP session	Written/ Viva voce	12	126
AS6.3	Describe the common complications encountered by patients in the recovery room, their recognition and principles of management	K	Lecture, Small group discussion, DOAP session	Written/ Viva voce	12	126
AS7.1	Visit, enumerate and describe the functions of an intensive care unit	S	Lecture, Small group discussion, DOAP session	Written/ Viva voce	13	129
AS7.2	Enumerate and describe the criteria for admission and discharge of a patient to an ICU	S	Lecture, Small group discussion, DOAP session	Written/ Viva voce	13	130
AS7.3	Observe and describe the management of an unconscious patient	S	Lecture, Small group discussion, DOAP session	Written/ Viva voce	13	130
AS7.4	Observe and describe the basic setup process of a ventilator	S	Lecture, Small group discussion, DOAP session	Written/ Viva voce	13	131
AS7.5	Observe and describe the principles of monitoring in an ICU	S	Lecture, Small group discussion, DOAP session	Written/ Viva voce	13	135
AS8.1	Describe the anatomical correlates and physiologic principles of pain	K	Lecture, Small group discussion, DOAP session	Written/ Viva voce	19	186
AS8.2	Elicit and determine the level, quality and quantity of pain and its tolerance in patient or surrogate	S	Lecture, Small group discussion, DOAP session	Written/ Viva voce	19	191

Competency Table

Number	COMPETENCY The student should be able to	Core (Y/N)	Suggested Teaching Learning method	Suggested Assessment method	Chapter	Page number
AS8.3	Describe the pharmacology and use of drugs in the management of pain	K	Lecture, Small group discussion, DOAP session	Written/ Viva voce	19	193
AS8.4	Describe the principles of pain management in palliative care	K	Lecture, Small group discussion, DOAP session	Written/ Viva voce	19	192
AS8.5	Describe the principles of pain management in the terminally ill	K	Lecture, Small group discussion, DOAP session	Written/ Viva voce	19	192
AS9.1	Establish intravenous access in a simulated environment	S	Small group discussion, DOAP session	Skill assessment	17	166
AS9.2	Establish central venous access in a simulated environment	S	Small group discussion, DOAP session	Skill assessment	17	169
AS9.3	Describe the principles of fluid therapy in the preoperative period	K	Lecture, Small group discussion, DOAP session	Written/ Viva voce	17	172
AS9.4	Enumerate blood products and describe the use of blood products in the preoperative period	K	Lecture, Small group discussion, DOAP session	Written/ Viva voce	18	179
AS10.1	Enumerate the hazards of incorrect patient positioning	K	Lecture, Small group discussion, DOAP session	Written/ Viva voce	20	198
AS10.2	Enumerate the hazards encountered in the perioperative period and steps/ techniques taken to prevent them	K	Lecture, Small group discussion, DOAP session	Written/ Viva voce	20	198

Competency Table

Number	COMPETENCY The student should be able to	Core (Y/N)	Suggested Teaching Learning method	Suggested Assessment method	Chapter	Page number
AS10.3	Describe the role of communication in patient safety	K	Lecture, Small group discussion, DOAP session	Written/ Viva voce	20	198
AS10.4	Define and describe common medical and medication errors in anesthesia	K	Lecture, Small group discussion, DOAP session	Written/ Viva voce	20	199

CHAPTER 1

Evolution of Anesthesiology as a Specialty

Mukul Chandra Kapoor

Learning Objectives

- History of anesthesia as a specialty
- Some interesting anecdotes from history
- Evolution of anesthesia techniques
- Evolution of anesthetic drugs
- Evolution of anesthesia machines

HISTORY

AS1.1: Describe the evolution of Anesthesiology as a modern specialty.

"Anesthesia is the most humane of all of man's accomplishments, and what a merciful accomplishment it was!" —Joseph Lewis

In ancient times, simple surgical procedures were performed after producing unconsciousness by crude methods. Methods used to facilitate surgery included making patients semi-conscious by alcohol ingestion, herbal mixture ingestion, hypnotism, witchcraft, blows to the head, carotid artery compression, and physical restriction by strongmen. Most methods were innocuous and ineffective. The effective ones were unsafe and often lethal. Most herbal mixtures used were concoctions of alkaloids extracted from plants, like opium poppy.

Barbaric surgeons performed surgery without analgesia or sedation. Major surgery was performed in dirty operating rooms without antisepsis while the patients were screaming and struggling against the knife.

One 19th-century renowned infamous surgeon, Robert Liston, claimed that he could take apart a man's leg in 30 seconds (**Fig. 1**). He accidentally amputated his assistant's fingers and slashed a spectator's coat during one such operation. The spectator died of fright, and both the assistant and the patient succumbed to gangrene.

Nitrous Oxide and Ether Rave Parties

Nitrous oxide and ether were used as recreational gases in the later part of the 18th

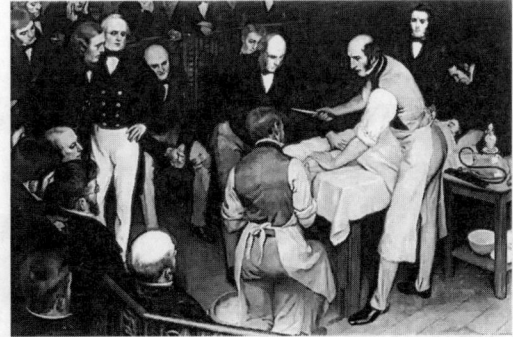

Fig. 1: Robert Liston performing his famed amputation.

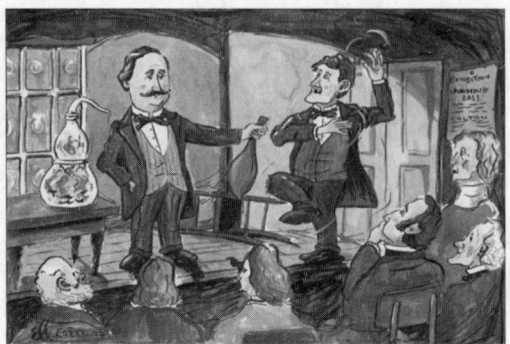

Fig. 2: Laughing gas Frolic Party.

century, when 'laughing gas parties' and 'ether frolics' were in vogue (**Fig. 2**). After inhalation of nitrous oxide, commercial demonstrations of expected abnormal behavior of people and its inhalation's euphoria led to Davy's coining of its name as 'laughing gas' in 1799. Davy also described that it eased the pain of his erupting wisdom tooth. Nitrous oxide was used successfully for an amputation performed painlessly by John Hunter, the 'father' of modern surgery, but its value was not appreciated then.

The Saga of Horace Wells

Horace Wells (**Fig. 3**), a Connecticut dentist, had sought ways of easing the pain of extracting the rotten teeth of patients. Horace Wells attended a "Grand Exhibition" of nitrous oxide by Gardner Q Colton. He noticed that a young man (Samuel Cooley), who had inhaled the gas, injured his shin yet did not display any apparent discomfort. Wells had one of his teeth removed by a colleague after inhaling the gas without experiencing pain. However, when Wells demonstrated a tooth extraction at the Harvard Medical School in 1845, the medical student volunteer cried in pain, and he was called a 'humbug.' Wells became a manic depressive soon after being dismissed as a charlatan.

William Thomas Green Morton

William Morton (**Fig. 4**), who had been Wells's student and colleague, and had helped with the demonstration, recognized that a 'better' agent was required. As a medical student at Harvard, Charles Jackson (**Fig. 5**), a chemistry teacher, majorly influenced him. Morton studied ether and tested it in animals and his patients. He proposed a demonstration of his method at the Massachusetts General Hospital. John Warren, a surgeon, invited him to demonstrate his technique on 16 October 1846. Before a large audience, Morton administered diethyl ether vapor to patient Gilbert Abbott while Warren excised the patient's neck tumor. The patient displayed no sign of pain or distress. Anesthesia was formally born with this first successful public demonstration. After the demonstration, Morton exclaimed, "Gentlemen, this is no humbug."

Considering the importance of this event, the hall where Morton demonstrated his discovery was later named **Ether Dome** (**Fig. 6**). The Ether Dome is today a National Historic Landmark and a popular tourist spot. Morton is recognized as the 'Father of Modern

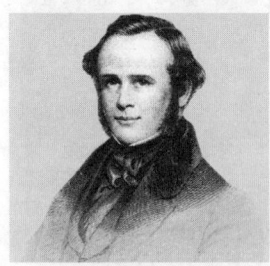

Fig 3: Horace Wells

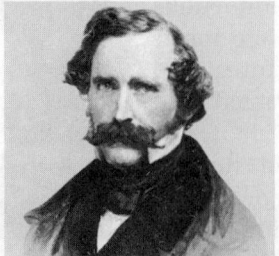

Fig 4: WTG Morton

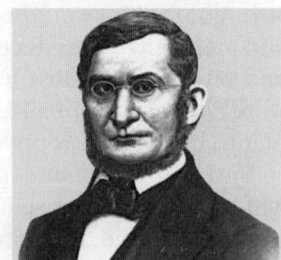

Fig 5: Charles Jackson

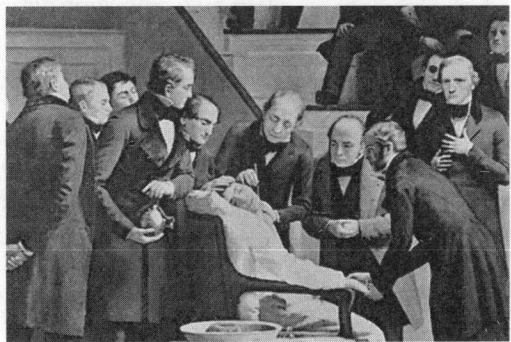

Fig. 6: Demonstration of ether at the ether dome.

word 'anaisthesis', which means loss of sensation, particularly to touch). A new term, "etherization," was coined.

The world celebrated the miracle of "painless" surgery. The news of pain-free surgery spread like wildfire across the globe, and soon, other agents like nitrous oxide and chloroform were used to administer anesthesia. These advances led to a series of discoveries and consequently heralded the development of complex surgical procedures supported by the newly discovered science of anesthesia.

Anesthesia,' and 16 October is celebrated internationally as World Anesthesia Day.

Controversy on Credit for the Discovery

Morton tried to patent the agent, but ethics prevented that. However, the scientific credit remained in dispute. The controversy between Morton, Jackson, and Wells over the primacy of the discovery raged. There is evidence that ether was used for surgery by others in 1842, but the practitioners did not communicate it. The 'Ether Monument' in Boston, to commemorate this epic event, thus does not mention the discoverer's name (**Fig. 7**).

The Name 'Anesthesia'

Anesthesia was suggested by Oliver Wendell Holmes Sr for the delirious state produced by ether (derived from the Greek

Global Spread of Anesthesia

The global spread of the news of the first successful anesthetic administration was fast considering the communication limitations of the times. The first anesthetics in Britain were administered on 19 December 1846 at two different sites.

Robert Liston, London's infamous and leading surgeon, demonstrated, in public, an amputation under ether on 21 December 1846. James 'Young' Simpson, an enthusiastic advocate of anesthesia, pioneered inhalation analgesia for women in labor despite religious and medical concerns regarding its safety and use. He also discovered the anesthetic properties of chloroform in 1847 while searching for a better drug.

The First Specialist Anesthetists

> **AS1.2:** Describe the roles of Anesthesiologist in the medical profession (including as a peri-operative physician, in the intensive care and high dependency units, in the management of acute and chronic pain, including labor analgesia, in the resuscitation of acutely ill).

Junior surgical team members administered anesthesia in the initial days. Their knowledge of physiology and pharmacology was limited. No standard equipment was available, and no drug dosages were defined. As a result, the mortality and morbidity associated with anesthesia were significant.

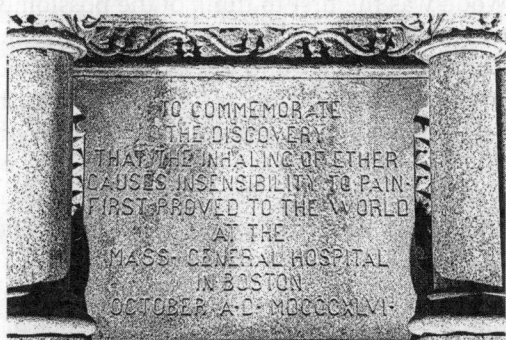

Fig. 7: The inscription on the ether monument in Boston.

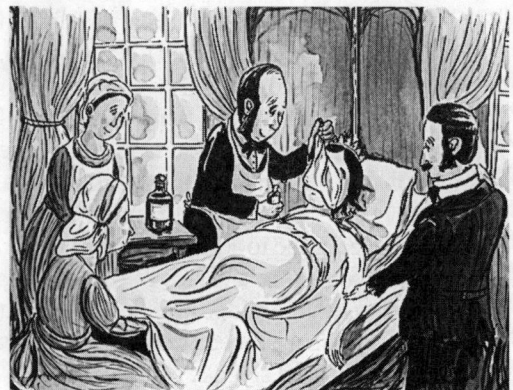

Fig. 8: A cartoon depicting chloroform administration to Queen Victoria. Note the handkerchief through which she inhaled.

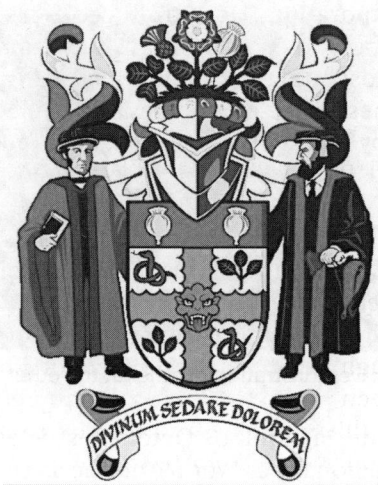

Fig. 9: The crest of the British Royal College of Anaesthetists with the two supporters of the arms.

Dr John Snow, a London-based physician, took the initiative to develop skills to deliver the anesthetics and published some instructional literature. In 1853, his eminence as a practitioner of anesthesia earned him an invite to administer labor analgesia with chloroform to Queen Victoria for the birth of Prince Leopold (**Fig. 8**). He administered chloroform again to the queen in 1857 for the birth of Princess Beatrice. Anesthesia thus received royal patronage. The royal seal of approval established chloroform as one of the blessings of the age.

Joseph Thomas Clover took over the mantle of John Snow after his death. Clover's significant contribution was to the administered anesthetic concentration and the monitoring of the patient. The British royal warrant designated the pioneer anesthetists, John Snow and Joseph Clover, as the 'supporters' of the arms of the College Crest of the Royal College of Anaesthetists. The motto on the scroll at the shield's base said in Latin '*Divinum Sedare Dolorem.*' meaning '*It is divine to appease the pain*' (**Fig. 9**).

The Resurgence of Nitrous Oxide

In the USA, Colton continued doing demonstrations of extracting teeth under the effects of nitrous oxide and established a commercial venture for dental extraction under the effects of the gas. This technique for dental extractions reached London in 1868. Clover found that simultaneous nitrous oxide use speeded up the induction of anesthesia with ether. The simultaneous use of nitrous oxide initiated combinations of several drugs rather than a more extensive and potentially toxic dose of one drug.

Discovery of Local Anesthesia

Nerve compression and application of ice to peripheries before surgery were used in the late 1700s to numb the areas for surgery. Alexander Wood was the first to think of the possibility of producing nerve blockade by direct drug injection around a nerve. He injected morphine around nerves as no drug with local anesthetic properties was discovered. Wood has been called the "father-in-law" of local anesthesia for giving the concept of local anesthesia without demonstrating it, as he lacked an agent that worked locally.

In 1847, James Young Simpson suggested that 'local' anesthesia could be more beneficial than general. In 1868, Sir Benjamin Ward Richardson discovered that spraying ether on a surface numbed the area by cooling it by evaporation. He introduced freezing of the part with an ether spray, and it became the most practical method of using local anesthesia. The ether spray was replaced in 1880 by ethyl chloride. This technique was termed '*Refrigeration*' or '*Freezing*' anesthesia.

Cocaine

In the 1700s and 1800s, South Americans routinely chewed Coca leaves for social, medicinal, recreational, and religious purposes. Although the stimulant effects of Cocaine had been known for years, the numbing effects of this South American alkaloid were first noted only in 1860. In 1884, Sigmund Freud published a review of the systemic effects of Cocaine which mentioned its numbing effect, but that went unnoticed.

Karl Koller

Karl Koller, a Vienna-based Ophthalmologist, was looking at ways to numb the eye for surgery. Koller experimented with several substances to numb the eye without success. Karl Koller had a eureka moment when he accidentally tasted a sample of cocaine given by Freud and realized that it numbed his tongue. He immediately prepared a suspension of cocaine crystals and experimented with its use on the cornea of a frog. The trials progressed quickly to clinical use, and Koller read his paper on local anesthesia with cocaine at a conference on September 15, 1884.

The discovery news spread globally within days, thanks to the recent innovation of the electric telegraph. Koller's work was translated and published in different parts of the world. His work was the trigger for developing regional/local anesthesia, and within months, most peripheral nerve block techniques were described.

Cocaine Goes into Disrepute

Cocaine was soon sold everywhere and in almost everything. The ingredients of the original recipe for coca-cola-included Coca leaves. Cocaine advertisements said it could "make the coward brave, the silent eloquent, and render the sufferer insensitive to pain." Had Cocaine been restricted to local anesthesia and few other medical uses, it would have become the 'wonder drug' of medicine. Medical literature published hundreds of case reports of "cocainism" - severe addictions with a damaging effect on nerves, hallucinations, delusions, and emaciation. Many addicts were medical practitioners who had experimented on themselves, including the luminary Sigmund Freud.

Newer Local Anesthetics

New anesthetic drugs were sought to replace cocaine. Ernest Fourneau synthesized Amylocaine in 1903, while Alferd Einhorn developed procaine in 1904. Procaine was safe and replaced cocaine to become the standard local anesthetic. In 1925, Karl Meischer synthesized dibucaine, and in 1928 Otto Eisleb synthesized tetracaine. Both were effective long-acting local anesthetics, but their systemic toxicity limited their use. In the mid-1940s, Nils Löfgren and Bengt Lundquist developed lignocaine. In 1957, Bo af Ekenstam synthesized mepivacaine and bupivacaine. To reduce systemic toxicity, purified S-enantiomers levobupivacaine and ropivacaine, rather than racemic mixtures, were introduced commercially in 1996.

DEVELOPMENT OF ANESTHETIC TECHNIQUES

Infiltration Anesthesia

In 1895, Karl Ludwig Schleich promoted infiltration anesthesia by cutaneous infiltration of a mixture of 0.2% sodium chloride with 0.02% cocaine. A large volume of dilute local anesthetic is needed to perform surface surgery. Schleich's technique is still relevant, particularly with the current enthusiasm for 'tumescent anesthesia.'

Conduction Block

The first conduction block, by injecting five drops of 2% cocaine solution close to a metacarpal branch of the ulnar nerve to remove a bullet from the patient's little finger, was by William Burke. However, the credit for realizing its potential goes to William Stewart Halsted and his associate John Hall of New York. In 1891, François-Franck was the first to apply the term 'block' to the infiltration of a nerve trunk, and it blocked both motor and sensory nerves, with sensory blockade becoming apparent more rapidly than the motor.

Additives to Local Anesthetics

In 1885, Corning believed that locally injected cocaine was removed by the capillary circulation and began researching means to prolong its action. He applied a compressive bandage tourniquet proximal to the injection site to prolong the anesthesia. Heinrich FW Braun added epinephrine to reduce the absorption of the drug (a chemical tourniquet). The term '*conduction block*' was also coined by Braun.

Intravenous Regional Anesthesia

August Karl Gustav Bier published the first report of intravenous regional anesthesia, still referred to as the infamous Bier block. Bier occluded the circulation in a segment of the arm with two tourniquets and injected a solution of dilute procaine through a venous cutdown in the isolated segment. The injected drug diffused through the limb producing direct vein anesthesia in just a few minutes.

Spinal Anesthesia

The mortality associated with general anesthesia was high with sparse knowledge of its safe administration. The first spinal anesthetic with cocaine was administered by J Leonard Corning, a neurologist, in 1885. The name *Spinal Anesthesia* too was coined by him. He hypothesized that the spinal blood vessels would carry the cocaine via communicating vessels into the spinal cord. There was no mention of cerebrospinal fluid or the insertion depth into the spinal space. Ironically, the first spinal anesthetic was administered six years before the first lumbar puncture.

Lumbar Puncture

The credit for the initial description and popularization of the lumbar puncture goes to Heinrich Irenaeus Quincke. In 1891, he used needles (with an internal diameter of 0.5–1.2 mm) to enter the subarachnoid space via a paravertebral approach. Bier and his colleague, August Hildebrandt, administered the spinal anesthetic to each other to demonstrate the effects. Both developed a severe headache that lasted for days. Spinal anesthesia was recognized after Bier published his well-known work in 1899 and displayed that it could produce a profound block with a minimum amount of the drug. After Bier's paper, interest in spinal anesthesia spread rapidly, and in the next two years, there were more than 1000 publications on spinal anesthesia.

Wooley and Roe Case

Two patients, Wooley and Roe, developed permanent painful spastic paresis after spinal anesthesia. In the legal trial of these cases in 1953, spinal anesthesia was implicated in the complication. This adversity severely impacted the popularity of spinal anesthesia. Fortunately, a follow-up analysis of over 10,000 spinal anesthetics failed to demonstrate any significant neurological disease and re-established it as a safe and effective means of providing anesthesia.

Epidural Anesthesia

Jean Enthuse Sicard, a neurologist, published the first report on epidural analgesia in 1901. He administered cocaine through the sacral hiatus to treat sciatica and tabes. Independently in the same year, Fernand

Cathelin used the same technique for surgical anesthesia. In 1921, the Spanish surgeon Fidel Pagés-Miravé used a lumbar epidural approach for surgery, but he, unfortunately, died in an accident before this was published. In 1931, Achille Dogliotti published the first report on identifying the epidural space and injection of local anesthetics. In 1947, Manuel Martinez Curbelo of Cuba used a Tuohy needle and a small ureteral catheter to provide continuous lumbar epidural analgesia. In 1943, John Bonica used the lumbar epidural for labor analgesia for his wife's complicated delivery.

Regional Anesthesia

In 1902, Harvey Cushing coined the name regional anesthesia to block a nerve plexus during general anesthesia. The work of Gaston Labat greatly facilitated the spread of regional anesthesia at the Mayo Clinic in Rochester, Minnesota. Most current techniques of regional anesthesia were devised in the early twentieth century.

Balanced Anesthesia

In 1902, Harvey Cushing advocated combining local with general anesthesia to decrease the stress of surgery. In 1926, Lundy used 'balanced anesthesia' for the triad of sleep, analgesic, and local anesthetic block. Balanced anesthesia today implies a triad of sleep produced by either inhaled or intravenous agents, profound analgesia, and muscle relaxation.

DEVELOPMENT OF ANESTHETIC AGENTS

Sodium Pentothal

Sodium thiopental was first used in humans on March 8, 1934, by Dr Ralph M Waters and rapidly became the ultrafast acting barbiturate of choice for induction of anesthesia. Thiopental went into disrepute for causing several anesthetic deaths in victims of the attack on 'Pearl Harbor.' Of the 344 wounded administered thiopentone, 331 survived. The mortality of the 13 victims was probably due to hypovolemic shock. It was thus not justified to blame thiopentone for the deaths. Thiopentone remained the primary anesthesia induction agent for a very long time. Propofol has replaced thiopentone as the primary induction agent in the last two decades.

Inhaled Anesthetics

The first generation of inhaled anesthetics (ether and chloroform) though safe to use, were comparatively crude and associated with multiple adverse effects. Several second-generation inhaled anesthetics (ethyl chloride, ethylene, propylene, and trichloroethylene) were tried to seek an ideal anesthetic agent. However, all of them were explosive, except trichloroethylene, and associated with hepatic and cardiac toxicity. Trichloroethylene decomposed to release phosgene (a poison) when warmed in the presence of soda lime. The third generation (methoxyflurane, halothane, enflurane, isoflurane, sevoflurane, and desflurane) are all fluorinated anesthetics. The newer agents are associated with early awakening, eye-opening, response to verbal command, and orientation to person, place, and time.

Muscle Relaxation

A significant challenge in thoracic and abdominal surgery was the requirement of high inhalation anesthetic concentrations for muscle relaxation, which resulted in cardiac/respiratory depression and delayed recovery. In 1942, Harold Griffith and Enid Johnson of Montreal, Canada, used South American arrow poison 'curare' to introduce neuromuscular blockade. This method required anesthetists to maintain the airway to allow mechanical lung ventilation for gas exchange.

Depolarizing neuromuscular blocker suxamethonium was described as early as

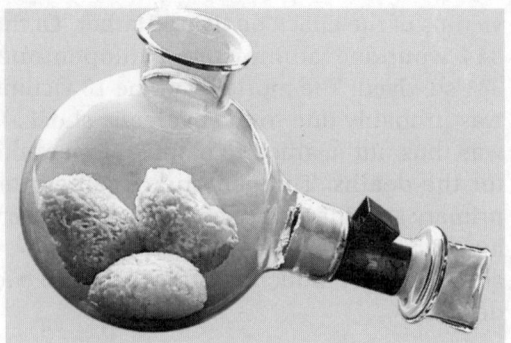

Fig. 10: Replica of Morton's two-necked glass globe containing an ether-soaked sponge.

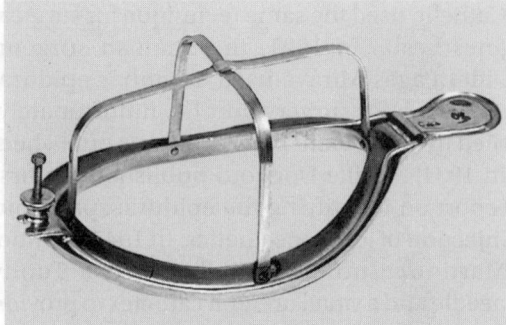

Fig. 11: Schimmelbusch mask.

1906 but came into medical use only in 1951. The adverse effects of the agent have limited its role in clinical practice. New short and long-duration non-depolarizing neuromuscular blocker agents replaced curare as the main relaxant in the 1980s.

DEVELOPMENT OF ANESTHESIA DELIVERY SYSTEMS

Early Anesthesia Delivery Systems

Anesthesia delivery systems had a humble beginning, like a handkerchief or a folded cloth. Labor analgesia was administered to Queen Victoria by pouring chloroform over a folded cloth. Morton's all-important presentation of anesthesia used "a small two-necked glass globe" containing an ether-soaked sponge, which he patented (**Fig. 10**). To overcome this patent restriction, clinicians poured ether directly onto a small bell-shaped sponge held firmly over the patient's nose and mouth.

Schimmelbusch Masks

The Schimmelbusch mask (**Fig. 11**) was a popular open breathing system until the 1950s in the western world (still used in some developing countries). The mask consists of a wireframe covered with several layers of gauze and applied to the patient's face over the mouth and nose. Its use involved pouring ether over the gauze, and the patient spontaneously inhales the vaporized ether.

Boyle's Machine

Henry Edmund Gaskin Boyle, a leading English anesthetist, invented the first commercially successful anesthesia machine in 1917. It was a modification of the American Gwathmey-Woolsey Nitrous Oxide-Oxygen apparatus. The Boyle machine (**Fig. 12**)

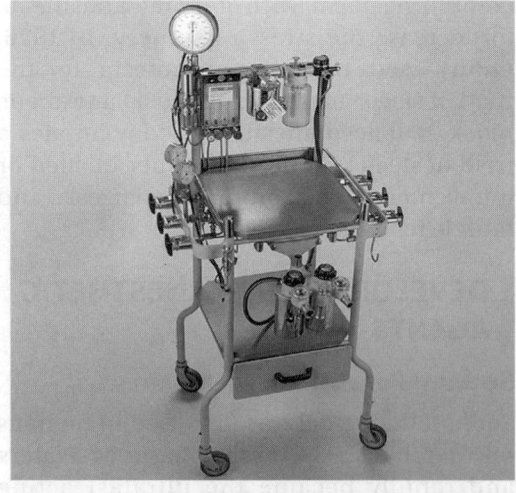

Fig. 12: Boyle's machine.

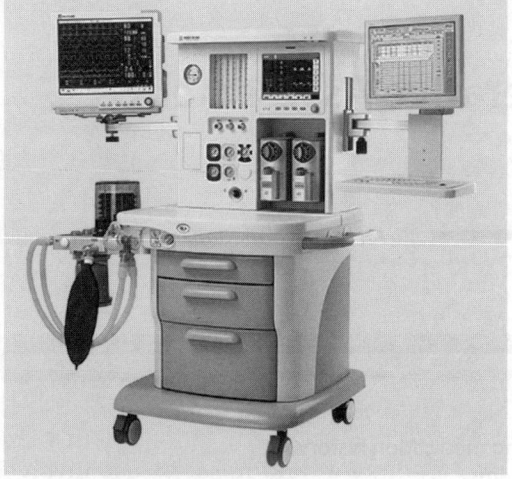

continued in production for over 50 years until the advent of the modern anesthesia machines with mechanical ventilators, vaporizers, and advanced monitoring. The current generation of advanced anesthesia delivery systems is called anesthesia workstations (**Fig. 13**).

Fig. 13: A modern anesthesia workstation.

MULTIPLE CHOICE QUESTIONS

1. **Nitrous oxide is called the 'laughing gas' because:**
   a. People start laughing after inhaling it
   b. People named it 'laughing gas,' the failure of the first public demonstration of its use
   c. People used to laugh at the abnormal behavior of people who inhaled it
   d. None of the above

2. **WTG Morton is called the 'Father of Modern Anesthesia' because:**
   a. He was the first to demonstrate the anesthetic effects of nitrous oxide
   b. He was the first to demonstrate the anesthetic effects of chloroform
   c. He was the first to demonstrate the anesthetic effects of cocaine
   d. He was the first to demonstrate the anesthetic effects of ether

3. **Karl Koller demonstrated the local anesthetic effects of drugs by using the following agent to numb the eye:**
   a. Cocaine   c. Procaine
   b. Lignocaine   d. Sensorcaine

4. **The first spinal anesthetic was administered by:**
   a. August Bier
   b. J Leonard Corning
   c. Heinrich Irenaeus Quincke
   d. John Snow

5. **The Schimmelbusch mask was:**
   a. A mask for the resuscitation of a newborn
   b. An open breathing system for anesthetic agent delivery
   c. Mask used to protect from airborne microbes
   d. Mask used in operating rooms to prevent infection

Answers
1. c   2. d   3. a   4. b   5. b

CHAPTER 2

Preoperative Assessment

Richa Jain, Kiran Mahendru, Anju Grewal

Learning Objectives

- Purpose of preoperative assessment
- Elicit and document appropriate history, including medication history
- Preoperative assessment of the major organ systems
- Preoperative investigations
- Risk assessment
- Determine the readiness for surgery and ASA grading
- Preoperative optimization
- Preoperative drug therapy
- Informed consent
- Preanesthetic counseling
- Premedication
- Preoperative medication
- Review preanesthetic check-up

INTRODUCTION

AS3.1: Describe the principles of preoperative evaluation.

Preoperative assessment is the clinical assessment performed before administration of any anesthetic and is referred to as a pre-anesthetic checkup (PAC). It aids the anesthesiologist in identifying preexisting medical diseases, assessing the patient's perioperative risk, preparing them for anesthesia, and formulating/tailoring the best anesthetic plan. This process is used to educate the patient about anesthesia and the perioperative period, answer all their queries and obtain written informed consent. It also serves as a medium to establish a good rapport between anesthesiologists with the patient.

OBJECTIVE OF PREANESTHETIC CHECKUP

AS3.2: Elicit, present and document an appropriate history including medication history in a patient undergoing surgery as it pertains to a preoperative anesthetic evaluation.

The goal of PAC is to reduce perioperative risk and morbidity, enhance the quality of patient care and outcome as well as reduce hospital costs. The information obtained during preoperative assessment helps identify the underlying basis for the surgery, determine the extent of co-morbidities, initiate interventions

Table 1: Summary of the preanesthetic assessment plan.

Age/gender/height/weight	Diagnosis/procedure/nature of surgery	Allergies/adverse reactions
Previous anesthetic/surgical history Malignant hyperthermia/adverse reactions Airway difficulty	**Current history** **Current medications** Over the counter, illicit drug **Fasting status**	**General physical examination** Vital signs including pain Venous access Pallor/cyanosis/clubbing/jugular veins Pedal edema Back and spine examination
Airway Previous history of difficult airway, sleep apnea **Examination:** To follow line of sight approach: Nasal patency, malar region, face, teeth, mouth opening, mallampati class, thyromental distance, neck circumference and mobility		**Cardiovascular** Congenital heart disease, hypertension, coronary heart disease, heart failure, cardiomyopathy, valvular disease, angina, dyspnea, orthopnea, exercise tolerance
Pulmonary Upper respiratory tract infections/pneumonia, tobacco smoking, asthma, COPD, cough, dyspnea, sleep apnea, O_2/inhaler/steroid use, pneumothorax		**Neurologic system** Stroke, seizures, syncope, head injury, raised ICP, altered mental status, headache, neuromuscular disease, spinal cord injury, paresthesia
GI/ Hepatic Jaundice, nausea/vomiting, cirrhosis, hepatitis, bowel obstruction, hiatus hernia, reflux, alcohol use		**Endocrine/metabolic** Diabetes, thyroid disease, rheumatoid arthritis, steroid use
Renal Insufficiency, failure, dialysis		**Infectious** COVID-19, HIV, influenza, TB, foreign travel.
Hematological Anemia, bleeding diathesis, transfusions, chemotherapy, coagulopathy		**Miscellaneous** Obesity, menstrual history/pregnancy, past major trauma, psychiatric illness, history of substance abuse or addictions

COPD: chronic obstructive pulmonary disease; ICP: increased intracranial pressure; TB: tuberculosis.

for preoperative optimization, and choose necessary preoperative testing. Preoperative evaluation primarily consists of history and physical examination pertinent to the patient and planned surgery. In addition to history and examination, reviewing previous anesthetic records is useful in detecting the problems encountered during anesthetic exposure and any adverse reactions to specific anesthetic agents. The evaluation must be complete and accurate to identify potential complications. The PAC document serves as a medico-legal document. **Table 1** summarizes the PAC plan routinely followed.

GENERAL CLINICAL ASSESSMENT

The PAC generally starts with the history of present illness, indication for surgery, and the planned procedure. Information regarding current and past medical problems, current medications, previous surgical procedures, previous anesthetic exposures, and any anesthesia-related complications are sought. It is important to elicit a history of allergy to any medication and substance or drug abuse. As part of general physical examination, heart/pulse rate (HR) with rhythm, blood pressure (BP), respiratory rate (RR), oxygen saturation by pulse oximetry (SpO$_2$), temperature, single breath holding time, degree of pain, weight, height, and BMI are determined. The presence of pallor, jugular venous distention, edema, cyanosis, clubbing, icterus, and lymphadenopathy are noted. Peripheral veins are inspected for intravenous accessibility, while the back and spine are also assessed for the presence of any obvious anatomical abnormality.

Airway

Assessment of the patient's airway is an integral part of the PAC to ensure safe airway management. It aims to predict the potential for difficulty with bag-mask ventilation, laryngeal mask airway insertion and ventilation, laryngoscopy, endotracheal intubation, front of neck access difficulty, and extubation when a patient is planned for general anesthesia. It intends to develop an airway management plan along with backup alternative plans ahead of time to avoid an unanticipated difficult airway.

Historical Evaluation

Information from focused history or medical records is evaluated about the airway. History of previous difficult intubation, surgical intervention on the airway or cervical spine, radiation, trauma, rheumatoid arthritis, diabetes mellitus, obstructive sleep apnea, snoring, and cervical spine disease are useful in predicting a difficult airway.

Focused Airway Examination

The evaluation of the airway follows the line-of-sight method, which involves examining the multiple airway features along the line of sight systematically from parts of the face, nose, mouth, and neck; and thereby recording all the variations from the normal as difficult or available (**Table 2**).

Modified Mallampati (MMP) class (**Fig. 1**) is assessed by asking the patient (in a sitting or upright position) to open his/her mouth and protrude the tongue maximally without phonation, with the observer being at eye level with the patient. This test gives an idea of the relationship between tongue size and the size of the oral cavity. It predicts how easily the

Table 2: Components of preoperative airway examination that suggest difficult airway.

Focused airway examination	Variation
Nose	Deformed, narrow nares/nasal passage, blocked nostril(s)
Malar region, cheeks	Deformed, masses, flowing beard
Mouth	Deformed, microstomia
Teeth	Edentulous, missing, bucked, loose irregular, overbite (maxillary incisors anterior to mandibular incisors) Inter-incisor distance <4 cm
Oral cavity	Mallampati Class > II, High arched, narrow, or cleft palate, space-occupying masses
Lower jaw	Receding, prognathic, injury, mass
Lower jaw subluxation	Inability to protrude mandibular incisors anterior to maxillary incisors
Mandibular space	Short chin (thyromental distance < 3 fingerbreadths), poor compliance, swelling
Neck	Short, thick, swelling, deformity, >40–42 cm of neck circumference and inability to palpate cricothyroid membrane
Head-neck range of movement	Limited to less than <90°

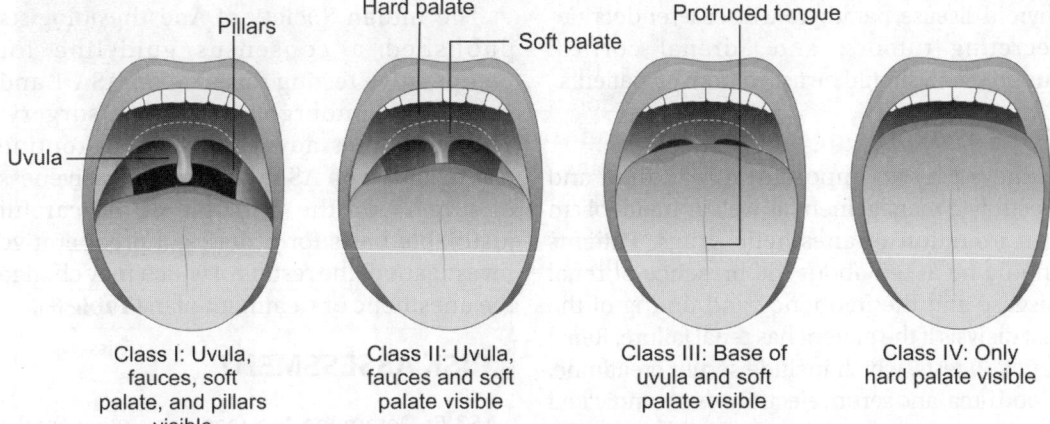

Fig. 1: Modified Mallampati classification.

tongue can be displaced by a laryngoscope blade during intubation. MMP > II indicates an anticipated difficult airway.

PREOPERATIVE ASSESSMENT OF ORGAN SYSTEMS

Once the general assessment is completed, the evaluation is focused on the heart, lungs, brain, and other organs affected by diseases reported by the patient.

Cardiovascular System

The cardiovascular system is assessed to identify signs and symptoms of uncontrolled hypertension, unstable cardiac diseases such as myocardial ischemia, congestive heart failure, and significant arrhythmias.

Symptoms of chest pain, palpitations, breathlessness on exertion, and syncope should be sought to exclude cardiovascular diseases. The auscultatory examination should assess for murmurs suggestive of valvular heart diseases, abnormal rhythm, abnormal heart sounds (third or fourth heart sound) suggestive of heart failure, and bruits over carotid arteries in patients with a history of stroke. Peripheral pulses are examined to exclude peripheral vascular disease or congenital heart diseases.

Pulmonary System

Patients are questioned regarding cough with or without expectoration, wheezing, difficult breathing, stridor, and snoring. History of current or recent upper respiratory tract infection, tuberculosis, asthma, and smoking is also obtained. The examination involves examining breathing patterns and accessory muscle use, auscultation to detect decreased or abnormal breath sounds, wheezing, and crepitations.

Neurologic System

Patients with pre-existing neurologic disorders risk aggravating their problems after anesthetic exposure. A history of stroke, symptoms of cerebrovascular disease, seizures, pre-existing neuromuscular disease, or nerve injuries should be sought in all patients. In healthy patients, a neurologic examination can be accomplished through simple observation, while it may be extensive in patients with coexisting diseases. Testing of muscle power, sensation, and reflexes may be important in patients for whom the anesthetic plan or surgical procedure may result in a change in condition.

Endocrine System

Questions directed to history or symptoms of endocrine diseases that may affect the perioperative course, such as diabetes mellitus, thyroid disease, parathyroid disease, endocrine-secreting tumors, and adrenal cortical suppression, should be asked from all patients.

Renal System

Kidneys play an important role in fluid and electrolyte management as well as metabolism and excretion of anesthetic drugs. Patients should be asked about the presence of renal disease and the frequency and timing of the last dialysis if the patient has renal failure. Renal function tests, which include serum creatinine, blood urea, and serum electrolytes, are indicated in patients with co-existing renal diseases.

Hepatic System

The liver is primarily responsible for plasma protein production, synthesis of coagulation factors, metabolism, and clearance of drugs. Patients with liver diseases should be enquired about history specific to its risk factors, such as previous blood transfusions, illicit drug use, or excessive alcohol intake. History of bruising or bleeding as coagulation disorders may discourage the choice of regional anesthesia. On physical examination, signs of underlying liver disease, such as jaundice, spider nevi, ascites, hepatosplenomegaly, or palmar erythema, should be assessed.

PREOPERATIVE TESTING

> **AS3.3:** Demonstrate and document an appropriate clinical examination in a patient undergoing general surgery.
> **AS3.4:** Choose and interpret appropriate testing for patients undergoing surgery.

The 2012 ASA Practice Advisory for Preanesthesia Evaluation states that routine preoperative tests should not be ordered in an asymptomatic patient. Selective preoperative tests may be ordered with the purpose of guiding or optimizing perioperative management. Specific information from the medical record, history, physical examination, and the type of invasiveness of the planned procedure and anesthesia help guide preoperative testing.

The Indian Society of Anesthesiologists published a consensus guideline for preoperative testing focusing on ASA 1 and 2 patients undergoing elective surgery. The guidelines advocate minimal routine testing based on ASA status and invasiveness of surgery on the principle of the careful justifiable basis for ordering a preoperative investigation, the results of which may change the anesthetic or treatment plan (**Table 3**).

RISK ASSESSMENT

> **AS3.5:** Determine the readiness for general surgery in a patient based on the preoperative evaluation.

Preoperative assessment of patients' risk for undergoing anesthesia enables improved understanding of their inherent risks by the patients and better clinical care by healthcare providers. Various indices and classification systems have been designed to assess and determine the perioperative risk to the patient.

Functional Capacity

Assessment of a patient's functional capacity is an integral component of preoperative clinical examination. It is an important determinant of perioperative risk for morbidity and mortality; and the need for further preoperative testing.

Metabolic Equivalent of Task (MET)

Functional capacity is typically quantified in terms of the metabolic equivalent of task (MET), where one MET is the basal rate of energy consumption at rest (3.5 mL/kg/min). Patients' MET can be clinically assessed using equivalent levels of exercise as in **Table 4**. The functional capacity can be classified as poor (less than 4 METS), average (4-7 METS), good (7-10 METS), excellent (higher than 10 METS), and unknown.

Duke Activity Status Index

The Duke's activity status index has been designed to ease and improve the preoperative

Table 3: Preoperative tests based on clinical considerations.

Preoperative test	Clinical consideration
Blood count	• Extremes of age • Liver or kidney disease • Anticoagulant use • Bleeding/hematologic disorder • Malignancy type • Invasiveness of procedure
Coagulation studies	• Liver or kidney disease • Bleeding disorder • Anticoagulant use • Chemotherapy
Serum chemistries (glucose, electrolytes, renal and liver function)	• Liver or renal disease, or perioperative risk of dysfunction • Diabetes • Diuretic, digoxin, or steroid use • Central nervous system disease • Endocrine disorders • Elderly • Malnutrition • Type and invasiveness of procedure
Chest X-ray	• Pulmonary disease or clinical manifestations • Unstable cardiovascular disease • Type and invasiveness of procedure
ECG	• Cardiovascular disease or clinical risk factors • Pulmonary disease • Type and invasiveness of procedure
Pregnancy test	Possible pregnancy
Urinalysis	• Specific procedures (e.g., prosthesis implantation, urologic procedures) • Urinary tract symptoms present

Table 4: Metabolic equivalents of functional capacity.

mETs	Equivalent level of Exercise
1	Eating, bathing, dressing
2	Walking down stairs or in your house, or cooking
3	Walking 200 yards on level ground
4	Raking leaves, gardening
5	Climbing 1 flight of stairs, walk up a hill, dancing or bicycling
6	Heavy carpentry using a push mower
7	Digging, spading soil, single tennis
8	Moving heavy furniture, rapidly climbing stairs or jogging slowly
9	Jumping rope slowly, sawing wood or moderate cycling
10	Swimming quickly, running or jogging briskly, bicycling uphill
11	Skiing cross country or playing full court basketball
12	Running rapidly for moderate or long distances

Revised Cardiac Risk Index (RCRI)

Lee's Revised Cardiac Risk Index (RCRI) is the most commonly used risk score for predicting the risk of perioperative cardiac complications in patients with heart disease scheduled for major non-cardiac operations. The complications include myocardial infarction, pulmonary edema, ventricular fibrillation or primary cardiac arrest, and complete heart block.

The six independent preoperative predictors of major cardiac complications are assigned one point each. The total score predicts the incidence of major adverse cardiac events (**Table 6**).

American Society of Anesthesiologists (ASA) Classification

The ASA physical status classification system (**Table 7**) is the most commonly used classification to predict perioperative risks. It evaluation of functional capacity. It is a brief self-administered questionnaire about activities of daily living, which determine the patient's functional capacity (**Table 5**).

Table 5: Duke activity status index.

Poor	1–4 MET	• Can you take care of yourself? • Eat, dress or use the toilet? • Walk indoors around the house? • Walk a block or two on level ground at 3.2 to 4.8 km per hour? • Do light work around the house like dusting or washing dishes?
Moderate	4–7 MET	• Climb a flight of stairs or walk up the hill? • Walk on level ground at 6.4 km per hour? • Run a short distance?
Good	7–10 MET	• Do heavy work around the house like scrubbing floors or lifting or moving heavy furniture? • Participate in moderate recreational activities like golf, bowling, dancing, double tennis, or football?
Excellent	>10 MET	Participate in strenuous sports like swimming, single tennis, football or basketball?

MET: metabolic equivalent of task

Table 6: Revised cardiac risk index.

High-risk surgery (intraperitoneal, intrathoracic, or suprainguinal vascular)	1
History of ischemic heart disease (history of myocardial infarction or a positive exercise test, current angina pectoris, ongoing nitrate therapy, or pathological Q waves in ECG)	1
History of congestive heart failure	1
History of cerebrovascular disease	1
Insulin-dependent diabetes mellitus	1
Serum creatinine >2 mg/dL	1

Risk of Major Cardiac Events (MACE) based on total RCRI score: Score 0: 0.4%; Score 1: 0.9%; Score 2: 6.6%; and Score >3–11%

is used to assess and communicate a patient's preanesthesia medical co-morbidities.

New York Heart Association (NYHA) Functional Classification

The NYHA functional classification system is used to classify the functional status of patients with heart disease based on limitations during physical activity (**Table 8**).

PREOPERATIVE OPTIMIZATION

The history and physical examination in PAC accurately predict the risk of anesthesia and the need to change the existing therapy or add a new one to optimize the patient for the upcoming surgical stress. Optimizing a patient's preoperative physical condition will also help to reduce postoperative morbidity and mortality. The disorders of different organ systems must be optimized preoperatively.

- **Cardiovascular system:** Hypertension is the most frequently encountered in PAC. The end-organ damage due to long-standing hypertension needs to be assessed. Elective surgery should be postponed if blood pressure exceeds 180/110 mm Hg. To reduce the risk of perioperative major cardiovascular complications, optimization of blood pressure using lifestyle modification and pharmacological therapy is recommended. Ischemic heart disease patients identified to have increased risk can be managed by either revascularization (surgical or percutaneous) or by optimization of medical management.
- **Respiratory system:** The main risk factors for postoperative pulmonary complications are obesity, pre-existing pulmonary disease, and advancing age. The most common respiratory diseases encountered during PAC are asthma, acute upper respiratory tract infection (URTI), and chronic obstructive pulmonary disease (COPD).

Table 7: ASA physical status classification with examples.

ASA Class	Definition	Adult examples including but not limited to:
ASA I	A normal healthy patient	Healthy, nonsmoking, no or minimal alcohol use
ASA II	A patient with mild systemic disease	Mild diseases only without substantive functional limitations. Current smoker, social alcohol drinker, pregnancy, obesity (30<BMI <40), well-controlled DM/HTN, mild lung disease
ASA III	A patient with severe systemic disease	Substantive functional limitations; One or more moderate to severe diseases. Poorly controlled DM or HTN, COPD, morbid obesity (BMI ≥40), active hepatitis, alcohol dependence or abuse, implanted pacemaker, moderate reduction of ejection fraction, ESRD undergoing regularly scheduled dialysis, history (>3 months) of MI, CVA, TIA, or CAD/stents
ASA IV	A patient with severe systemic disease that is a constant threat to life	Recent (<3 months) MI, CVA, TIA or CAD/stents, ongoing cardiac ischemia or severe valve dysfunction, severe reduction of ejection fraction, shock, sepsis, DIC, ARD or ESRD not undergoing regularly scheduled dialysis
ASA V	A moribund patient who is not expected to survive without the operation	Ruptured abdominal/thoracic aneurysm, massive trauma, intracranial bleed with mass effect, ischemic bowel in the face of significant cardiac pathology or multiple organ/system dysfunction
ASA VI	A declared brain-dead patient whose organs are being removed for donor purposes	

CAD, coronary arterial disease; CVA, cerebrovascular accident; MI, myocardial infarction; TIA, transient ischemic attack.

* Although pregnancy is not a disease, the parturient physiologic state is significantly altered from when the woman is not pregnant, hence the assignment of ASA 2 for a woman with uncomplicated pregnancy.

**The addition of "E" denotes emergency surgery: (An emergency is defined as existing when a delay in treatment of the patient would lead to a significant increase in the threat to life or body part)

Table 8: New York Heart Association classification.

Functional capacity	Objective assessment
NYHA Class I	No limitation of physical activity. Ordinary physical activity does not cause fatigue, dyspnoea, palpitations or angina pain
NYHA Class II	Slight limitation of physical activity. Ordinary physical activity causes fatigue, dyspnoea, palpitations or angina pain
NYHA Class III	Marked limitation of physical activity. Less than ordinary activity causes fatigue, dyspnoea, palpitations or angina pain. Asymptomatic at rest
NYHA Class IV	Inability to do any physical activity without discomfort. Symptoms at rest

- *URTI*: In a patient with upper respiratory tract infection, ascertain if surgery is urgent. Patients with clear systemic signs of infection such as fever, purulent rhinitis, productive cough, and wheeze should be scheduled after about six weeks, so the URTI settles down. Patients with asthma are at increased risk of severe bronchospasm perioperatively.
- *Optimization of respiratory tract*: Chest physiotherapy, antibiotic therapy,

and bronchodilator therapy during the preoperative period improve the reversible components of asthma. Anti-inflammatory and bronchodilator therapy should be continued and the last dose administered before induction of anesthesia. In selected patients, a preoperative course of oral corticosteroids may be useful to improve overall lung function. In a patient with COPD, preoperative pulmonary optimization includes smoking cessation, administration of antibiotics for purulent sputum, bronchodilators, chest physiotherapy, incentive spirometry, deep breathing, and postural drainage.
- **Central nervous system:** Patients with a history of seizures should continue anti-epileptic drug therapy till the day of surgery. A patient with an intracranial tumor or head injury should be assessed for increased intracranial pressure, and pharmacological optimization should be done using mannitol and steroids to decrease the pressure.
- **Kidney:** In a patient with chronic renal disease, the main aim is to prevent the onset and consequences of renal failure. Preoperative medication must be individualized. Nephrotoxic drugs should be avoided. Patients on hemodialysis should undergo dialysis during the 24 hours preceding elective surgery.
- **Electrolyte balance:** Derangement in electrolytes and acid-base levels should be corrected preoperatively. Serum potassium should not exceed 5.5 mEq/L on the day of surgery.
- **Blood:** Hemoglobin is evaluated preoperatively and optimized using recombinant human erythropoietin therapy if the patient is anemic. In case a coagulopathy is detected preoperatively, it should be corrected. The international normalized ratio (INR) should be less than 1.5 before acceptance for surgery.
- **Liver:** Risk stratification is done using scores like the model for end-stage liver disease (MELD) or Child-Turcotte-Pugh (CTP). In patients not suitable for preoperative optimization, alternatives to surgery and workup for transplantation can be done.
- **Endocrine system:** The most common endocrine disorder encountered during PAC is diabetes mellitus. Adequate sugar control is a prerequisite before taking up a patient with diabetes mellitus for surgery. Hemoglobin A1C (glycosylated Hb) level is an independent predictor of poor postoperative outcomes. Hyperglycemic patients must be optimized with oral hypoglycemic agents or insulin, depending on the patient's characteristics and sugar level.

Patients with hypothyroidism/hyperthyroidism should be optimized using appropriate drugs like thyroxine and propyl thiouracil to make the patient clinically and biochemically euthyroid. Adequate thyroid control prevents complications of myxedema coma and thyroid storm in the perioperative period.

PREOPERATIVE DRUG THERAPY

Many patients are on drug therapy for various medical conditions. Drug therapy for various comorbidities should be carefully evaluated. Special attention is needed to assess geriatric patients who may be receiving poly-pharmacy. Some essential drugs need to be continued perioperatively without any interruption. Certain drugs have potential interactions with anesthetic agents, so their intake may need to be stopped, replaced, or their dose adjusted before surgery.

During the preoperative assessment, thorough documentation of all the drugs used with their indication, duration of treatment, doses, frequency, and patient compliance is a prerequisite. The aptness of the regime with special consideration for drug interactions and adverse drug events must be carefully evaluated and modified if needed.

INFORMED CONSENT AND COUNSELING

Patient autonomy is an integral part of the patient care pathway. The patient should be the prime decision-maker for the course of treatment. Patients should be adequately informed about the treatment options available, advantages, associated risks, alternatives to therapy if present, and outcomes of denying the same.

"Consent" is the patient's concordance for a health care professional to provide the treatment. It is the legal permission to carry out the required procedures after discussing the pros and cons. Informed written consent is a legal necessity before the conduct of all major diagnostic, anesthesia, and surgical procedures. Any lapse in taking valid consent is treated as deliberate assault in a court of law.

Principles for a Valid Consent

1. Consent must be obtained by a doctor before starting a treatment or procedure.
2. It should be taken well before the procedure so that patient is not pressurized to sign.
3. Consent should be confirmed before starting the procedure.
4. The consent is valid for an indefinite period unless there is a change in the patient's condition or proposed procedure.
5. Consent should be signed by the patient only except for a minor (<18 years of age) or an incompetent adult.
6. A patient competent to provide valid consent is more than 18 years of age and has a sound mind.
7. If the patient is incompetent, the consent can be taken from a surrogate decision-maker who is a next of kin or caregiver.
8. A child > 12 years of age can give valid consent for medical examination (Indian Penal Code section 89).
9. Consent should be free, i.e., should not be given under any influence, fraud, or coercion.
10. The doctor must disclose the information related to the patient's condition, treatment benefits, adverse events, alternatives, if any, risk of refusing treatment, and cost of treatment.
11. The patient should be encouraged to ask questions and clear all queries.
12. Consent should be procedure-specific, like consent for a diagnostic procedure cannot be considered valid for treatment. Blanket consent, which does not specify the procedure, is invalid.
13. Consent obtained during the time of surgery is invalid.
14. Whenever a blood transfusion is anticipated, written consent should be taken before the surgery.
15. New consent is required for a repeat procedure. Prior consent is not valid.
16. Surgical consent does not cover anesthesia care. It should be taken by the anesthesia provider should explain the necessary procedure and the risks involved.
17. Competent patients have the right to refuse treatment even in life-threatening conditions. In these cases, it is important to document the informed refusal
18. The consent should always be signed by the doctor and a witness. Missing signatures make the consent invalid.
19. The consent should be properly documented.
20. A patient can withdraw the consent anytime.
21. In medical emergencies, lifesaving treatment can be given without consent, but the surgeon should document that the intervention is lifesaving and sign it.

PREMEDICATION

AS3.6: Choose and write a prescription for appropriate premedications for patients undergoing surgery.

Premedication is the administration of drugs before induction of anesthesia. It is no longer administered routinely. A premedicated patient must be monitored for the side effects

Table 9: Premedication: Indications and drugs used.

Indication for using premedication	Drugs used
Anxiolysis	• Benzodiazepines: Midazolam, alprazolam • α2 agonists: Dexmedetomidine, clonidine
Analgesia	• Opioids: Fentanyl, morphine • NSAIDs: Diclofenac, ketorolac
Decrease gastric secretions, increase gastric pH	• H_2 receptor antagonist: Ranitidine • Proton pump inhibitors: Pantoprazole
Increase gastric motility	• Prokinetics: Metoclopramide
Decrease salivary gland and mucosal gland secretions	• Anticholinergics: Atropine, glycopyrrolate
Prophylaxis against PONV	• 5HT3 receptor antagonist: Ondansetron • D2 receptor antagonist: Metoclopramide, haloperidol • H1 receptor antagonist: Promethazine • Muscarinic cholinergic type 1 receptor antagonist: Scopolamine • Steroid receptor: Dexamethasone • Neurokinin type 1 receptor antagonist: Aprepitant

NSAIDs: non-steroidal anti-inflammatory drugs

of the drug used while in the ward, during transport to the operation theatre, and in the preoperative waiting area. The practice of anesthesiology is constantly evolving, and with increasing knowledge of the appropriate use of pharmacological support, the use of premedication is revamping.

Purposes of Premedication

The main purposes of premedication are:
- To present a tranquil and anxiety-free patient for surgery
- To decrease the hazards of anesthesia and surgery.

The other uses of premedication can be
- Prevent postoperative pain
- Prophylaxis against postoperative nausea and vomiting (PONV)
- Decrease perioperative shivering
- Decrease postoperative pruritus
- Decrease gastric secretions
- Prevent allergic reactions
- Suppress reflex responses to surgical stimulus
- Decrease anesthetic drug requirement.

The drugs used for premedication and their indication are listed in **Table 9**. The premedication drug may be administered orally, intramuscular, intravenous, intranasal, or rectally. The following should be considered before administration of premedication— patients' age, physical status, level of anxiety, type, and timing of surgery.

REVIEW PAC

Current accreditation guidelines mandate that the PAC of all patients must be reviewed just before surgery to ensure safe administration of anesthesia. The review PAC is designed to verify the time of intake of the last meal or oral fluids to verify the nil-per-oral status before induction of anesthesia. Important biochemical parameters must be reviewed and all salient features verified. The consent documents must be reviewed. Premedication, if given, must be documented. In patients with comorbid diseases likely to alter the biochemical homeostasis, the results of investigations on the morning of surgery must be reviewed. Hemodynamic parameters and oxygen saturation must be reassessed.

CHAPTER 2 ◆ Preoperative Assessment

MULTIPLE CHOICE QUESTIONS

OSCE
A 70 years old male patient with a history of bronchial asthma, diabetes mellitus, and coronary artery disease has come for pre-anesthetic evaluation for planned hernia surgery. He had an episode of bronchospasm about one month back. He can climb one flight of stairs. Presently he has a history of productive cough. He does not have a history of angina. His blood pressure is 180/110 mm Hg. He is on regular salbutamol inhaler therapy three times daily and takes Metoprolol 50 mg daily. His blood sugar (fasting) is 180 mg/100 mL.

1. **His functional ASA class would be:**
   a. ASA II
   b. ASA III
   c. ASA IV
   d. ASA V

2. **For his preoperative optimization, he would be advised:**
   a. Addition of steroids to control his asthma
   b. Not advised as he will not be accepted for surgery under general anesthesia
   c. Chest physiotherapy, antibiotic therapy, and bronchodilator therapy
   d. None of the above

3. **Given his hypertension:**
   a. He should be referred to internal medicine/cardiology for evaluation and optimization
   b. He should be prescribed additional antihypertensives and taken up for surgery after a week
   c. He can be taken up for surgery with upgraded monitoring after explaining due risk
   d. He should be advised against surgery and conservative treatment

4. **A good predictor of safe outcomes for surgery in patients with diabetes mellitus is:**
   a. Fasting blood sugar level
   b. Glycosylated hemoglobin in the normal range
   c. The patient is on oral anti-glycemic agents and not on insulin therapy
   d. All of the above

5. **All of the following are valid for 'Informed Consent' *except*:**
   a. Consent must be taken by a doctor before surgery
   b. The Consent document must be in a language the patient understands
   c. Consent must be procedure specific
   d. Consent is a must even in life-saving surgery

6. **Premedication is administered to:**
   a. Reduce anxiety
   b. Reduce the requirement for anesthetic agents
   c. Reduce response to surgical stimulus
   d. All of the above

Answers
1. b
2. c
3. a
4. b
5. d
6. d

CHAPTER 3

Airway

Deepak Pahwa

Learning Objectives

- Basic anatomy of the airway
- Mask ventilation, including triple airway maneuver
- Endotracheal intubation
- Laryngoscopes
- Endotracheal tube
- Overview of common supraglottic devices
- Difficult airway
- Emergent tracheostomy

INTRODUCTION

AS4.2: Describe the anatomy of the airway and its implications for general anesthesia.

The word 'airway' means passage for air to flow into our lungs. The airway not only provides a passage for airflow into our lungs but also warms and humidifies the air we breathe. The hairs present in the nose have a layer of mucus that prevents dust, pollen, and other allergens from reaching the lungs. Airway plays a major role in phonation, speech, swallowing, and producing cough.

The knowledge of the airway is essential because many clinical situations can lead to loss of airway patency (obstructive sleep apnea), blunting or loss of airway reflexes (head injury, brain tumors), or result in hypoventilation (general anesthesia). Optimal airway management during such difficult clinical situations is essential to prevent death or hypoxic brain injury to the patient.

For understanding, the airway can be divided into two parts—the upper airway and the lower airway. The upper airway extends from the external nares to the larynx to the level of the cricoid cartilage. The lower airway includes the structures in the airway beyond the cricoid cartilage.

ANATOMY OF THE UPPER AIRWAY

Nose

The nasal cavity starts at the level of external nares and extends to the nasopharynx. It is divided into two nasal fossae by a midline nasal septum. The nasal septum is formed by the septal cartilage in the inferior half, while the ethmoid and the vomer bones form the superior half of the nasal septum. Superior, middle, and inferior turbinates (bony structures covered by mucosa) form the lateral wall of the nasal cavity. The turbinates divide the nasal fossae into superior, middle, and inferior meatuses (**Fig. 1**). The paranasal

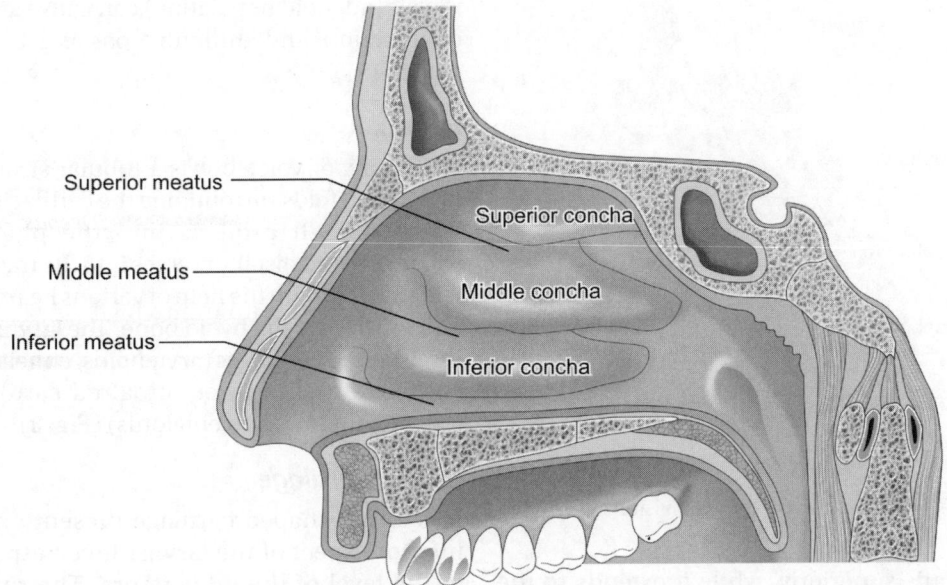

Fig. 1: Lateral wall of the nasal cavity.

sinuses drain into the nose through the ostia on the lateral wall of the nasal cavity.

Blood Supply

The nose gets its arterial supply from:
- Ophthalmic artery (ethmoid branches)
- Maxillary artery (greater palatine and sphenopalatine branches)
- Facial artery (superior labial and lateral nasal branches).

Clinical Significance

Head injury or facial trauma can cause damage to the cribriform plate, which separates the nasal cavity from the brain. Administration of positive pressure mask ventilation to such patients can transmit bacteria or other impurities from the nasal cavity into the brain and cause meningitis or sepsis. Airway devices introduced through the nasal cavity can enter the subarachnoid space in these patients. Nasotracheal tubes, when placed, pass between the floor of the nasal cavity and the inferior turbinate. Repeated attempts at nasotracheal intubation can lead to damage to the lateral wall of the nasal cavity. Vasoconstrictor nasal drop use is recommended to reduce the vascularity of the nose before attempting the insertion of any airway device in the nose.

Pharynx

The pharynx is a tubular structure connecting nasal and oral cavities to the larynx and the esophagus. It extends from the base of the skull and ends at the level of the inferior border of the cricoid cartilage. It is divided into three parts - the nasopharynx, the oropharynx, and the laryngopharynx (**Fig. 2**).

The nasopharynx extends from the base of the skull to the soft palate. The superior and posterior walls of the nasopharynx contain the adenoid tonsils. The oropharynx starts from the posterior border of the soft palate and extends to the superior border of the epiglottis. The base of the tongue lies anterior to the oropharynx. The lateral walls of the oropharynx are formed by the tonsillar pillars, which contain palatine tonsils. The boundaries of the hypopharynx are the upper border of the

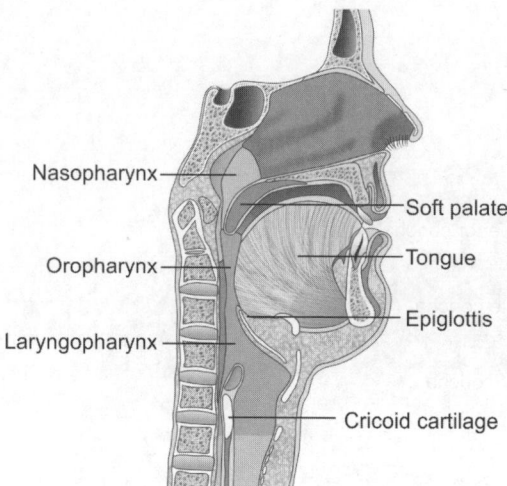

Fig 2: Pharynx and its divisions.

epiglottis superiorly, while it extends to the lower border of the cricoid cartilage anteriorly and the C6 vertebra posteriorly.

Clinical Significance

Loss of tone of pharyngeal musculature can cause airway obstruction during anesthesia. A triple airway maneuver (described later in the chapter) helps relieve it. Hypertrophy of tonsils (adenoid or palatine) can cause airway obstruction and difficulty passing airway devices.

Larynx

The larynx or voice box is a tubular structure of mucosal folds surrounding the cartilaginous framework. It projects into the pharynx superiorly and distally merges into the trachea. It is attached with the help of various ligaments and muscles to the hyoid bone. The larynx has three paired cartilages (arytenoids, cuneiform, corniculate) and three unpaired cartilages (cricoid, thyroid, and epiglottis) (**Fig. 3**).

Cricoid Cartilage

It is a ring-shaped cartilage present on the inferior aspect of the larynx. It corresponds to the level of the C6 vertebra. The ring of the cricoid cartilage is signet-shaped with a broad posterior portion and a narrow anterior portion. It is the only tracheal cartilage that completely encircles the trachea.

Clinical Significance

As the cartilage is present on the posterior part, compression of the cricoid can occlude

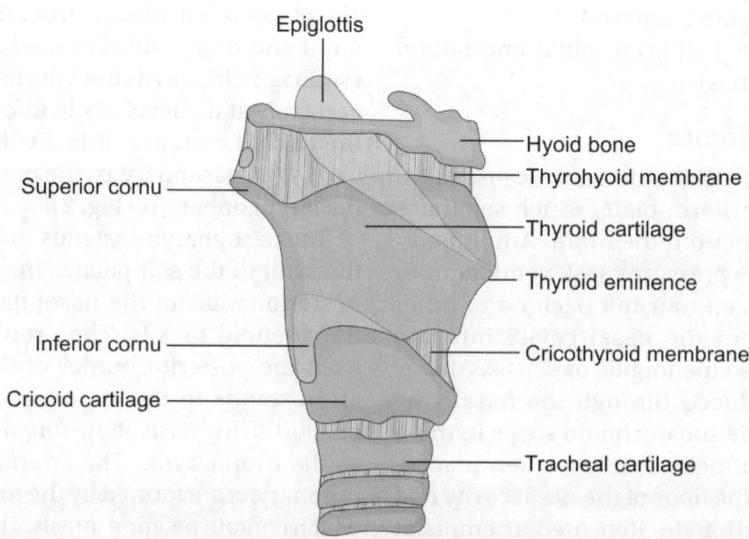

Fig. 3: Larynx and its cartilages.

the esophageal lumen. Cricoid pressure is thus used to prevent regurgitation of stomach contents during mask ventilation in patients with full stomachs.

Thyroid Cartilage

The thyroid cartilage is the largest of the cartilages present in the larynx. It has two laminae. Posteriorly the two laminae are separate, while anteriorly, they are connected at an acute angle, forming Adam's Apple. Adam's Apple is more prominent in males because of the more acute angle at which the laminae join. A 'V-shaped' notch is present above the superior margin of the thyroid cartilage. The thyroid cartilage is attached to the cricoid cartilage by the cricothyroid membrane in the midline and cricothyroid muscles laterally.

Clinical Significance

Cricothyrotomy is the emergency placement of a cannula through the cricothyroid membrane in difficult airway situations when other means to provide oxygen to the patient have failed.

Epiglottis

The epiglottis is the leaf-shaped cartilage attached to the inner surface of the thyroid cartilage in the midline. It projects posterosuperior from its attachment to cover the opening of the larynx. Epiglottis is attached to the hyoid bone through the Hyoepiglottic ligament. Median and lateral glossoepiglottic folds are the mucosal reflections of the epiglottis anteriorly.

Clinical Significance

The epiglottis serves an important function of protecting the airway. During deglutition, it projects posterosuperior and covers the opening of the larynx to prevent food particles from entering the larynx. A large epiglottis may obstruct the laryngeal view during laryngoscopy for tracheal intubation, particularly in infants and children. Miller laryngoscope blades are used to overcome this difficulty.

Arytenoid Cartilage

These are paired pyramidal structures present in the posterior larynx. The upper part of the arytenoid cartilage lies at the level of the false cords, while the vocal processes at the base provide attachment to the vocal ligaments.

Corniculate and Cuneiform Cartilages

These are the small cartilages in the aryepiglottic folds, with the cuneiform cartilage lying anteriorly and the corniculate cartilage lying posteriorly.

When viewed from above during direct laryngoscopy (**Fig. 4**), the uppermost structure that is visible is the epiglottis. It forms the

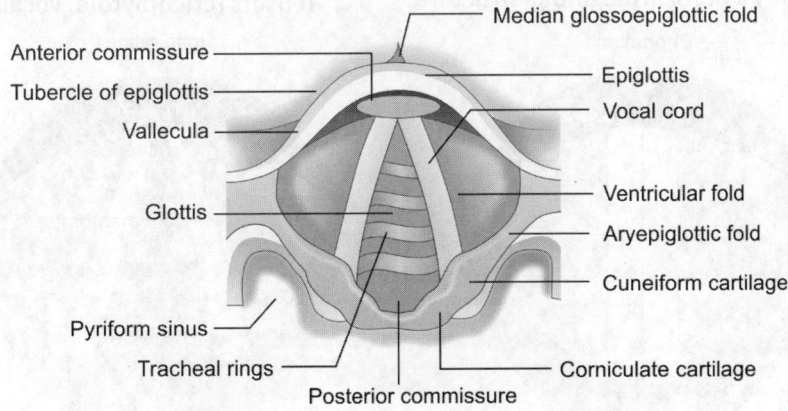

Fig. 4: Laryngoscopic view of the glottis.

upper anterior boundary of the laryngeal inlet. Aryepiglottic folds arise from the lateral margins of the epiglottis and run back towards the inter arytenoid notch posteriorly, forming the posterior border of the laryngeal inlet.

Vocal Cords

Two parallel mucosal folds run in the anterior to the posterior direction along the lateral aspect of the endolarynx, forming false and true vocal cords superiorly and inferiorly, respectively. True vocal cords are engaged in the generation of voice and have fine medial edges, while the false cords have a blunted medial margin. A thin cleft 'ventricle' lies between the true and the false cords. True vocal cords attach anteriorly to the inner surface of the angle of the thyroid cartilage, forming an anterior commissure. While posteriorly, they are attached to the vocal process through vocal ligaments at the lowermost part of the arytenoid cartilage. True vocal cords divide the larynx into three parts:

1. Supraglottis/vestibule (area above the vocal cord)
2. Glottis (space between the vocal cords)
3. Subglottis (part of the larynx lying below the true vocal cords).

Bones of the Larynx

The hyoid is the only bone in the larynx. The larynx is mainly a fibrocartilaginous structure attached to the hyoid bone through the thyrohyoid membrane and muscle. The hyoid bone helps in anchoring the larynx during respiration and phonation.

Muscles of the Larynx

The larynx is involved in the very delicate and complex function of phonation. This can be achieved because of several small muscles attached to the larynx. These can be divided into extrinsic—which attach the larynx to the surrounding structures, thus helping in the movement of the larynx; and the intrinsic muscles, which are connected to the laryngeal cartilage and help in the movement of the glottis and the laryngeal inlet. The movement of the larynx during phonation and inspiration is shown in **Figure 5**.

The extrinsic muscles can be either elevators or depressors of the larynx:
- *Elevators*: These include stylopharyngeus, stylohyoid, geniohyoid mylohyoid, thyrohyoid, and digastric muscles.
- *Depressors*: These include sternohyoid, sternothyroid, and omohyoid muscles.

The intrinsic muscles include:
- Muscles acting on the vocal cords
    - Abductors (posterior cricoarytenoid)
    - Adductors (lateral cricoarytenoid, interarytenoid, thyroarytenoid)
    - Tensors (cricothyroid, vocalis)

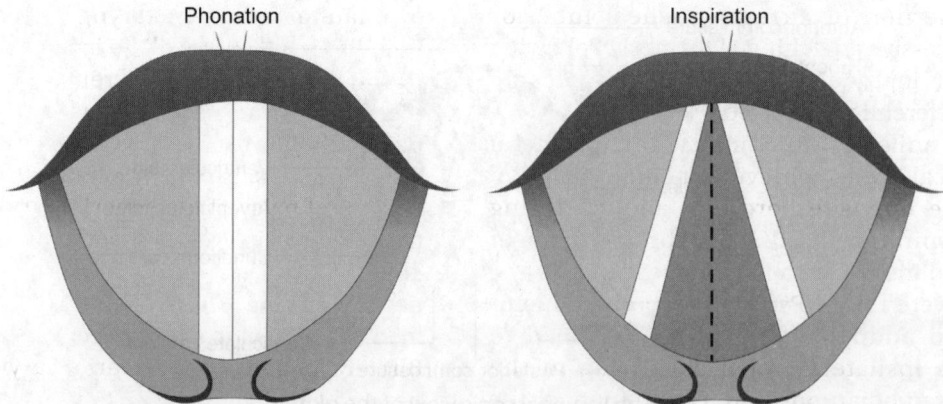

Fig. 5: Position of the vocal cords during normal phonation and inspiration.

- Muscles acting on laryngeal inlet
  - Openers of the laryngeal inlet (thyroepiglottic part of the thyroarytenoid)
  - Closers of the laryngeal inlet (interarytenoid, aryepiglottic).

Nerve Supply of Larynx

The motor supply to all the muscles moving the vocal cords is by the recurrent laryngeal nerve except the cricothyroid, which is from the external laryngeal branch of the superior laryngeal nerve. The sensory supply above the glottis is by the internal laryngeal nerve, which is a branch of the superior laryngeal nerve, while below the glottis, it is from the recurrent laryngeal nerve.

Applied Anatomy

- *Laryngospasm*: Stimulation of the internal branch of the superior laryngeal nerve in the supraglottic region can produce closure of the glottis resulting in laryngospasm. This is commonly triggered by vocal cord injury (commonly after laryngoscopy without achieving adequate depth of anesthesia or without administering muscle relaxants to the patient), the presence of secretions over the cords, irritants, anxiety, allergens, and acid reflux.
- *Vocal cord palsy* (**Fig. 6**): Injury to the recurrent laryngeal nerve (RLN) may occur during surgeries on the thyroid and the parathyroid glands, trauma, malignancy, insertion of an endotracheal tube, or excessive stretching of the neck. Following RLN injury, abductors of the vocal cords are preferentially affected.
- In unilateral RLN injury, the ipsilateral vocal cords achieve a median position. The opposite cord will abduct during inspiration, and both cords will meet midline during phonation.
- Severe trauma may affect both abductor and adductor fibers. This will lead to the ipsilateral vocal cord lying in the paramedian position. On phonation, the opposite cord crosses the midline and closes the glottis, while during inspiration, it abducts completely.
- Bilateral abductor palsy can be seen if RLN is injured on both sides. The glottis gets closed and results in severe respiratory distress due to bilateral unopposed adduction of the cords. When there is complete palsy of bilateral recurrent laryngeal nerves, both the vocal cords will lie in a cadaveric position, and the glottis remains open (See **Fig. 6**). Therefore, bilateral complete paralysis of the recurrent laryngeal nerve is less dangerous than incomplete paralysis.
- Unilateral palsy of the superior laryngeal nerve leads to ipsilateral cricothyroid palsy. The ipsilateral cord assumes an abducted position leading to hoarseness and difficulty in raising the pitch of the voice.
- Bilateral palsy of the superior laryngeal nerve is quite rare.

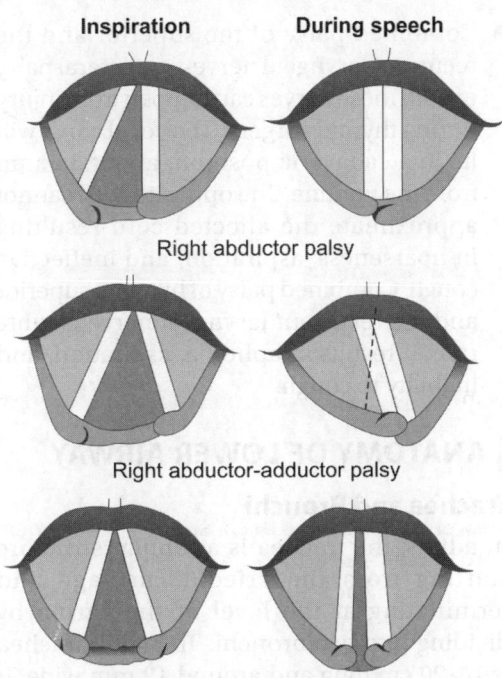

Fig. 6: Position of the vocal cords in different types of laryngeal nerve palsy.

- Combined palsy of the superior and the recurrent laryngeal nerve—unilateral palsy of both these nerves can happen from injury during thyroid surgery. The vocal cords will lie in a cadaveric position, about 3.5 mm from the midline. The opposite cord cannot approximate the affected cord resulting in hoarseness, aspiration, and ineffective cough. Combined palsy of bilateral superior and the recurrent laryngeal nerve is quite rare. It results in aphonia, aspiration, and inability to cough.

ANATOMY OF LOWER AIRWAY

Trachea and Bronchi

In adults, the trachea is a tubular structure starting from the cricoid cartilage and terminating at the level of the carina by dividing into two bronchi. The adult trachea is 10–20 cm long and around 12 mm wide. It has around 16–20 cartilaginous rings, which are deficient posteriorly. From the sixth ring onwards, the trachea lies intrathoracic.

Clinical Significance

The length of the adult trachea increases by up to 2 cm during neck extension. This can cause the distal tip of the endotracheal tube to come out of the trachea while extending the neck of the patient. Similarly, during flexion of the neck, the endotracheal tube can move deeper by 2 cm, resulting in endobronchial migration of the tip of the endotracheal tube. Therefore one should be vigilant about the position of the tube whenever the neck of the patient is moved.

Some patients have 'Stove Pipe' deformity of the trachea wherein tracheal rings are complete and are not deficient posteriorly. This condition may be associated with an increased risk of difficult endotracheal intubation.

Bronchi and Bronchioles

The trachea bifurcates into the right and left main stem bronchi. The right main stem bronchus is shorter, wider, and steeper as compared to the left main stem bronchus. The right and left main stem bronchi branch into three and two lobar bronchi, respectively. These bronchi are further divided into medium and small bronchi and then into bronchioles. Small bronchi, less than 0.8 mm in diameter, are called bronchioles. They are devoid of cartilage in their walls. Bronchioles further divide into terminal bronchioles and respiratory bronchioles, which bear alveoli.

The bronchi are surrounded by irregular cartilaginous rings. These rings disappear as the diameter of the airways approaches 0.6 mm. These rings are surrounded by smooth muscles and a fibroelastic sheath. The fibroelastic sheath provides strength to the airway while the smooth muscles help in changing the diameter of the airway. The tone of smooth muscles is under the control of the vagus nerve. The absolute thickness of the muscular layer decreases as one moves distally to the bronchioles, but its relative thickness in proportion to the wall of the bronchioles increases. Therefore, the smaller bronchioles close off earlier during bronchospasm.

UPPER AIRWAY OBSTRUCTION

It is essential to understand the anatomical relationship between various structures present in the upper airway and their role in maintaining the patency of the airway. The tongue is connected with the help of the genioglossus muscle to the mandible. Hyoid bone provides attachment to the muscles in the suprahyoid (mandible, tongue) and the infrahyoid (larynx, sternum, clavicle) regions.

Epiglottis is connected to the hyoid bone by the hyoepiglottic ligament and the thyroid cartilage by the thyroepiglottic ligament. This muscular hammock around the hyoid bone, the platysma, and the deep cervical fascia can be stretched using the airway maneuver (**Fig. 7**). The maneuver causes anterior displacement of the tongue-hyoid-thyroid-

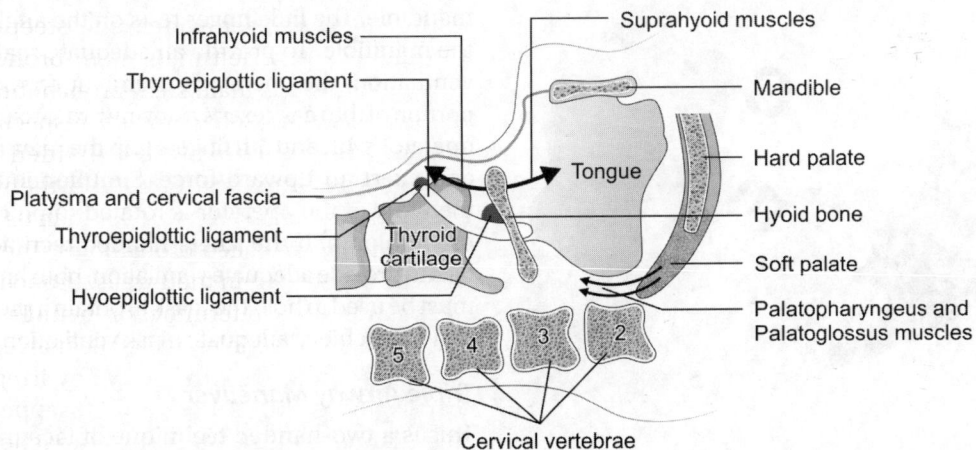

Fig. 7: Muscle hammock formed by bones, muscles, ligaments, and cervical fascia of the upper airway to maintain the airway patency.

epiglottis complex and helps open the airway. The hyoid bone, along with the hyoepiglottic and thyroepiglottic ligament, acts as a lever and helps open the epiglottis.

On the other hand, the soft palate is attached only to the adjoining soft tissue structures (palatoglossus, palatopharyngeus, and tensor palati muscles), which are not amenable to manipulation. the soft palate does not respond to airway manipulation because of this relationship. Only the tongue and epiglottis respond to airway manipulation.

AIRWAY MANAGEMENT

In patients with acute respiratory failure, noninvasive management of the airway is the most time-critical step. Face mask ventilation is the most important component of noninvasive management of the airway. Every clinician should know and develop skills to provide face mask ventilation to the patients if required. Face mask ventilation remains the essential skill to rely on in case of failed attempts at advanced airway insertion despite the easy availability of advanced airway devices like endotracheal tubes and supraglottic airway devices.

Face Mask Design and Parts

Any face mask designed for resuscitation or anesthesia purposes is attached with a positive pressure generating device to provide ventilation to the patient. A face mask has three parts: body, seal, and connector (**Fig. 8**). The body of the face mask should preferably be made of transparent plastic to detect secretions/regurgitation. The body forms the main structure of the mask. It has a slot-connector at the top for attaching the positive pressure generating device. The rim of the body of the mask forms the seal of the mask, and this is usually filled with air to facilitate an effective seal.

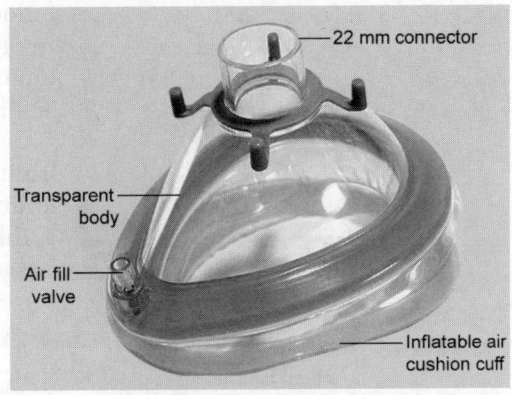

Fig. 8: Face mask and its parts.

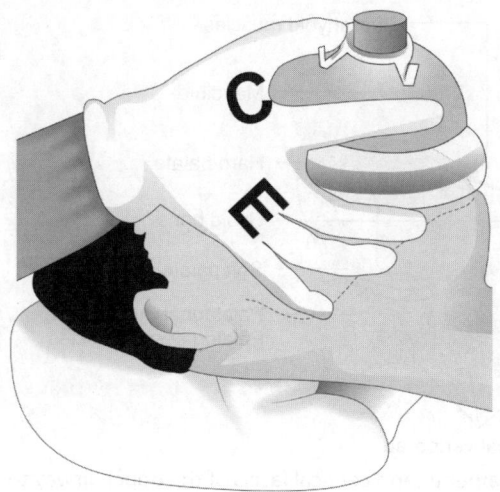

Fig. 9: 'CE' technique of holding a face mask.

Holding the Face Mask

The face mask must form a tight seal around the face to allow for effective ventilation of the patient. Face masks can be held using a one-handed or two-handed technique. The most commonly used technique is the one-handed CE technique (**Fig. 9**). In this, the thumb and index fingers of the operator form a "C" shaped grip around the mask's body while the balance three fingers spread along the ramus of the mandible. The little finger rests on the angle of the mandible. To provide an adequate seal for ventilation, the operator's thumb at the nasal portion of the mask exerts a downward force. The operator's 4th and 5th fingers grip the mandible and exert an upward force. Simultaneously, the wrist of the operator is rotated to pull the mandible up. If the single-handed technique fails to provide adequate ventilation, both hands must be used to hold the mask to obtain a proper seal and achieve adequate mask ventilation.

Triple Airway Maneuver

This is a two-handed technique of face mask ventilation where the operator uses both his hands to provide chin lift, head extension, and jaw thrust along with opening the mouth of the patient (**Fig. 10**). It is considered the best technique to relieve airway obstruction in a patient.

Endotracheal Intubation

It is defined as the insertion of an endotracheal tube into the trachea to provide ventilation or any other lung therapy. Endotracheal intubation not only provides a conduit for providing ventilation to the patient but also secures and protects the airway from

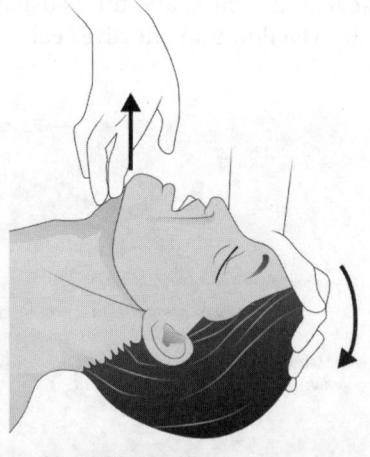
Head tilt-chin lift

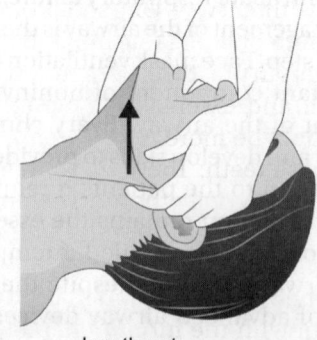
Jaw-thrust

Fig. 10: Triple airway maneuver: Head extension with jaw thrust and chin lift.

aspiration, secretions, isolation of the lungs, and administration of medications.

Indications for Endotracheal Intubation
- Securing the airway during anesthesia
- Medically unstable patients, including patients with respiratory failure, shock, or requiring CPR.
- To protect their airway from aspiration as in comatose patients or patients with head injury with GCS less than or equal to 8.
- To facilitate elective mechanical ventilation support.
- To facilitate cardiopulmonary support in patients with multiple organ failure.
- To facilitate invasive ventilation in the case of noninvasive ventilation is unsuccessful.

AIRWAY ASSESSMENT

Before attempting endotracheal intubation, any medical practitioner should take a thorough history and examine the patient to look for any signs that may indicate difficulty in intubating the patient. One should always ask the patient about any previous anesthesia exposure and if there was any difficulty with intubation. Several tests have been described in the literature to identify patients with the possibility of difficult intubation.

Measuring Various Airway Distances

The first step in airway assessment is a physical examination of the airway. One should look for adequate mouth opening (at should be more than two fingers in breadth), neck movements (both flexion and extension), thyromental distance (should be more than 6.5 cm), buck teeth, and loose teeth. These measurements should be combined with the most commonly used airway assessment tool, the modified Mallampati classification. This classification is based on the view of the upper airway of a sitting patient with the mouth opened wide and the tongue sticking out (described in Chapter 2).

LARYNGOSCOPY AND INTUBATION

Proper position of the patient is mandatory for laryngoscopy and intubation. This includes increasing the bed height so that the patient's forehead lies at the level of the xiphoid process of the anesthesiologist. The patient's neck is then flexed at the cervical spine, and the head is extended at the atlantooccipital joint to give a sniffing position. The head can be flexed by placing a 10 cm thick pillow below the head. This position helps align the oral, laryngeal, and pharyngeal axes (**Fig. 11**).

Intubation Process

The patient should ideally be pre-oxygenated by administering 100% oxygen through a tight-fitting face mask for 3 min. This helps increase the oxygen reserves of the lungs and helps in increasing the duration for which the body can sustain without oxygen desaturation. Preoxygenation is especially indicated in anticipated difficulty intubation patients, pregnant patients, obese patients, and patients with coexisting lung diseases. After preoxygenation, the patient is administered narcotics, a sedative induction agent, and skeletal muscle relaxants to blunt the airway

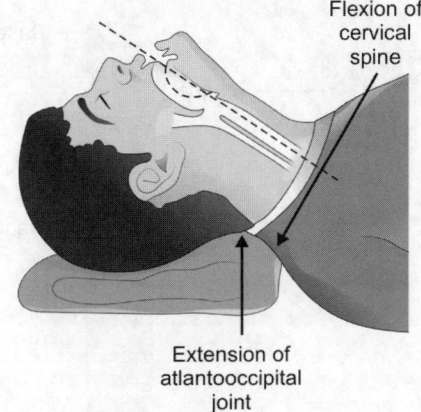

Fig. 11: Sniffing position for laryngoscopy and intubation.

reflexes. The patient is then mask ventilated till the time the drugs given to the patient take effect (except in rapid sequence intubation, which is indicated in patients at high-risk of aspiration, and such patients are not mask ventilated). This is followed by laryngoscopy for endotracheal intubation.

Laryngoscopy

Direct laryngoscopy is commonly used to facilitate tracheal intubation. To visualize the glottis, three upper airway axes (oral, pharyngeal, and laryngeal) should be in line. This is facilitated by the sniffing position as described above. After giving a sniffing position, the patient's neck is extended using the operator's right hand while the little finger and medial border of the operator's left hand open the mouth of the patient by pushing the mandible caudally. The laryngoscope (**Fig. 12**) blade is introduced into the oral cavity, the tongue pushed to the left side, and the lower jaw lifted, pulling the laryngoscope anteriorly and caudal by moving the upper arm and shoulder rather than the wrist. The glottic opening is visualized, and an appropriately sized endotracheal tube is inserted through the

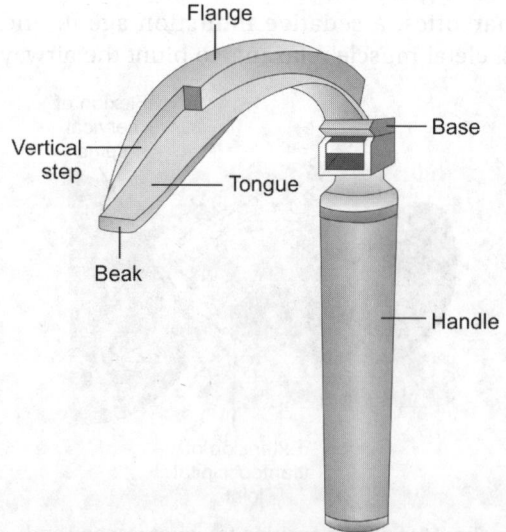

Fig. 12: Laryngoscope with Macintosh blade.

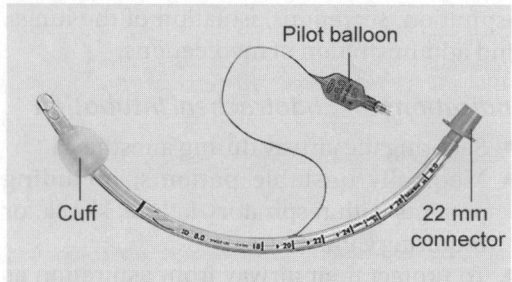

Fig. 13: Endotracheal tube.

glottic opening under constant visualization. The development of video laryngoscopes has improved the visualization of the cords, especially in patients with the anterior larynx. The video laryngoscopes provide a vision 30–60° anterior to the line of sight.

Endotracheal Intubation

The endotracheal tubes (ETT) are curved, plastic, single lumen tubes (**Fig. 13**). The ETTs have a 15 mm adapter attached at the proximal end for connecting the breathing circuit; a high volume low, pressure cuff; a beveled tip that facilitates passage of the tube through the glottic opening, and an extra opening in the distal end of the sidewall of the tube called 'Murphy's eye' for providing an extra port for ventilation. The most commonly used ETTs are the cuffed tubes, forming a seal along the tracheal wall, which helps reduce the risk of aspiration and adequately deliver tidal volume into the lungs. Cuffless ETTs are commonly used in neonates and infants. The cuff in the ETT should be inflated, with a small volume of air, to a pressure of less than 25 cm H_2O to seal the airway around the tube. ETTs come in various sizes, usually described in their internal diameter. ETT with an internal diameter of 7 mm is commonly used in females, while 8 mm ETT is used in males.

Laryngeal Mask Airways

As the name suggests, the laryngeal mask airway is a minimally invasive device that

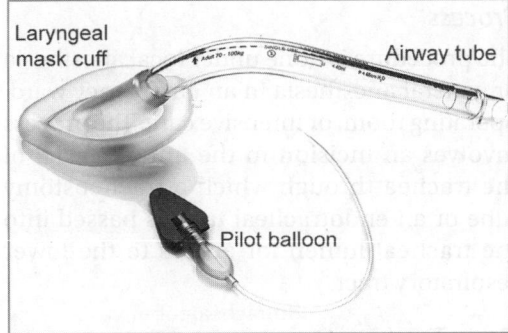

Fig. 14: Laryngeal mask airway.

has an inflatable mask that fits against the epiglottic tissue and has tubing attached to it that exits through the mouth (**Fig. 14**). One can connect the breathing circuit to the tube, and thus laryngeal mask can also be used to provide positive pressure ventilation. It was developed by Archie Brain as an alternative to both endotracheal intubation and face mask ventilation.

Uses of Laryngeal Mask Airway

- In anesthetized low-risk patients with minimal risk of gastric aspiration and undergoing elective, short-duration surgeries. These include orthopedic, plastic, and urology surgeries.
- To maintain airway while giving anesthesia for diagnostic radiological procedures.
- For securing the airway in pediatric patients undergoing minor procedures under anesthesia, for example, lumbar puncture, bone marrow aspiration, biopsy.
- As an advanced airway device to secure the airway during cardiopulmonary resuscitation.
- They have a definitive role in difficult airway algorithms. Their use is recommended in failed bag-mask ventilation to provide rescue breaths and as a conduit for placement of an endotracheal tube in case of unanticipated difficult intubation.
- As a conduit during flexible bronchoscopy or laryngoscopy.
- In expected difficult intubation to provide ventilation or as a conduit for passing endotracheal tubes.
- The second-generation laryngeal mask airways are increasingly used for laparoscopic and other short surgical procedures.

MANAGING DIFFICULT AIRWAY

When an airway is difficult to secure, one can use several devices to provide ventilation and oxygen to the patient. If one cannot mask-ventilate the patient using a single hand, one can use both hands while an assistant can compress the reservoir bag to ventilate the patient. The other option is to use an oropharyngeal or a nasopharyngeal airway. An oropharyngeal airway (**Fig. 15**) has a plastic body, a flange, a tip, and a channel for airflow. It opens the airway by preventing the tongue from approximating the pharyngeal wall and covering the epiglottis. The size of the oropharyngeal airway is determined by keeping the airway against the patient's mouth so that the flange lies at the level of lips while the tip lies at the level of the angle of the mandible.

When faced with unanticipated difficult intubation where one is not able to place an ETT and also unable to ventilate the patient with a laryngeal mask airway, one can use a special airway device called Combitube (**Fig. 16**) which can be inserted even by a novice and can tide over the crisis. This tube has two

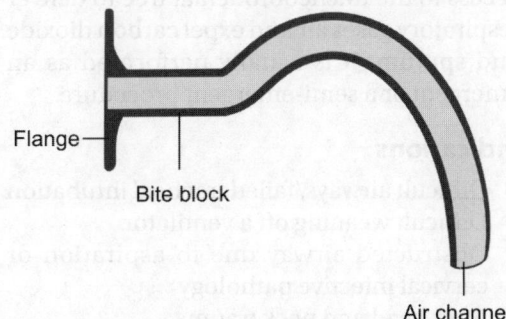

Fig. 15: Oropharyngeal airway.

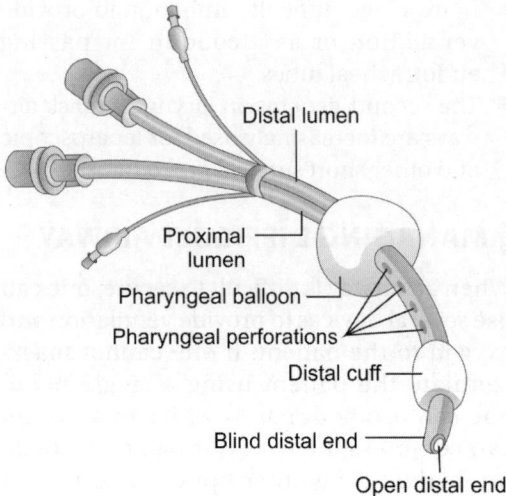

Fig. 16: Combitube.

lumens and two inflatable cuffs, a distal low volume and a proximal large volume inflatable cuff. The tube is entered blindly through the patient's mouth. If the tube enters the trachea, ventilation is achieved through the distal lumen like a normal ETT. Still, if the tube enters the esophagus, the ventilation is achieved through the ports proximal to the distal cuff. The only disadvantage of combitube is that it is not available in pediatric sizes.

EMERGENT TRACHEOSTOMY

Tracheostomy is a surgical procedure to create a surgical airway. A tracheostomy provides access to the tracheobronchial tree to deliver respiratory gases air and expel carbon dioxide and sputum. It is usually performed as an emergent or a semi-emergent procedure.

Indications
- Difficult airways/failed tracheal intubation
- Difficult weaning off a ventilator
- Obstructed airway due to aspiration or cervical infective pathology
- After head and neck trauma
- Lethal neurologic insult

Process
The procedure is done under local anesthesia or general anesthesia in an emergency ward, operating room, or intensive care. The process involves an incision in the anterior wall of the trachea through which a tracheostomy tube or an endotracheal tube is passed into the tracheal lumen for access to the lower respiratory tract.

Open Tracheostomy
A skin incision is made in the midline anterior neck. The incision is extended through the platysma muscle to expose the strap muscles. The strap muscles are retracted to expose the cricoid cartilage and thyroid gland. The thyroid isthmus is identified and ligated, if necessary. The second and third tracheal rings are identified, and an incision is made between the rings. A tracheostomy tube is placed through this incision. Hemostasis is ensured, and the incision is closed with the tube in situ.

Percutaneous Tracheostomy
This method uses a dilatational process via a modified Seldinger technique and is better performed under bronchoscopic guidance. It is currently considered the standard of care for the emergent airway. A 2–3 cm vertical incision in the neck overlies the trachea and below the cricoid cartilage. The paratracheal tissue is dissected bluntly until the trachea is palpable. An introducer needle is inserted through the anterior wall of the trachea at the level of the second tracheal ring. Placement of the needle bevel in a downward position helps to direct the guidewire into the distal trachea. The needle over the wire is removed, and the track is serially dilated with different-sized dilators. Keeping the wire and the protective sheath in place, a tracheostomy tube is passed into the trachea over the wire and protective sheath (**Fig. 17**). The percutaneous technique is easily performed at the bedside,

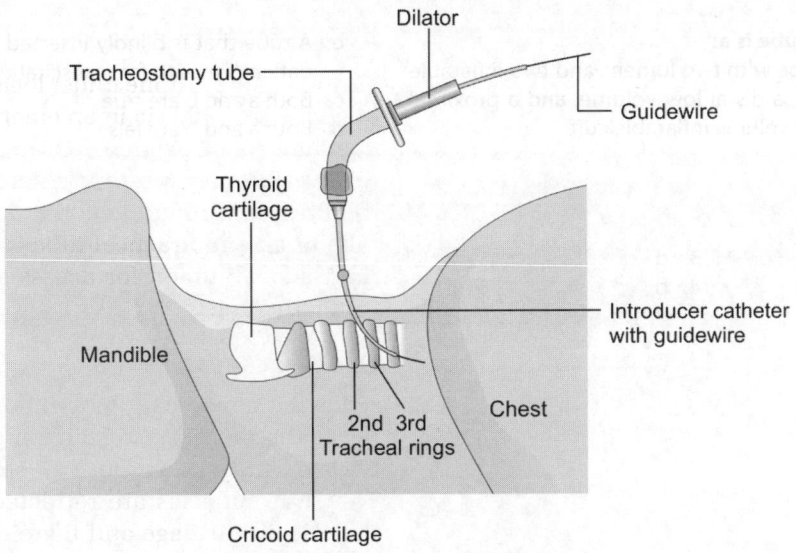

Fig. 17: Percutaneous tracheostomy.

avoiding the transport of potentially critically ill patients. It is associated with less blood loss and lower infection rates than the open technique.

MULTIPLE CHOICE QUESTIONS

1. **The cartilage compressed to occlude the esophagus and prevent regurgitation in patients with a full stomach is:**
   a. Thyroid cartilage
   b. Cricoid cartilage
   c. Epiglottis
   d. Corniculate cartilage
2. **The muscles responsible for the movement of the vocal cords are all *except*:**
   a. Posterior cricoarytenoid
   b. Interarytenoid
   c. Sternothyroid
   d. Cricothyroid
3. **In bilateral abductor palsy:**
   a. The glottis gets closed
   b. There is severe respiratory distress
   c. There is aphonia
   d. All of the above
4. **Triple airway maneuver is a:**
   a. Three-prong method to clear the airway after aspiration
   b. The two-hand technique of face mask ventilation relieves airway obstruction in a patient
   c. Three steps for tracheal intubation
   d. None of the above
5. **The commonly used airway assessment tool based on the view of the upper airway of a sitting patient with the mouth opened wide and the tongue sticking out is the:**
   a. Modified Mallampati classification
   b. Guedel's classification
   c. Safar's classification
   d. Modified ASA classification
6. **A laryngeal mask airway is a:**
   a. A mask-shaped device to cover the face for delivery of anesthetic gases
   b. Mask with gauze cover to deliver on which chloroform or ether is poured for anesthesia
   c. A minimally invasive device with an inflatable mask that fits against the epiglottic tissue and has tubing attached to it that exits through the mouth
   d. A device used to overcome the obstruction in patients with laryngeal masks

7. **Combitube is a:**
   a. A tube with two lumens and two inflatable cuffs, a distal low volume, and a proximal large volume inflatable cuff
   b. A tube that is blindly inserted through the patient's mouth for resuscitation
   c. Both a and b are true
   d. Both a and b are false

Answers
1. b
2. c
3. d
4. b
5. a
6. c
7. c

CHAPTER 4

General Anesthesia

Parul Gupta, Rakhee Goyal

Learning Objectives

- Principle of general anesthesia
- Balanced anesthesia
- Process of general anesthesia (induction, intubation, maintenance, recovery, and tracheal extubation)
- Modes of ventilation in general anesthesia

INTRODUCTION

General anesthesia (GA) is the term familiar to most people, but there are more myths than facts, more fear than assurance. GA is a process to render a patient unconscious and still during the period of surgery, with no recall (amnesia) or awareness of this time and no sensory, motor, or autonomic response to any stimulation. GA is a state of controlled unconsciousness. During a GA, drugs send the patient to sleep, become unaware of surgery, become immobile, and have no pain while surgery is carried out. GA is used to make surgery safer or more comfortable for the patient.

Early anesthesia was all about ether and chloroform. Still, modern anesthesia has come a long way not only to facilitate surgeries and interventions and provide analgesia but also to optimize the patient as a whole and vital organ support throughout the surgical procedure.

How does GA work?

It is not clear exactly how GA works, but it is known that anesthetics stop the transmission of neural signals to the brain. The general anesthetics reduce nerve transmission at synapses between nerves, i.e., the sites at which neurotransmitters are released. The exact mechanism of this synaptic neurotransmission inhibition is not yet fully understood. Volatile anesthetic agents are more soluble in lipids than in water. They primarily affect the function of ion channel and neurotransmitter receptor proteins in the membranes of nerve cells, which have high-lipid content.

Balanced Anesthesia

Besides unconsciousness, the other key elements include muscle relaxation, analgesia, and reversibility of the whole process at the termination of surgery. They are commonly referred to as the 'Triad of Balanced Anesthesia' (**Fig. 1**). The synchronization of these elements makes it possible to have balanced anesthesia wherein optimal doses of different drugs that act on different receptors can be used safely to provide suitable conditions to facilitate surgery.

Need for General Anesthesia

General anesthesia can be given to any patient for any surgery except when the patient does

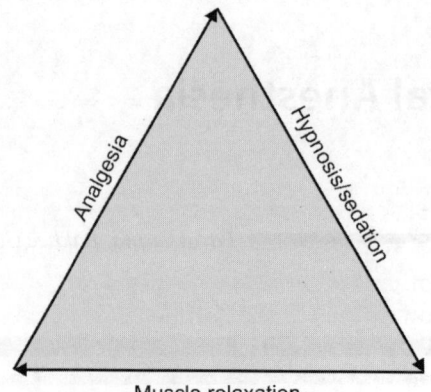

Fig. 1: Balanced anesthesia triad.

not consent or needs to be optimized. The most common site for administration of GA is the operating room (OR). Still, with the latest equipment, monitoring devices, and trained personnel, it can even be administered in nonoperative room settings like radiology suites and outpatient settings. The indications of GA are:
- Procedures requiring muscle relaxation
- Presence of contraindications for regional anesthesia
- Hemodynamic fluctuations anticipated
- Surgeries involving significant blood loss
- Uncooperative patient
- Patient's request for GA.

Before GA

A detailed preanesthetic assessment and written informed consent are mandatory before accepting a patient for GA. The patients are accepted in the American Society of Anesthesiologists (ASA) physical status grades I to VI with or without 'E' depending on their overall health condition and comorbidities, with higher grades being at higher risk than the lower ones, and 'E' denoting emergency scenarios. The details of the preanesthetic assessment are described in Chapter 2.

Once accepted for GA and written informed consent is obtained from the patient, the process of GA is conducted in the designated operating room that is well-equipped and staffed as per national guidelines. This process commonly runs through four phases, namely induction, intubation, maintenance, and reversal.

PROCESS OF GA

The triad of general anesthesia involves the administration of a hypnotic agent, mostly an analgesic, and may or may not include a muscle relaxant depending upon the surgical needs. There is no common recipe for every patient. Rather, the GA is tailored and titrated according to the surgery and patient-related factors and the amount of pain and surgical stimulation anticipated.

Premedication

AS4.3: Observe and describe the principles and the practical aspects of induction and maintenance of anesthesia.

The induction phase may be preceded by a premedication phase in certain cases, but mostly it is synced together. The aim is to allay the patient's anxiety and facilitate a smooth transition to unconsciousness. Benzodiazepines like midazolam are given as premedication because of their anxiolytic properties and the ability to cause anterograde amnesia. With the advent of enhanced recovery from surgery protocols, traditional premedication is generally no longer recommended. Premedication is now restricted to essential drugs, the patient is already being administered (such as anti-hypertensives, anti-epileptics, etc.) or needed to prevent certain adverse effects of anesthetic agents (such as drugs to prevent postoperative nausea and vomiting and hypersensitivity response).

Induction of GA

The induction of anesthesia means transitioning from an awake to an unconscious state. The endpoint of induction can be faintly defined and is associated with multi-system and physiological effects. Before initiating the induction of GA, standard ASA monitors are applied, which include noninvasive blood pressure, pulse oximeter, and electrocardiogram. Apart from these, ventilation, temperature, and urine output are also measured for patients under GA.

Preoxygenation

The patient is preoxygenated with 100% oxygen before induction of GA to denitrogenate the lungs and fill the patient's functional residual capacity with oxygen. Preoxygenation provides a safety reserve to prevent oxygen desaturation during periods of inadequate ventilation for laryngoscopy and intubation and difficult facemask holding, especially in patients with compromised respiration and circulation.

Inhalation Induction

General anesthesia can be induced through inhalation of an inhalation agent (like sevoflurane). Inhalation induction is a routine practice in children who do not have intravenous access. The child inhales a high concentration of the volatile agent while breathing spontaneously. Intravenous (IV) access is taken once the patient is asleep.

Intravenous Induction

Intravenous agents are the most commonly used for induction of GA. Propofol, thiopentone, etomidate, and ketamine are the agents used for IV induction. Propofol is the most popular and extensively used IV agent. It has a rapid onset, profound sedation, quick recovery, anti-emetic property, and is easily available. Propofol causes pain on injection, which can be prevented by injecting it into a larger vein, injection in running intravenous fluids or injecting lignocaine IV before propofol injection. A calculated dose of induction agent according to the patient's weight is injected (1–3 mg/kg), and further titrated doses are administered based on the effect.

Etomidate is a cardiostable agent and is ideal for patients with cardiovascular disorders. Its use is restricted to critically balanced cardiac patients because it can cause adrenal insufficiency, pain on injection, and thrombophlebitis.

Many barbiturates have been used for the induction of GA. Thiopentone was the most used barbiturate used and popular barbiturate. Its use has declined recently and is now limited to a certain category of patients like those undergoing electroconvulsive therapy.

Ketamine is also used for induction of GA at a dose of 1 mg/kg in patients with compromised hemodynamics. It also offers an advantage for patients with severe atopic disease, bronchial asthma, and children with congenital cyanotic heart diseases.

Opioids

An opioid dose is given as a part of the induction sequence. Besides being analgesic agents, preinduction opioids reduce the total dose of the induction agent required and reduce the stress response associated with induction and intubation. The most commonly used opioids are morphine and fentanyl. Morphine is a long-acting opioid with the histamine-releasing property. Fentanyl (1–2 mcg/kg) is a faster and short-acting opioid and is currently the opioid of choice. It is more potent than morphine.

Dissociative Anesthesia

Ketamine causes dissociative anesthesia and can be used as a sole agent for GA. It causes analgesia and bronchodilatation as well. Although it is a circulatory stimulant, it should be avoided in catecholamine-depleted patients. Its common side effects include agitation, hallucinations, and delirium. A small dose of benzodiazepine can be given before ketamine to prevent these side effects. Ketamine is usually used in the dose of 2 mg/kg for induction of dissociative anesthesia, and repeat titrated boluses are given for the maintenance of anesthesia. Ketamine is also used in a dose of 0.5 mg/kg for analgesia.

Rapid Sequence Induction/Intubation (RSI)

A modified induction/intubation process is used when rapid intubation of the trachea is required to reduce the risk of aspiration as in cases of a full stomach, intestinal obstruction, emergencies, obstetric patients, or if the patient has a history of gastroesophageal reflux disease. After preoxygenation, rapid induction and muscle paralysis are achieved using a rapid-acting neuromuscular blocker. Without a bag and facemask ventilation, the trachea is intubated. This rapid sequence helps secure the airway and reduces the risk of gastric insufflation and regurgitation.

Muscle Relaxation

Muscle relaxants are required to facilitate intubation and to provide surgical relaxation. The details of the neuromuscular blocking agents used as muscle relaxants are described in Chapter 7. Adequate muscle relaxation is required for endotracheal intubation. Laryngoscopy and tracheal intubation is done after muscle relaxation is achieved.

The onset of action of different neuromuscular blocking agents is different. In case neuromuscular monitoring is used, laryngoscopy and intubation are done after all twitches are lost in the 'Train-of-Four' (TOF) monitor.

Airway Management

On induction of GA, airway muscles lose their tone leading to the collapse of the upper airway and loss of airway reflexes. Chin lift, jaw thrust, and airways (oral and nasopharyngeal) can be used to maintain airway patency. Airway maintenance during anesthesia can be done with a supraglottic airway device or an endotracheal tube. Airway management is described in detail in Chapter 3.

Under direct under vision facilitated by direct laryngoscopy, the endotracheal tube (ETT) is inserted. Confirmation of proper tube placement can be done by chest auscultation, chest rise, and condensation on the endotracheal tube lumen. However, the appearance of a capnograph trace is the gold standard for the correct placement of the ETT in the trachea. The ETT can be inserted orally or nasally, depending on the surgical requirement. In patients with thoracic surgery, a double-lumen tube may be used for isolating and ventilating the two lungs separately through different channels (one-lung anesthesia).

Laryngoscopes are available with different shapes and sizes of blades. Macintosh (curved) and Miller (straight) blades are the most commonly used (**Fig. 2**). The portable video-laryngoscope or a fiberoptic bronchoscope can be used for difficult airways. Video laryngoscope use is specially indicated in patients with anterior larynx, limited mouth openings, and in patients with airway lesions as it provides a 30° to 60° anterior view.

Supraglottic airway devices like laryngeal mask airway (LMA) can also be used to ventilate patients under GA. Muscle relaxation may or may not be required for its placement. It seats in the posterior pharynx and seals the supraglottic airway to permit tracheal ventilation. A supraglottic device may not prevent aspiration if it does not provide a definitive seal. Supraglottic airway devices can be used as rescue airway devices

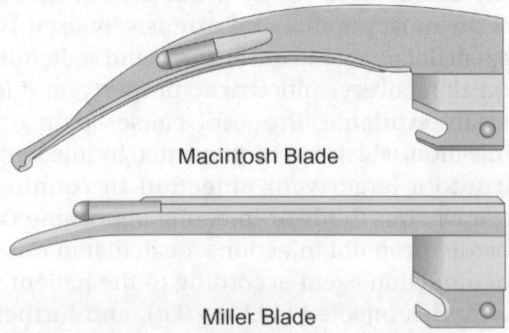

Fig. 2: Types of commonly used Laryngoscope blades.

in difficult airways, difficult mask ventilation, and difficult intubations.

Maintenance of Anesthesia

Anesthesia is maintained using an inhalation volatile agent or an intravenous agent (continuous infusion). During the maintenance phase, hypnosis, sedation, and muscle relaxation need to be maintained using inhalation agents or intravenous agents. It is also essential to maintain the patient's hemodynamics and blood gas homeostasis (described in Chapter 10). The patient is also exposed to cold operating room temperatures, so body temperature must be maintained. The measures to ensure patient safety are described in Chapter 20.

Inhalation Anesthesia

Volatile agents are more commonly used and are delivered through calibrated vaporizers mounted on the anesthesia machine. Inhalation agents include nitrous oxide (gas at room temperature) and volatile agents (halothane, isoflurane, sevoflurane, and desflurane which are in the form of liquids but delivered as vapors to the patients). The pharmacological properties of inhalation agents currently in use are described in Chapter 5.

The delivered concentrations of the inhaled agents are measured by the gas analyzers in the anesthesia gas monitor. End-tidal concentration of the volatile agents indicates the concentration of volatile agents achieved in the patient's blood and reflects the depth of anesthesia. Depth of anesthesia can also be monitored with a bispectral index (BIS) monitor, which monitors the EEG activity of the patient and by monitors using evoked sensory potentials. Minimal alveolar concentration (MAC) is the alveolar concentration of a volatile agent that prevents movement in 50% of healthy volunteers to a standard surgical stimulus (e.g., skin incision). The MAC varies between different agents and is inversely related to their potency. MAC is also affected by various pharmacological and physiological variables.

Intravenous Anesthesia

Total intravenous anesthesia (TIVA) can also be used to maintain anesthesia. Propofol with or without dexmedetomidine, midazolam, and muscle relaxants can be given through a continuous infusion without using volatile agents. The choice of maintenance agents depends upon the type of surgery and patient-related factors.

Controlled Mechanical Ventilation (CMV)

In case muscle relaxants are used during the maintenance phase, intermittent positive-pressure ventilation (IPPV) supports respiration. Different modes of ventilation which can be used are volume-controlled ventilation (VCV), pressure-controlled ventilation (PCV), and pressure-controlled ventilation - volume guaranteed (PCV-VG). In VCV, the desired tidal volume generated for delivery is set on the machine along with the respiratory rate. The airway pressure is variable (depends on the lung compliance of the patient). In PCV, the airway pressure generated is set and regulated, and the volume delivered by the ventilator is variable. In PCV-VG, the ventilation mode is PCV, but the set volume is guaranteed. Most modern anesthesia workstations have these ventilation modes to facilitate appropriate ventilation for exchanging breathing gases. Usually, the VCV mode is used for healthy adults, and PCV and PCV-VG modes are used in children.

Lung-protective Ventilation

Use of lung-protective ventilation is recommended with appropriate positive end-expiratory pressure (PEEP) and low tidal volumes (6–8 mL/kg) to prevent atelectasis, barotrauma, volutrauma, and postoperative pulmonary infections.

Opioid-free Anesthesia (OFA)

The opioid addiction epidemic in the western world has triggered a need to restrict the use of opioids in medical therapy. With the availability of potent non-opioid analgesics and multimodal analgesia methods, there is a trend to move towards OFA. Multimodal analgesia includes using non-steroidal anti-inflammatory drugs (NSAIDs), ketamine, paracetamol, and regional anesthetic blocks.

Enhanced Recovery After Surgery (ERAS)

To improve patient outcomes, reduce patient length of stay, and thereby reduce the cost of surgery, ERAS is getting very popular. Anesthesia for ERAS is managed in such a way as to promote early mobilization with the use of short-acting agents to ensure a quick recovery and early discharge from the hospital. Multimodal analgesia is used to reduce the after-effects of drugs. Different ERAS protocols for different surgeries have been defined. The results of these protocols are very promising, and their use has reduced the length of hospital stay and improved patient outcomes.

Monitoring During GA

Throughout the conduct of GA, monitoring of oxygenation, ventilation, vitals, fluid balance, urine output, and blood loss should be done to ensure hemodynamic stability and patient safety. The details of the modes of monitoring are described in Chapter 9.

Emergence from Anesthesia

At the end of the surgery, the maintenance agent should be discontinued. After discontinuation of inhalation agents, their end-tidal concentration must be monitored. The patient will awaken only after most of the agent has been washed out of the body. To wash off inhalation agents, there is a need to administer higher fresh gas flows. A patient will wake up only when the concentration of an agent has fallen to about 0.2 MAC. NSAIDs and anti-emetics should be given before the end of the GA for adequate analgesia and prevention of postoperative nausea and vomiting (PONV).

Reversal of Neuromuscular Blockade

Upon completion of the surgery, the neuromuscular blockade has to be reversed. Reversal of neuromuscular block can be achieved by administration of its competitive antagonist anti-cholinesterase agent. Neostigmine is the most common drug used. Neostigmine must be given with an anticholinergic agent (atropine or glycopyrrolate) to prevent bradycardia and other muscarinic effects of the drug. A new cyclodextrin derivative drug, Sugammadex, has been recently introduced for early reversal of the steroidal neuromuscular blocking agents.

Tracheal Extubation

A safe tracheal extubation requires a lot of skill and experience and is perhaps more challenging than induction and intubation. Several physiological changes occur with the patient transitioning from a deep to the lighter plane of anesthesia. Many potential complications can occur during this period, like bronchospasm, agitation, etc. A quick oral toilet should be done using a suction before extubation to clear any secretions. The trachea should be extubated once the patient meets the extubation criteria, i.e., the patient is awake, breathing spontaneously with adequate tidal volume, and protective reflexes have returned. Tracheal extubation may be done in a deeper plane for a few patients (e.g., reactive airway disease) to reduce the risk of coughing and laryngospasm associated with awake extubation. Deep plane extubation is also favored for certain neurosurgical and cardiac patients to prevent sudden surges in intracranial pressure and systemic blood pressure. Deep plane extubation is, however, associated with the risk of aspiration. It is vital to verify that the patient can maintain a clear airway after tracheal extubation.

Postoperative Care

The postanesthesia care unit (PACU) is a transition place from the operating room to the ward. The patient is monitored here for any immediate postoperative surgical or anesthetic complications. The potential complications which can occur include hypoxemia, nausea, vomiting, pain, hemodynamic instability, and surgical problems. PONV is the most common complication seen. It can be prevented by avoiding nitrous oxide and volatile agents, using propofol infusion, timely antiemetic prophylaxis, minimizing the use of opioids, and maintaining adequate hydration. All patients should be monitored closely in the PACU and discharged only when fulfilling the discharge criteria. Details of postoperative care are described in Chapter 12.

MULTIPLE CHOICE QUESTIONS

1. **Balanced anesthesia is the triad of:**
   a. Unconsciousness, inhalational anesthetic agents, and benzodiazepines
   b. Unconsciousness, muscle relaxation, and analgesia
   c. Hypnosis, sedation, and muscle relaxation
   d. Sedation, immobility, and unconsciousness

2. **The alphabet 'E' as a suffix to the ASA functional class denotes:**
   a. A grade slightly higher than the numerical class written
   b. Denotes emergency
   c. Denotes extra risk factors
   d. All of the above

3. **The patient is preoxygenated with 100% oxygen before induction of GA to:**
   a. Denitrogenate the lungs
   b. To increase the oxygen saturation of the patient
   c. To ease the anxiety of the patient
   d. To help induction of anesthesia

4. **The following agents are used for induction of anesthesia *except*:**
   a. Dexmedetomidine
   b. Propofol
   c. Thiopentone
   d. Etomidate

5. **All these are common adverse effects of ketamine used for dissociate anesthesia *except*:**
   a. Agitation
   b. Bronchospasm
   c. Hallucinations
   d. Delirium

6. **The gold standard method of confirming the correct placement of an endotracheal tube is:**
   a. Chest auscultation
   b. Chest rise on ventilating the lung
   c. The appearance of a capnography trace
   d. Fogging on the endotracheal tube

7. **In enhanced recovery after surgery (ERAS) involves:**
   a. Use of multimodal analgesia techniques
   b. Use of short-acting anesthetic agents to ensure a quick recovery and early discharge
   c. Reduces cost of surgery
   d. All of the above

8. **The phases of general anesthesia include all *except*:**
   a. Muscle relaxation
   b. Induction
   c. Intubation
   d. Reversal

Answers
1. b
2. b
3. a
4. a
5. b
6. c
7. d
8. a

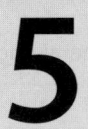

Pharmacology of Anesthetic Agents

Tushar Chokshi

Learning Objectives

- Basic pharmacology of drugs used in anesthesia
- Induction agents
- Sedatives
- inhalation agents
- Analgesics
- Opioids

INTRAVENOUS AGENTS

AS4.1: Describe and discuss the pharmacology of drugs used in induction and maintenance of general anesthesia (including intravenous and inhalation induction agents, opiate and nonopiate analgesics, depolarizing and nondepolarizing muscle relaxants, anticholinesterases).

PROPOFOL

Propofol was invented in 1977 and came into clinical use in 1989. It is considered a 'Switch on - Switch off' anesthetic. It has only hypnotic and anesthetic properties but has no analgesic properties. It is available as a milky white solution in a 1% (10 mg/mL) and a 2% (20 mg/mL) formulation. It is also called Milk of Amnesia. Propofol solution contains soya oil, medium-chain triglycerides (MCT), glycerol, egg lecithin, sodium hydroxide, oleic acid, and water for injection.

Mechanism of Action

It acts by increasing gamma-amino-butyric acid (GABA)-mediated inhibitory tone in the central nervous system (CNS). It decreases the rate of dissociation of the GABA from the receptor, thereby increasing the duration of the GABA-activated opening of the chloride channel with resulting hyperpolarization of the cell membrane. The endocannabinoid system may contribute significantly to propofol's anesthetic action and its unique properties. It causes a prominent reduction in the brain's information integration capacity.

Pharmacokinetics

- Formula: $C_{12}H_{18}O$
- Molar mass: 178.275 g.mol^{-1}
- Protein binding: 95–99%
- Metabolism: Liver glucuronidation
- Onset of action: 15–30 seconds
- Elimination half-life: 1.5–31 h
- Duration of action: 5–10 min
- Excretion: Renal
- Renal clearance: 120 mL/min

Administration of Drug

It is preferably administered in a large vein. Administer 2 mL lidocaine before to prevent injection pain, or add 2 mL lidocaine can be added to 20 mL propofol. Propofol should be titrated (approximately 20–40 mg propofol every 10 seconds) against the patient's response until clinical signs show the onset of anesthesia (**Table 1**).

Clinical Use

Its use is indicated in:
- Initiation and maintenance of sedation in Monitored anesthesia care
- Combined sedation and regional anesthesia
- Induction of general anesthesia
- Maintenance of general anesthesia
- Intensive care unit (ICU) sedation
- Lie detector test.

Contraindications

Documented hypersensitivity, egg allergy, soybean/soy allergy.

Cautions to Use

Bronchial asthma, long-term NSAIDs use, severe hypovolemia or shock, EF < 30% with cardiac disease, severe hepatic dysfunction, severe renal impairment, long-term infusion, GI bleeds, ulcers, perforation, pregnancy and lactation.

Adverse Effects

Hypotension, apnea lasting 30–60 seconds, abnormal movements, injection site burning/pain, respiratory acidosis, hypertriglyceridemia, rash and itching, arrhythmia, bradycardia, decreased cardiac output, bronchospasm, edema, phlebitis, allergic reaction, pancreatitis, asystole/cardiac arrest, seizures.

ETOMIDATE

Etomidate was invented by Janssen Pharma in 1964 and was first introduced as an anti-fungal agent. It was approved as an intravenous (IV) anesthetic agent in 1972. It is available as a milky white [MCT/long-chain triglycerides (LCT) preparation] or clear solution in 2 mg/mL in a 10 mL vial. It is a preferred drug in hemodynamically unstable patients for induction of anesthesia and patients with heart disease as it does not reduce the systemic vascular like other induction agents.

Mechanism of Action

Etomidate stimulates GABA receptors in the CNS and depresses the reticular activating system. It contains a carboxylated imidazole ring [R-1-ethyl-1-(a-methyl benzyl) imidazole-5-carboxylate] that interacts with GABA receptors to block neuroexcitation and causes sedation, hypnosis, and anesthesia without analgesia.

Administration of Drug

It is preferably administered in a large vein. Never dilute etomidate. Administer 2 mL lidocaine before the drug. The first dose must be completed within one arm-brain circulation (60–90 sec). As a continuous infusion, the dose is 0.04–0.05 mg/kg/h with continuous monitoring. Etomidate decreases the level of circulating cortisol when given to the critically ill, so 100–200 mg hydrocortisone can be given before etomidate infusion (**Table 2**).

Pharmacokinetics

- Onset of action: Within 30 to 60 sec
- Peak effect: In 1 min
- Duration: 3 to 5 min (terminated by redistribution)
- Protein binding: 76%
- Metabolism: By hepatic and plasma esterase
- Distribution half-life: 3 min (anesthesia)
- Redistribution half-life: 30 min (sedation)
- Elimination half-life: 3 h (drowsiness)

Table 1: Induction and maintenance dose of propofol as per age and functional status.

	Induction dose	Maintenance dose
Children	3–3.5 mg/kg	0.125–0.3 mg/kg/min
Adult	2–2.5 mg/kg	0.1–0.2 mg/kg/min
Geriatric	1–1.5 mg/kg	0.05–0.1 mg/kg/min
ASA III-IV	1 mg/kg	0.05 mg/kg/min

Table 2: Induction dose of etomidate as per age and functional status.

	Induction Dose
Children	0.1-0.3 mg/kg
Adults	0.3-0.4 mg/kg
Geriatric/Pregnancy/Adrenal Compromise	0.2 mg/kg

Clinical Use

Its use is indicated in:
- Sedation and conscious sedation
- Hypnosis
- Lie-detector test
- Anesthesia induction agent
- Etomidate speech and memory test (eSAM).

Contraindications

Proven sepsis with unstable hemodynamics, compromised adrenal function, hypersensitivity of etomidate, children less than ten years of age, pregnancy, and geriatric patients.

Adverse Effects

Transient injection site pain in about 80% of patients, skeletal muscle movements, mainly myoclonic (peripheral limb movements) in about 30% of patients, opsoclonus (uncontrolled eye movements), adrenal suppression in about 10% of patients, hiccups, and apnea up to 90 seconds, less frequently, nausea, vomiting, laryngospasm, snoring, arrhythmia and hypercarbia.

SODIUM THIOPENTAL (PENTHOTAL)

Pentothal or Thiopentone was discovered in 1930 and clinically used in 1934 for the first time. It is a popular anesthesia induction agent. It is a rapid-onset short-acting barbiturate. The drug went into disrepute after it was falsely implicated in the death of soldiers after the Pearl Harbor attack. It remained the most popular anesthetic for several decades after that. It is available as a yellowish hygroscopic powder stabilized with anhydrous sodium carbonate as a buffer. It is prepared for IV use by reconstitution with an appropriate diluent (sterile water and 0.9% sodium chloride).

Mechanism of Action

Barbiturates are relatively non-selective compounds that bind to an entire superfamily of ligand-gated ion channels, of which the $GABA_A$ receptor is representative.

Pharmacokinetics

- Protein binding: 80%
- Metabolism: Liver (mainly) and renal excretion
- Metabolites: Pentobarbital (active)
- Onset of action: 30–45 sec
- Elimination half-life: 5.5–26 h
- Duration of action: 5–10 min

Administration of Drug

It is prepared as a 2.5% solution (25 mg/mL) and is administered in a dose of 3-4 mg/kg. The dose requirement in non-premedicated children is 5-6 mg/kg. In convulsive states, administration of 75-125 mg is recommended to control seizures. For narcoanalysis and narcosynthesis in psychiatric disorders, a slow infusion of 100 mg/min is commonly used.

Clinical Use

Its use is indicated in:
- Sole anesthetic agent
- Induction of anesthesia
- Supplement regional anesthesia
- Hypnosis during balanced anesthesia
- Anti-convulsant
- Control increased intracranial pressure
- Narcoanalysis and narcosynthesis in psychiatric disorders
- To induce a medical coma/euthanasia
- Truth serum tests.

Contraindications

Hypersensitivity to barbiturates, acute intermittent porphyria, severe cardiovascular disease, hypotension/shock, and Addison's disease.

Adverse Effects

Respiratory depression, myocardial depression, arrhythmia, prolonged somnolence and recovery, sneezing/coughing/shivering, bronchospasm/laryngospasm, anaphylactic/anaphylactoid reactions, and immune hemolytic anemia.

Accidental Arterial Injection

Accidental intra-arterial injection can cause artery spasm, severe pain, blanching of the upper limb, and gangrene. A dilute solution of papaverine, 40 to 80 mg, or 10 mL of 1% procaine, is injected into the artery to relieve the smooth muscle spasm.

KETAMINE

Ketamine was invented in 1962 and approved for clinical use in 1970. It is used for dissociative anesthesia. It is a rapid-acting general anesthetic that produces profound analgesia. Normal pharyngeal-laryngeal reflexes are maintained with slightly enhanced skeletal muscle tone. It is a cardiovascular and respiratory stimulant with transient/minimal respiratory depression. It increases blood pressure, salivation, bronchodilation, hallucination, agitation, and catatonia.

Mechanism of Action

Ketamine interacts with N-methyl-D-aspartate (NMDA) receptors, opioid receptors, monoaminergic receptors, muscarinic receptors, and voltage-sensitive Ca ion channels. It does not interact with GABA receptors and selectively depresses the thalamo-neocortical system before significantly obtunding the more ancient cerebral centers and pathways (reticular-activating and limbic systems).

Pharmacokinetics

- Bioavailability 93–100%
- Protein binding 53.5%
- Distribution half-life 1.95 min
- Elimination half-life 186 min
- Elimination by mainly in urine 91%
- Water and lipid soluble.
- Oral ketamine is broken down by bile acids and undergoes hepatic metabolism.

Administration of Drug

It can be administered IV, intramuscular (IM), infusion, oral, nasal, intratracheal, per-rectal, sublingual, and topical gel. The effect of an IV injection starts in 2 min and lasts for about 25 min. The effect of IM injection starts in 5 min and lasts for 4–6 h. The oral dose-effect starts in 30 min and lasts for four hour (**Table 3**).

Clinical Use

Its use is indicated in:
- Induction of general anesthesia
- Total IV anesthesia (TIVA)
- Analgesic supplement
- Relieve bronchospasm
- Induction of anesthesia in severe hypotensive states.

Table 3: Dose of Ketamine as per indication of use.

	Dose
Dissociative anesthesia	1–2 mg/kg IV
Partially dissociative anesthesia	0.4–0.8 mg/kg IV
Analgesia	0.1–0.3 mg/kg IV
Procedural sedation (IV)	1–2 mg/kg IV
Procedural sedation (IM)	4–8 mg/kg IM
Postoperative infusion	0.1–0.2 mg/kg/h IV

Contraindications

Angina, stroke, very high blood pressure, psychiatric disorders, uncontrolled epilepsy, raised intraocular pressure, eye injury, acute porphyria, and age less than 3 months.

Adverse Effects

Increases heart rate and blood pressure, increases intracranial pressure, transient redness of the skin, increased salivation, and vomiting, pain eruptions or rashes at the injection site, tonic-clonic movements, double vision, involuntary eye movements, increased bronchial secretions, anaphylaxis, dependence, cognitive deficits, and emergence delirium.

MIDAZOLAM

Midazolam was patented in 1974 and approved for clinical use in 1982. It is the most commonly used benzodiazepine as it is shorter acting, potent, and causes less pain at the injection site. In 2018, midazolam was approved as a "truth serum medication."

Mechanism of Action

Midazolam binds to the GABA receptor and enhances the affinity of GABA for its receptor site on the same receptor complex. The pharmacodynamic consequence includes anti-anxiety effects, sedation, and reduction of seizure activity. It has no analgesic effect.

Pharmacokinetics

- Bioavailability: By IV 100%, oral 40%, IM 90%, nasal 78%, and buccal 90%
- Protein binding: 97%
- Onset of action: Within 5 min (IV), 15 min (IM), 20 min (oral), 10 min (Buccal)
- Elimination half-life: 1.5–2.5 h
- Duration of action: 1–6 h
- Excretion: Kidney
- Metabolism: Hepatic hydroxylation by cytochrome P450 3A4 enzyme system.

Table 4: Dose of midazolam as per mode of administration.

	Dose
Oral pediatric dose	0.25–0.5 mg/kg
IV sedation	0.01–0.05 mg/kg IV
IV maintenance dose	0.05–0.1 mg/kg/h IV
IM sedation	0.02–0.05 mg/kg
Rectal dose	0.4 mg/kg
Nasal	5 mg spray in 1 nostril
Geriatric dose	0.01–0.02 mg/kg IV

Administration of Drug

It can be administered by oral, IV, IM, nasal, buccal, and rectal routes. It is more potent and has a shorter duration of action than diazepam. Midazolam nasal spray is the only FDA-approved nasal option for treating seizure clusters. It is available as an injection, syrup, tablet and buccal form. The IV/IM preparation is available as 1 mg/mL and 5 mg/mL. The syrup is available as a 2 mg/mL solution (**Table 4**).

Clinical Use

Its use is indicated in:
- Preoperative sedation/anxiolysis/amnesia
- Nonoperating room anesthesia (NORA)
- Adjuvant in TIVA and opioid-free anesthesia
- To reduce the dose of induction agent of general anesthesia
- Continuous IV infusion for sedation in ICU
- As oral/nasal/rectal premedication in pediatric patients
- Acute management of seizures and schizophrenia

Adverse Effects

Apnea, bradypnea, myoclonic jerks, variable blood pressure readings, drowsiness, headache, hiccups, nausea, vomiting, and confusion.

Overdose

It is a medical emergency. Antidote is flumazenil (0.01 mg/kg IV).

DEXMEDETOMIDINE

Dexmedetomidine was approved for use in 2000 for ICU sedation. It is α_2-adrenergic receptor agonist. It has sedative, anxiolytic, sympatholytic, and analgesic-sparing effects and causes minimal depression of respiratory function. It supplements analgesia and is said to decrease opioid requirements by 50%.

Patients receiving dexmedetomidine are sedated but arousable, i.e., conscious sedation. There is bradycardia and transient hypertension followed by hypotension after its administration due to its peripheral vasoconstrictive and sympatholytic action. Overdose may cause 1st or 2nd degree AV Block. It is used in pediatric TIVA with ketamine.

Mechanism of Action

Dexmedetomidine induces sedation by decreasing the activity of noradrenergic neurons in the locus ceruleus in the brain stem, thereby increasing the activity of inhibitory gamma-aminobutyric acid (GABA) neurons in the ventrolateral preoptic nucleus. It is highly selective for α_2-receptors with an α_2:α_1 ratio of 1620:1.

Pharmacokinetics

- Bioavailability: IV preparation is 100%, IM 70%, buccal and nasal 80%, and Oral 20%.
- Protein binding: 94%
- Onset of action: within 1 min
- Duration of action: 15–20 min
- Metabolism: Metabolized in the liver into inactive metabolites by glucuronidation and hydroxylation
- Elimination half-life: 2 hours
- Excretion: Renal mainly.

Clinical Use

Its use is indicated in:
- Preanesthetic sedation (IM/IV)
- Induction and maintenance of anesthesia
- Adjuvant in TIVA

Table 5: Dose of Dexmedetomidine as per indication of use.

	Dose
Adult ICU sedation	Initial bolus: 1 mcg/kg IV infusion over 10 min Maintenance dose: 0.2–0.7 mcg/kg/h IV infusion
Adult procedural sedation	Initial bolus: 1 mcg/kg IV infusion over 10 min Maintenance dose: 0.2–1.0 mcg/kg/h IV infusion
Geriatric ICU sedation	Initial bolus: Not given Maintenance dose: 0.2–1.0 mcg/kg/h IV infusion
Adult procedural sedation	No guidelines but reduced dosage recommended

- Adjuvant in central neuraxial and regional anesthesia
- Postoperative analgesia and sedation
- ICU sedation

Relative Contraindication

Infusion more than 24 h, preexisting severe bradycardia, bradyarrhythmia, ejection fraction <30, and partial/complete atrioventricular block.

Administration of Drug

It can be administered IV, IM, oral, nasal, nerve blocks, intrathecal, and transdermal as a gel. It is administered as an infusion prepared in 0.9% sodium chloride in water. The drug is currently approved only for ICU and procedural sedation. It is used off-label by other routes, e.g., intrathecal in a dose of 0.1 mcg/kg and buccal/nasal in a dose of 1 mcg/kg (**Table 5**).

INHALATION AGENTS

NITROUS OXIDE

Nitrous oxide was first synthesized in 1772 by Joseph Priestley. It was coined the name "Laughing Gas" by Humphry Davy, as it was used to entertain the guests at 'Frolic Parties.' Breathing pure nitrous oxide causes hypoxia (oxygen insufficiency) and even causes death by asphyxiation. At room temperature, it is a colorless gas with a slight metallic scent and taste. Though it is nonflammable, it supports combustion. It was the most popular inhalation agent until the invention of modern anesthetic agents.

A very typical and important feature of inhaled nitrous oxide is the 'second-gas' effect. Nitrous oxide diffuses more rapidly across alveolar membranes than nitrogen, and its rapid uptake from the alveoli causes the remaining alveolar gases to be concentrated. This accelerates the uptake of volatile agents into the blood and speeds the onset of anesthesia. The reverse occurs at the end of anesthesia as nitrous oxide enters the alveoli very rapidly, diluting the concentration of other gases in the alveoli. The resultant lowering of oxygen concentration within the alveoli, with the patient breathing air, may cause diffusion hypoxia.

Nitrous oxide can interfere with vitamin B12 metabolism, which is necessary for DNA production and cellular reproduction. Its use may be avoided during the first trimester of pregnancy and in children less than 3 years of age. Nitrous oxide has significant global warming potential as a greenhouse gas.

Mechanism of Action

The exact mechanism of action of nitrous oxide is unknown, but it is thought to affect the pain centers of the brain and spinal cord. It is also thought to affect the Gamma Amino Butyric Acid (GABA) cells inhibiting the nerve cells to cause drowsiness and sleep. It has an inhibitory action at N-methyl-D-aspartate (NMDA) glutamate receptors but has stimulatory activity at dopaminergic, adrenergic, and opioid receptors.

Pharmacokinetics

- Boiling point: –88.5°C
- Critical temperature: 36.5°C
- Molecular weight: 44
- Blood-gas coefficient: 0.47
- Oil-gas coefficient: 1.4
- Minimum alveolar concentration (MAC)*: 105 vol%

Administration of Drug

Nitrous oxide is administered as a vapor in the anesthetic gas mixture. The gas is stored as a liquid, and vapor present over the liquid is added to the gas mixture through a calibrated flowmeter tube. Nitrous oxide is stored in gas cylinders mounted on the anesthesia workstation. It may also be delivered to the anesthesia workstation through a medical gas pipeline system. Oxygen concentration in the gas mixture with nitrous oxide must not be below 30%. 50:50 nitrous oxide and oxygen mixture in cylinders (Entonox) are commercially available in some parts of the world. This entonox mixture is used for analgesia during childbirth.

Clinical Use

Nitrous oxide inhalation causes intoxication, euphoria, dysphoria, spatial disorientation, temporal disorientation, and reduced pain sensitivity. It is a weak anesthetic but a good analgesic agent. It is a vasodilator.

Adverse Effects

The common adverse effects are dizziness, fatigue, headache, excessive sweating, and shivering. One of the most important adverse effects is postoperative nausea and vomiting, which makes it a major contributor to anesthetic morbidity. The emetogenic effects of nitrous are thought to be caused by changes in middle ear pressure, bowel distension, and activation of dopaminergic neurons.

---

*The minimum alveolar concentration (MAC) value is defined as the concentration of an inhalation anesthetic agent in the lung alveoli required to prevent movement in response to a surgical stimulus in 50% of patients.

Expansion of Air-filled Spaces

The higher solubility of nitrous oxide vis-a-vis nitrogen causes rapid expansion of nitrogen-containing spaces when nitrous oxide is administered. Pressure or volume changes due to this expansion may have deleterious consequences, as seen in pneumothorax, bowel obstruction, and middle ear disease.

ISOFLURANE

Isoflurane was invented in the early 1970s and was approved for the induction and maintenance of general anesthesia in 1979. Isoflurane is a halogenated ether compound and is nonflammable. It carries a strong, pungent odor that makes it difficult to use for inhalation induction of general anesthesia. It vaporizes readily but is a liquid at room temperature. It is not used for mask induction in pediatric patients, and it is associated with a higher incidence of airway hyperreactivity.

Mechanism of Action

It produces anesthesia by inhibiting neurotransmitter-gated ion channels such as GABA, glycine, and N-methyl-D-aspartate (NMDA) receptors in the central nervous system (CNS) to produce amnesia and sedation. It also acts on sites within the spinal cord to inhibit NMDA-type glutamate and glycine receptors and thus help reduce skeletal muscle motor function. It inhibits conduction in activated potassium channels. It inhibits plasma membranes Ca^{2+}-ATPase in a dose-related manner to alter the neuronal calcium homeostasis by increasing the fluidity of the lipid membrane. Isoflurane reduces junctional conductance by decreasing gap junction channel opening times and increasing gap junction channel closing times.

Pharmacokinetics

- Boiling point: 48.5°C
- Mol Wt: 184.5
- Vapor pressure: 238 mm Hg at 20°C
- Blood-gas coefficient: 1.43
- Oil-gas coefficient: 90.8
- MAC: 1.15 vol%
- Metabolism: Liver (0.2%)

Administration of Drug

Isoflurane is administered as a vapor in the anesthetic gas mixture. The vaporization of the drug takes place in a calibrated isoflurane-specific vaporizer in the anesthesia workstation. It has a shelf-life of 5 years when stored between 15–30°C in an amber-colored glass bottle.

Clinical Use

Pharyngeal and laryngeal reflexes are obtunded by isoflurane, a profound respiratory depressant. As the anesthetic dose increases, tidal volume decreases, but the respiratory rate remains unchanged. Blood pressure decreases and progressive increases in depth of anesthesia it corresponding decreases further. Cardiac output is maintained primarily through increased heart rate, compensating for a reduction in stroke volume. Isoflurane is a vasodilator, and it thus reduces systemic vascular resistance. It is also a coronary arteriolar dilator and diverts blood from collateral-dependent myocardium to normally perfused areas (coronary steal).

Adverse Effects

Dose-dependent extensions of effects like respiratory depression, hypotension, arrhythmias; postoperative shivering, nausea, vomiting, ileus, malignant hyperthermia, elevated carboxyhemoglobin levels, hepatic dysfunction, and hepatitis.

SEVOFLURANE

Sevoflurane was invented in 1971 and has been in clinical use since 1990. It is an ether derivative inhalation anesthetic agent used for the induction and maintenance of general anesthesia. It is a volatile, nonflammable, and nonirritant compound with low solubility and blood-gas partition coefficient. It has a good safety record, and together with desflurane, it is replacing traditionally used volatile agents in modern anesthesia practice. It is considered a 'greenhouse gas' as it does not destroy the ozone layer. It, however, has a high oil-gas coefficient and thus gets trapped in body fat stores in long-duration anesthetics.

Mechanism of Action

The exact mechanism of action is not known. Sevoflurane acts as a positive allosteric modulator of $GABA_A$ receptors in neurons and recombinant receptors. It also acts as an NMDA receptor antagonist, potentiates glycine receptor currents, and inhibits nAChR and 5HT3 receptors.

Pharmacokinetics

- Boiling point: 58.6°C
- Molecular weight: 200.05
- Vapor pressure: 157 mm Hg at 20°C
- Blood-gas coefficient: 0.68
- Oil-gas coefficient: 47
- Metabolism: Liver through cytochrome P450(CYP)2E1 (2% metabolized)
- MAC: 2.1 vol%

Clinical Use

It is the preferred agent for mask induction as it is less irritating to the respiratory tract. It has got fast onset and offset and has no analgesic effect. It is one of the most common inhalation anesthetic agents and can be used across all ages. Sevoflurane reduces peripheral vascular resistance causing mild hypotension and a mild fall in cardiac output. It increases heart rate at low concentrations, but heart rate normalizes at higher concentrations.

Administration of Drug

Sevoflurane is administered as a vapor in the anesthetic gas mixture. The vaporization of the drug takes place in a calibrated vaporizer in the anesthesia work station. It has a shelf-life of 24 months when stored below 25°C and not exposed to light (in amber-colored glass bottles).

Degradation Products

Degradation products of sevoflurane, inorganic fluoride ions, and haloalkene degradation product compound A, can cause nephrotoxicity. Fluoride ions are produced by the metabolism of sevoflurane and can reach high concentrations after prolonged anesthesia. Compound A is produced by sevoflurane exposure to strong alkalis (KOH and NaOH) in carbon dioxide absorbers (soda-lime and baralyme). Compound A has been reported to be nephrotoxic in rats but not in humans.

Adverse Effects

- In adults: Hypotension, nausea, and vomiting
- In elderly: Bradycardia, hypotension, and nausea
- In children: Agitation, cough, vomiting, and nausea; depression of cardiovascular function in a dose-related fashion.

DESFLURANE

Desflurane was invented in 1970 and approved for clinical use in 1987. It is considered the most ideal inhalation anesthetic agent available today. The unique feature of desflurane is that it is a halogenated inhaled anesthetic with low solubility in blood and body tissues. Thereby, its uptake, distribution, and elimination are very rapid. It undergoes negligible metabolism, and so exhibits negligible toxic effects.

Mechanism of Action

Desflurane is a fluorinated ether with properties of a general anesthetic and muscle relaxation. Desflurane is known to act as a positive modulator of the $GABA_A$ and glycine receptors and as a negative modulator of the nicotinic acetylcholine receptor, affecting other ligand-gated ion channels. Desflurane appears to act on the lipid matrix of the neuron membrane and disrupt neuronal transmission in the brain.

Pharmacokinetics

- Boiling point: 22.8°C
- Molecular Weight: 168.04
- Vapor pressure: 88.5 mm Hg at 20°C
- Blood-gas coefficient: 0.42
- Oil-gas coefficient: 19
- MAC: 6 vol%
- Metabolism: Not metabolized

Clinical Use

Desflurane causes dose-dependent tachycardia and hypertension with depression in myocardial contractility and decreased systemic vascular resistance. It causes dose-dependent cerebral vasodilatation, increases cerebral blood flow, cerebral blood volume, and intracranial pressure, and decreases cerebral oxygen consumption. It is a potent respiratory depressant, decreases tidal volume, increases respiratory rate, and is an irritant to the airway. Its use is contraindicated for the inhalation induction and maintenance of anesthesia in nonintubated pediatric patients because of a high incidence of upper airway adverse events, including coughing, laryngospasm, and secretions with the use of high MAC of the agent.

Desflurane has the most rapid onset and offset among volatile anesthetics due to its low solubility in blood. The low-fat solubility of desflurane prevents its accumulation in the slow compartment in overweight patients and long procedures. Its benefits include rapid and predictable emergence and early recovery. Its use promotes the early return of protective airway reflexes. In addition, the use of desflurane promotes rapid transfer of patients from the operating theatre to the recovery area, which has a positive impact on patient turnover.

Administration of Drug

Desflurane is administered as a vapor in the anesthetic gas mixture. Desflurane requires the use of a temperature-controlled (electrically heated), pressure-regulated vaporizer as it vaporizes at room temperature. This vaporizer pressurizes desflurane to roughly two atmospheres of pressure and warms it to 40°C, allowing optimal control of desflurane delivery. It has a shelf-life of 3 years when stored in amber-colored glass bottles or aluminum bottles and kept upright with the cap firmly in place.

Adverse Effects

Desflurane is a potent vasodilator that may cause a concomitant increase in heart rate. Cardiac output is usually preserved. Desflurane dilates cerebral arteries and reduces cerebral metabolic rate, and increases intracranial pressure. Rapid increases in desflurane concentration can cause a transient elevation in heart rate and blood pressure secondary to catecholamine release. Desflurane decreases the ventilatory response to carbon dioxide.

OPIOIDS

MORPHINE

Morphine is an opiate found in opium, the juice secreted by the seedpods of poppies. It was first isolated between 1803 and 1805 by German pharmacist Friedrich from the poppy straw of the opium poppy. Opiates (narcotic analgesics) are considered as 'gold standard' for analgesic therapy, and of the opioids, morphine is considered to be the 'standard' opioid analgesic. To illustrate their potency, all analgesics are compared to morphine. Morphine is the most commonly used agent in pain management in surgery and for almost every kind of pain.

By decreasing pain, morphine decreases the activation of the autonomic nervous system, and thus it is used in myocardial infarction. The venous dilatation effect of morphine also helps reduce the preload of the compromised heart after myocardial infarction. Morphine, however, is addictive and prone to abuse. When morphine is used for a long time, it may become habit-forming, causing mental or physical dependence. The antidotes to morphine (and all opioids) are naloxone and naltrexone.

Mechanism of Action

Morphine and all other opioids block pain transmission by their effect on the opioid receptors (μ, δ, and κ) in the central nervous system (CNS) and peripheral neural and non-neural tissue. The periaqueductal grey, locus ceruleus, rostral ventral medulla, and substantia gelatinosa of the dorsal horn have high concentrations of opioid receptors.

Within the CNS, activation of μ-opioid receptors in the midbrain is thought to be a major mechanism of opioid-induced analgesia. Opioids help reduce nociceptive transmission from the periphery to the thalamus. μ-opioid receptors are associated with analgesia, sedation, euphoria, physical dependence, and respiratory depression. κ-opioid receptors are associated with spinal analgesia, miosis, and psychotomimetic effects, while δ opioid receptors play a role in analgesia.

Pharmacokinetics

- Bioavailability: 20-40% (oral), 36-71% (rectally), 100% (IV/IM), 80-90% (Epidural/Spinal)
- Protein binding: 30-40%
- Metabolism: Hepatic 87% is excreted in 72 h.
- Elimination half-life: 120 min
- Onset of action: 1-2 min (IV), 15 min (IM), 20 min (PO)
- Duration of action: 3-4 h (IV/IM), 20-24 h Spinal/Epidural
- Excretion: Renal 90% (70-80% with 48 h), Biliary 10%
- Dose: The dosing regimen for each patient must be formulated individually, considering the prior analgesic treatment experience. The usual starting IV dose in adults is 0.1-0.2 mg/kg every four h.

Clinical Use

Morphine is used to treat both acute and chronic severe pain, pain due to myocardial infarction, and labor pains. It is used to treat acute pulmonary edema. It is administered as an adjuvant in central neuraxial blockade for perioperative analgesia. The use of oral fentanyl is usually restricted to chronic cancer pain and palliative care.

Administration of Drug

In clinical practice, morphine can be administered via oral, intravenous routes, subcutaneous, transdermal, sublingual, intramuscular, epidural, intrathecal, and intra-articular routes. It has a low-lipid solubility and penetrates the blood-brain barrier slowly and thus has a relatively slow onset of effect. About 40-60% of orally ingested morphine fails to reach the systemic circulation as it has a significant first-pass metabolism in the liver, where morphine is metabolized, predominantly by glucuronidation, to active metabolites excreted in the urine. It is often necessary to provide relatively frequent doses of morphine for optimal and consistent plasma and effect-site concentration of morphine.

It is available for intravenous and intramuscular use at 10 and 15 mg per mL. Oral preparations are available as 10, 15, 30, and 60 mg tablets. Rectal Suppository is available in preparations of 5, 10, 20, and 30 mg. It is also available as a solution and extended-release capsule.

Adverse Effects

Nausea, vomiting, constipation, lightheadedness, dizziness, drowsiness, diaphoresis, urinary retention, headache, dry mouth, pruritus, tolerance, and myoclonus. An IV injection may cause pain, redness, itching, or swelling. Morphine overdose may lead to slow, shallow, or irregular breathing; cold, clammy skin; miosis; bradycardia; and blurred vision. Morphine causes histamine release, and so its use is a relative contraindication in allergy, acute bronchial asthma and upper airway obstruction.

FENTANYL

Fentanyl was invented by Paul Janssen in 1960 and approved for clinical use in 1968. Fentanyl is a potent synthetic opioid similar to morphine but produces analgesia to a greater extent. It is 100 times stronger than morphine. Today, it is the most widely used opioid. Opioid epidemic with fentanyl is very common, and hyperalgesia is common with Fentanyl. Fentanyl is commonly used in ICUs for sedation owing to its versatility in titrating its IV infusion dose. Unlike morphine, fentanyl causes minimal histamine release. Fentanyl may induce chest wall rigidity.

Mechanism of Action

The mode of action is similar to that of other opioids. Biochemically, it is a μ-selective opioid agonist. It can activate other opioid system receptors such as δ- and κ-receptors to produce analgesia. Dopamine is increased in the reward areas of the brain, which elicits exhilaration and relaxation effects, and is responsible for the addiction to the drug. fentanyl crosses the blood-brain barrier and the placenta.

Pharmacokinetics

- Bioavailability: 100% (IM), 100% (IV), 9% (transdermal), 89% (intranasal), 65% (buccal), 54% (sublingual), 55% (inhaled)
- Protein binding: 80–85%
- Metabolism: Hepatic 90% (99% of the drug is metabolized to nor fentanyl by cytochrome P450)
- Elimination half-life: 8–10 h
- Onset of action: 60 sec (IV)
- Duration of action: 30–60 min (IV/IM)
- Excretion: Renal 75% within 72 h

Administration of Drug

Fentanyl is available as 50 mcg/mL preparation for IV/IM use. The dose of the drug administered depends on its intended use.
- *Premedication:* 50–100 mcg/dose IM or slow IV 30–60 min before surgery and when used as an adjunct to regional anesthesia: 25–100 mcg/dose slow IV over 1–2 min.
- *General anesthesia:* Minor surgical procedures 0.5–2 mcg/kg/dose IV; major surgery 2–20 mcg/kg/dose initially; 1–2 mcg/kg/h maintenance infusion IV.
- *Analgesia:* 1–2 mcg/kg IV bolus or 25-100 mcg/dose pro-re-nata (PRN - meaning as needed) or 1–2 mcg/kg/h by continuous IV infusion or 25–200 mcg/h; Severe pain: 50–100 mcg/dose IV/IM every 1-2 h.
- *Patient-controlled anesthesia (PCA):* 10 mcg/mL IV preparation; 20 mcg demand dose with 5–10 min lockout time interval and base rate of ≤50 mcg/h.

Clinical Use

Fentanyl is used as an analgesic agent during general anesthesia (induction and maintenance) for inpatient and outpatient procedures, for continuation as an analgesic in the postoperative period and intensive care. It is an analgesic component of total intravenous anesthesia (TIVA) and monitored-anesthesia-care in adult patients. Fentanyl is also used in neuroleptanalgesia. It is also used in breakthrough pain in patients with acute and chronic pain as a sedative in ICU.

Adverse Effects

Fentanyl's side effects are similar to those of other opioids, i.e., euphoria, confusion, respiratory depression, drowsiness, nausea, vomiting, visual disturbances, dyskinesia, hallucinations, delirium, muscle rigidity, constipation, sedation, urinary retention, paralytic ileus, confusion, and hallucinations. Fentanyl is contraindicated in patients who are on MAO-inhibitors.

REMIFENTANIL

Remifentanil was approved for clinical use in 1996. It is a potent, ultra short-acting synthetic opioid. It is used during surgery as an analgesic and an adjunct to anesthetic agents. It is also used for sedation combined with other medications. It is commonly used in combination with propofol for TIVA. Its analgesic effect is stronger than morphine but not fentanyl.

The primary advantage of remifentanil is a reduction in pharmacokinetic variability, and thus it offers a predictable duration. The drug is cleared by enzymatic hydrolysis by nonspecific esterases. The total remifentanil clearance is 30–50% of cardiac output and is unaffected by variables such as bolus versus infusion, hepatic or renal function, gender, and drug interaction. Remifentanil is used for cases requiring intense analgesia for a short period, e.g., a painful procedure accompanied by very little postoperative pain.

Mechanism of Action

It has a similar mechanism of action as other opioids. It is a µ-receptor opioid agonist which inhibits ascending pain pathways and produces analgesia. It is a respiratory depressant and sedative, increasing the pain threshold.

Pharmacokinetics

- Bioavailability: 100%
- Protein binding: 70%
- Onset: 1–3 min
- Elimination half-life: 3–10 min
- Metabolism: Cleaved by nonspecific plasma and tissue esterases
- Duration of effect: 3–4 min
- Excretion: Urine

Administration of Drug

Remifentanil is available as a powder for injection of 1 mg, 2 mg, or 5 mg in a vial. It is prepared for IV by adding 1 mL of diluent reconstituting solution per mg of remifentanil and shaken well to dissolve. It is then diluted to a final concentration of 25, 50, or 250 mcg/mL before administration. Remifentanil is given by continuous infusion. Bolus doses for loading before the infusion are unnecessary because a continuous infusion approaches steady-state concentrations in 10 min. Infusions of 0.05–0.1 mcg/kg/min and a small dose of benzodiazepine are effective in most cases.

The dose of the drug administered depends on its intended use.

- *Induction of anesthesia:* 0.5–1 mcg/kg/min IV until after intubation
- *Maintenance of anesthesia:* 0.25–0.5 mcg/kg/min IV; bolus of 0.5–1 mcg/kg may be administered every 2–5 min in case the depth of anesthesia is light, or there is an episode of intense surgical stress.
- *Conscious analgesia:* 1 mcg/kg IV bolus, followed by 0.05–0.2 mcg/kg/min IV
- *Postoperative analgesia:* 0.025–0.2 mcg/kg/min IV

Clinical Use

Remifentanil is a rapid- and short-acting opioid analgesic during craniotomies, spinal surgery, cardiac surgery, and bariatric surgery. A large opioid dose blunts the hemodynamic responses to painful stimuli and greatly reduces the need for other drugs such as propofol or volatile anesthetics. During general anesthesia, it may be used without undue lengthening of emergence times. In cardiac surgery, it helps in intraoperative control of stress responses and rapid recovery. Remifentanil may increase patients' safety by eliminating the risk of delayed respiratory depression.

Adverse Effects

Nausea, vomiting, respiratory depression, bradycardia/tachycardia, hypertension/hypotension, skeletal muscle rigidity, postoperative pain, shivering, pruritus, apnea, hypoxia, dizziness, addiction, abuse, and misuse.

MULTIPLE CHOICE QUESTIONS

1. **The following anesthesia induction agent is called 'switch off-switch on' anesthetic:**
   a. Thiopentone
   b. Ketamine
   c. Etomidate
   d. Propofol
2. **Propofol is associated with all *except*:**
   a. Reduced incidence of nausea and vomiting
   b. Pain during injection
   c. A milky solution as it is in an oil solvent base
   d. Decreases the level of circulating cortisol
3. **Ketamine is associated with:**
   a. Profound analgesia
   b. Loss of normal pharyngeal-laryngeal reflexes
   c. Cardiovascular and respiratory depression
   d. All of the above
4. **Conscious sedation can be administered with:**
   a. Midazolam
   b. Remifentanil
   c. Propofol
   d. Dexmedetomidine
5. **The property of the 'second-gas' effect of nitrous oxide means that:**
   a. It can be used with any other inhalational agent as a second gas
   b. It diffuses more rapidly across alveolar membranes, and its rapid uptake causes the remaining alveolar gases to be concentrate
   c. As the second gas, it enhances the hypnotic effect of the other inhalational agents
   d. It can cause hypoxia when administered with oxygen
6. **Which of the following is a property of Desflurane?**
   a. It is non-irritant to the respiratory tract
   b. It has the most rapid onset and offset among volatile anesthetics due to its low solubility in blood
   c. It has a sweet ethereal odor
   d. None of the above
7. **Opioids block pain transmission by:**
   a. Their effect on the opioid receptors (μ, δ, and κ) in the central nervous system
   b. Inactivation of μ-opioid receptors in the midbrain
   c. Enhancing nociceptive transmission from the periphery to the thalamus
   d. Blocking nerve transmission in the periaqueductal grey
8. **Remifentanil is a:**
   a. Potent, ultra-short-acting synthetic opioid
   b. Potent ultra-long-acting opioid
   c. Potent medium-duration opioid
   d. None of the above
9. **The adverse effects of morphine include all *except*:**
   a. Nausea and vomiting
   b. Constipation
   c. Dryness of skin
   d. Urinary retention

Answers
1. d
2. d
3. a
4. d
5. b
6. b
7. a
8. a
9. c

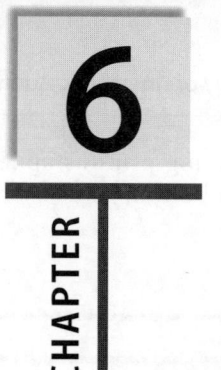

6

Structure of Neuromuscular Junction and Neuromuscular Transmission in Skeletal Muscles

Archana Puri, Mukul Chandra Kapoor

Learning Objectives

- Neuromuscular junction
- Neuromuscular transmission
- Types of neuromuscular blockers
- Pharmacology of common neuromuscular
- Reversal of neuromuscular blockade
- Anticholinesterases
- Residual neuromuscular blockade

NEUROMUSCULAR JUNCTION

The neuromuscular junction (NMJ) is a simple synapse connection between the terminal end of a motor nerve and a muscle (skeletal/smooth/cardiac). However, it is complex in its structure and function. It is the site for transmitting action potential from the nerve to the muscle. It is responsible for converting electrical impulses generated by the motor neuron into electrical activity in the muscle fibers. The NMJ is a very small structure (~30 microns long) compared to the muscle fibers it innervates. Typically, one skeletal muscle fiber has one NMJ where the motor axon joins the muscle fiber.

Anatomy

A motor unit is a single motor neuron and the muscle fibers it innervates. The structure of NMJ can be functionally divided into three parts: a presynaptic part (presynaptic terminal), the postsynaptic part (motor endplate), and an area between the nerve terminal and motor endplate (synaptic cleft). The functional anatomy of the NMJ is displayed in **Figure 1**.

Presynaptic Terminal

The long processes of neurons that travel from the spinal cord to skeletal muscles are called 'axons.' A myelinated motor neuron, on reaching the target muscle, loses its myelin sheath to form a complex of 100–200 branches called 'axon terminals.' The nerve endings of these branches that contact the muscle surface are called synaptic boutons or terminal boutons. The synaptic boutons are small bulbous swelling (called 'synaptic end bulb'). Each synaptic end bulb contains many synaptic vesicles, which contain the chemical neurotransmitter acetylcholine (ACh). Each synaptic vesicle (SV) stores around 5000–10000 molecules of ACh. The amount of ACh stored in each SV is referred to as 'quanta.' The SVs are arranged in clusters alongside small, thick, electron-dense patches of the membrane,

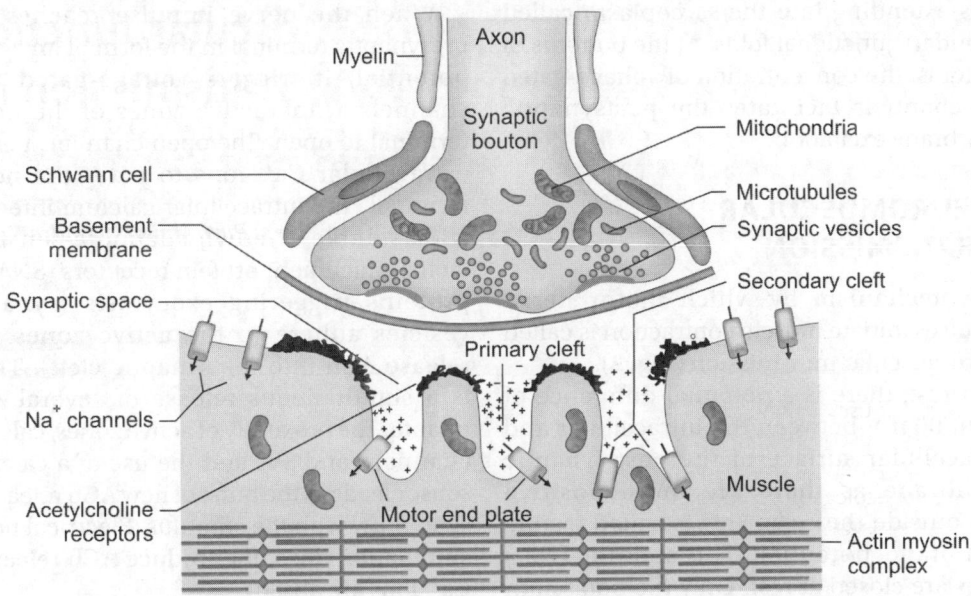

Fig. 1: Diagrammatic representation of the structure of neuromuscular junction.

and these sites are called active zones. The active zone contains many proteins and rows of voltage-gated calcium (Ca) channels. The nerve terminals have a complex mechanism for synthesis, exocytosis, and recycling of these synaptic vesicles. Non-myelinating Schwann cells called perisynaptic or terminal Schwann cells cover the NMJ and are thought to play a role in synapse formation, maintenance, and repair.

Synaptic Cleft

The synaptic cleft is a microscopic gap between the presynaptic terminal and the postsynaptic motor end plate. This cleft is filled with an extracellular matrix called the synaptic basal lamina. The basal lamina is composed of laminins and various collagens. The nerve and muscle are held in tight alignment by protein filaments of the basal lamina. The enzyme acetylcholinesterase (AChE), which breaks down the chemical transmitter acetylcholine, is attached to the basal lamina.

Motor End Plate

The motor end plate is part of the sarcolemma of the muscle cell, which is in closest proximity to the synaptic end bulb and forms the postsynaptic part of NMJ. The sarcolemma is a fine transparent tubular sheath that envelops the muscle fiber and is the thickened portion of the muscle plasma membrane. Sacrolemma is folded to form crypts called junctional folds. The synaptic boutons do not penetrate the motor endplate but fit into these folds. Junctional folds have nicotinic ACh receptors (AChR), which are ACh-gated ion channels. The shoulders of the folds are densely populated with AChRs. It is estimated that about 5 million AChRs are present in each junction. These channels open up when ACh binds to these receptors allowing the influx of extracellular sodium ions into the muscle membrane. This influx of positive charge creates an endplate potential which generates and transmits the action potential. Motor nerve terminals are embedded in the primary cleft. There are also several muscle membrane folds extending into the sarcoplasm called secondary junctional folds. At the bottoms of the folds, the concentration of voltage-gated Na⁺ channels facilitates the postsynaptic membrane excitation.

NEUROMUSCULAR TRANSMISSION

The mechanism by which motor nerve impulses initiate muscle contraction is called neuromuscular transmission (**Fig. 2**).

At rest, there is a potential difference of about 90 mV between the intracellular and extracellular surface of the post-synaptic membrane as there are more positive ions outside the cells. This is called resting membrane potential. The sodium (Na⁺) pores are closed at rest. Only the potassium (K⁺) ions permeate due to the concentration gradient (as K⁺ inside the cells is higher (about 150 mMol) as compared with K⁺ outside the cells (about 5 mMol). This movement of K⁺ continues till equilibrium is attained.

When the nerve impulse reaches the presynaptic terminal in the form of an action potential, it triggers voltage-gated Ca^{2+} channels at the active zones of the nerve terminal to open. The open channels permit extracellular Ca^{2+} ions to enter the nerve terminal. The intracellular calcium interacts with soluble N-ethylmaleimide-sensitive factor attachment protein receptors (SNARE) proteins triggering exocytosis (synaptic vesicles adhere to the active zones and release ACh into the synaptic cleft). There is a simultaneous release of several ACh quanta. The proximity of active zones, calcium channels, and SVs and the use of a calcium sensor leads to the burst of new ACh release in synchrony with the stimulus. Electrical nerve stimulation does not produce ACh release if Ca^{2+} ions are absent.

ACh released binds to the ACh binding site located at the interfaces of the AChR, triggering a conformational change to open the channel. There is an influx of positively charged ions across the channel to generate a change in the

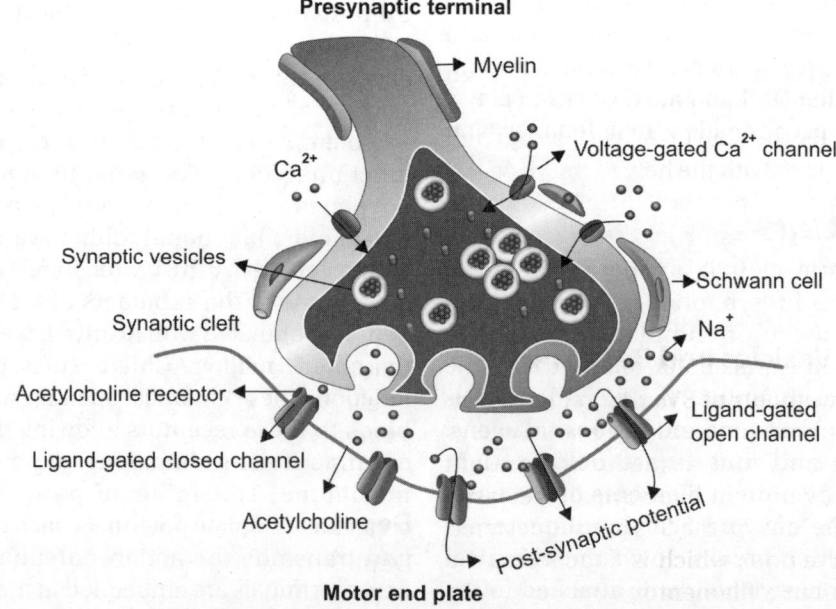

Fig. 2: Physiology of neuromuscular transmission.

membrane potential and thereby triggering an endplate potential. These small-amplitude potentials are called miniature endplate potentials. These potentials have only one-hundredth the amplitude of the evoked potential produced, which leads to muscle contraction. The evoked endplate potential produced spreads from the motor endplate to the rest of the sarcolemma, resulting in the contraction of the muscle.

Post-tetanic Potentiation

The calcium influx continues until the membrane potential returns to normal by outward movement of potassium from the nerve cell. Calcium in the nerve cannot be excreted if the nerve is stimulated repeatedly. After a tetanic stimulation, increasing calcium in the nerve ending causes post-tetanic potentiation of contraction. A stimulus applied to the nerve during this time causes the release of more than the normal amount of acetylcholine to cause a characteristic increase in the size of the twitch.

Acetylcholine

ACh is the neurotransmitter at NMJ. ACh is synthesized from acetyl coenzyme A and choline with the help of the enzyme choline-acetyl-transferase (ChAT). ACh is packed into synaptic vesicles with the help of the vesicular acetylcholine transporter (VAChT). Multiple synaptic vesicles pool in the presynaptic terminal near the release sites called active zones.

Synaptic Vesicles and Recycling

There are two pools of SVs that release ACh: a releasable pool and a reserve pool. The SVs in the releasable pool is smaller and present in the active zones. ACh is normally released by these SVs. Most of the SVs are sequestered in the reserve pool, which is attached to the cytoskeleton in a filamentous network. ACh molecules that do not react immediately with a receptor or those released after binding to the nAChRs are destroyed almost instantly by acetylcholinesterase, located in the synaptic cleft and the extra-junctional area. The enzyme is secreted from the muscle but remains attached to it by thin stalks of collagen. The action of ACh is short-lived because it is destroyed in less than 1 ms after its release. About half of the released ACh is hydrolyzed before even reaching the receptor. ACh molecules unbinding from the postsynaptic receptors invariably encounter acetylcholinesterase and are destroyed. Normally, a molecule of ACh reacts with only one receptor before it is hydrolyzed into choline and acetate. Choline is taken up by the nerve terminal and re-used for the synthesis of ACh.

NEUROMUSCULAR BLOCKERS

Neuromuscular blocking agents (NMBA) are among the most commonly used drugs during general anesthesia and intensive care. They facilitate endotracheal intubation, provide skeletal muscle relaxation during surgery and facilitate mechanical ventilation in intensive care. NMBAs compete with ACh and interfere with the transmission of nerve impulses resulting in skeletal muscle relaxation. Based on their mode of action, NMBAs are classified as:
1. *Depolarizing NMBA*: Blockers are depolarizing when they elicit action potential and desensitize the effector site to further stimulation.
2. *Nondepolarizing NMBA*: Blockers are said to be nondepolarizing when they do not elicit any action potential at the effector site and produce their effect by competing with ACh to bind to the AChRs.

Depolarizing Neuromuscular Block

Depolarizing NMBAs simulate the effect of ACh but block neurotransmission after initial stimulation. The only depolarizing agent in clinical use is suxamethonium. Two molecules of acetylcholine bonded together and thus mimics the effects of ACh at the AChR. Suxamethonium binds to the nicotinic AChR and opens the channel to depolarize the endplate. Depolarization block is also called Phase I and is usually preceded by muscle fasciculation due to repetitive firing and release of ACh.

In contrast to ACh, which gets fragmented by acetylcholinesterase, suxamethonium has a biphasic action: an initial contraction followed by relaxation because the endplate is continuously depolarized. Recovery from Phase I block occurs when suxamethonium diffuses away from the synaptic cleft. The depolarizing NMBs are not eliminated from the synaptic cleft until after they are eliminated from the plasma. The clearance of the drug from the body determines the duration of the block. It is metabolized by plasma cholinesterase (also known as pseudocholinesterase).

Phase II Block: Prolonged exposure of the NMJ to suxamethonium can result in a Phase II block. Phase II block occurs after repeated boluses of suxamethonium. In patients with atypical plasma cholinesterase, it can develop after a single dose of the drug. The block is characterized by fade of the train-of-four (TOF) twitch response, tetanic fade, and post-tetanic potentiation, which are characteristics of a nondepolarizing block.

Depolarizing Neuromuscular Blocking Agents

Suxamethonium (Succinyl Choline or Scoline)
Suxamethonium is prepared by joining two molecules of ACh and is also called acetylcholine. It has a rapid onset of action (30-60 sec) and an ultra-short duration of action (less than 10 min). It is fragmented by the pseudocholinesterase enzyme present in plasma. It is administered in a dose of 1-1.5 mg/kg intravenous. For rapid sequence intubation and cesarean section, it is administered in a dose of 2 mg/kg to achieve dense muscle relaxation. The adverse effects of the agent are bradycardia, fasciculations, hyperkalemia (caution in burns, spinal cord injury, massive trauma, Guillain Barre syndrome, and renal failure), muscle pains (due to muscle tissue damage by fasciculations), malignant hyperthermia, increased intraocular pressure, increased gastric pressure, and histamine release.

Nondepolarizing Neuromuscular Block

Nondepolarizing NMBAs antagonize the action of ACh competitively at the postsynaptic nicotinic receptor and do not produce conformational changes in the receptor, unlike depolarizing NMBAs. They impair or block neurotransmission by competing with ACh to bind to the AChRs. Their binding to the AChRs is dynamic, with repeated association and dissociation. The efficacy of the block depends on the relative concentrations of the NMBAs and their comparative affinities for the receptor. Acetylcholinesterase enzyme metabolizes ACh and removes it from the receptor site permitting nondepolarizing NMB to inhibit transmission. If an anti-acetylcholinesterase, such as neostigmine, is added, the cholinesterase cannot destroy acetylcholine. The concentration of ACh in the cleft increases the competition in favor of ACh. Thus, cholinesterase inhibitors reverse the neuromuscular paralysis produced by nondepolarizing NMBs by this mechanism. The quantification of neuromuscular block is expressed as depression of the single twitch height. It becomes evident when 70-80% of AChRs are occupied by non-depolarizing NMBAs, and for a complete block, at least 92% of the AChRs must be occupied. Non-depolarizing block manifests as a reduction in twitch height with successive stimuli (TOF fade) along with tetanic fade and post-tetanic potentiation.

Table 1: The onset, duration, and dosage of nondepolarizing neuromuscular blocking agents.

Neuromuscular blocker	ED95 (mg/kg)	Intubating dose (mg/kg)	Onset of action (min)	Duration of action (min)
Pancuronium	0.06–0.07	0.1	3–5	60–90
Vecuronium	0.05–0.06	0.08–0.1	3–5	20–35
Atracurium	0.25	0.4–0.5	3–5	20–35
Cis-atracurium	0.05	0.1	3–5	2–35
Rocuronium	0.3	0.6-1.2	1–2	20–35
Gantacurium	0.19	0.4-0.6	1.3–2.1	4–10

Nondepolarizing Neuromuscular Blocking Agents

Curare (Tubocurarine) was the first nondepolarizing NMBA to be used clinically. Curare was used by hunters on arrows to paralyze animals. Tubocurarine had a long onset of action and a prolonged duration of effect. It caused marked histamine release and thus hypotension, with compensatory tachycardia. It is no longer used clinically.

The nondepolarizing NMBAs currently in clinical use are all quaternary ammonium compounds. The common NMBAs used today are vecuronium, atracurium, cis-atracurium, rocuronium, and pancuronium. The dose of an NMBA required to produce 95% depression of twitch height is referred to as its ED95 dose. Normally the intubating dose of an NMBA is two or three times its ED95 dose. The onset, duration, and dosage of nondepolarizing NMBA are listed in **Table 1**, while their important pharmacological characteristics are listed in **Table 2**.

MONITORING NEUROMUSCULAR BLOCKADE

The train-of-four (TOF) monitor is commonly used to measure neuromuscular blockade. The details of neuromuscular monitoring are described in Chapter 9.

ANTAGONISM OF NEUROMUSCULAR BLOCK

The common way to overcome the effects of nondepolarizing NMBAs is to increase the amount of competing ACh. An increase in the number of molecules of ACh in the synaptic cleft increases the probability that agonist molecules occupy the available AChRs and

Table 2: Important pharmacological characteristics of nondepolarizing neuromuscular blocking agents.

Neuromuscular blocker	Chemical structure	Primary elimination	Histamine release	Vagal effect
Pancuronium	Steroid	Renal	No	Marked
Vecuronium	Steroid	Biliary	No	None
Atracurium	Benzylisoquinoline	Ester hydrolysis in plasma	Yes	None
Cis-atracurium	Benzylisoquinoline	Ester hydrolysis in plasma	No	None
Rocuronium	Steroid	Biliary	No	Mild
Gantacurium	Benzylisoquinoline	Ester hydrolysis in plasma	Yes	None

Table 3: Cholinesterase inhibitor drugs and their recommended doses for reversal of neuromuscular blockade.

Cholinesterase inhibitor	Dose (mg/kg)
Neostigmine	0.04–0.08
Pyridostigmine	0.1–0.25
Edrophonium	0.5–1.0
Physostigmine	0.01–0.03

Table 4: Commonly used anticholinergics and their recommended doses to antagonize cholinesterase inhibitors.

Anticholinergic	Dose (mcg/kg)
Glycopyrollate	0.05
Atropine	0.014 mcg/kg

the receptors in 'reserve' AChR. ACh must wait for the antagonist (nondepolarizing NMBA) to dissociate spontaneously before it can compete for the freed site. The nondepolarizing NMBAs bind to the receptor for about 1 ms, which is longer than the normal lifetime of ACh. The destruction of ACh normally takes place so quickly that most of it is destroyed before any significant number of antagonist molecules have dissociated from the receptor. Delaying the metabolism of ACh in the junction by administration of a cholinesterase inhibitor allows it to be available when the antagonist dissociates from the receptors.

The cholinesterase inhibitor drugs clinically available and their recommended doses are shown in **Table 3**. Using cholinesterase inhibitor agents is associated with muscarinic side effects such as bradyarrhythmia, salivation, bronchospasm, excitation, pupillary dilatation, increased bladder tone, and intestinal spasm. To reverse neuromuscular blockade by non-depolarizing NMBAs, cholinesterase inhibitors must be administered in conjunction with anticholinergic agents. Commonly used anticholinergics and their recommended doses to antagonize cholinesterase inhibitors are shown in **Table 4**.

Sugammadex: Recently, a γ-cyclodextrin compound, sugammadex, has been developed for early reversal of neuromuscular blockade by steroidal NMBAs. This cyclodextrin molecule engulfs and envelopes the nondepolarizing NMB agent molecules to prevent them from binding to the AChRs. Sugammadex is, however, useful to reverse the blockade of only rocuronium and vecuronium. Sugammadex 1.0 mg/kg adequately reverses an NMB at threshold 'Train of Four' count of four but without preventing recurarization.

RESIDUAL NEUROMUSCULAR BLOCKADE

A residual neuromuscular block is a common complication after general anesthesia. Patients usually demonstrate small degrees of residual paralysis. This muscular weakness is associated with impaired pharyngeal function, increased risk of aspiration, weakness of upper airway muscles, and airway obstruction. The hypoxic ventilatory response may be attenuated, and the patient has unpleasant symptoms of muscle weakness. Indiscriminate and long-duration administration of NMBAs intraoperative leading to residual NMB is an important risk factor in anesthetic-related morbidity and mortality. Incomplete neuromuscular recovery may result in acute respiratory events (hypoxemia and airway obstruction), longer post-anesthesia care unit stay, delays in tracheal extubation, and an increased risk of postoperative pulmonary complications. Most NMBAs tend to cumulate in the circulation with prolonged use, so it is important to restrict the amount of NMBA used in prolonged surgeries.

Residual neuromuscular blockade is an important patient safety issue that affects postoperative outcomes. It is managed with tracheal re-intubation and maintaining ventilation till the return of adequate muscle power. It is best prevented by using restricted doses of NMB and meticulous neuromuscular monitoring and tracheal extubation after the TOF ratio is at least 0.9.

MULTIPLE CHOICE QUESTIONS

1. Neuromuscular junction is:
   a. A simple synapse connection between the terminal end of a motor nerve and a muscle
   b. Responsible for converting electrical impulses generated by the motor neuron into electrical activity in the muscle fibers
   c. The site for transmitting action potential from the nerve to the muscle
   d. All of the above

2. Which of the following is true for a synaptic vesicle?
   a. Each synaptic vesicle stores around 500–1000 molecules of acetylcholine
   b. The synaptic vesicles are arranged in a chain alongside the junctional membrane
   c. The active zone contains many voltage-gated potassium channels
   d. None of the above

3. When the nerve impulse reaches the presynaptic terminal in the form of an action potential.
   a. It triggers voltage-gated Ca^{2+} channels at the active zones of the nerve terminal to open
   b. The open channels permit extracellular Ca^{2+} ions to enter the nerve terminal
   c. There is a release of several acetylcholine quanta
   d. All of the above

4. Depolarizing neuromuscular blocking agents:
   a. Elicit action potential and desensitize the effector site to further stimulation
   b. Cause an initial muscle contraction followed by relaxation by maintaining the endplate in a depolarized state
   c. They are not eliminated from the synaptic cleft until they are eliminated from the plasma
   d. All of the above

5. Prolonged exposure of the neuromuscular junction to suxamethonium can result in a Phase II block. Which of the following is correct about Phase II block?
   a. Phase II block is characterized by a complete block on stimulation by a 'Train of Four'
   b. Phase II block can be reversed by Neostigmine
   c. Phase II block can occur after repeated boluses of suxamethonium
   d. All of the above

6. Nondepolarizing neuromuscular blocking agents.
   a. Produce conformational changes in the receptor
   b. Antagonize the action of acetylcholine competitively at the postsynaptic receptor
   c. Their effect is not antagonized by cholinesterase inhibitors
   d. Act by enveloping the acetylcholine molecules

7. To reverse neuromuscular blockade by nondepolarizing neuromuscular blocking agents, cholinesterase inhibitors must be administered in conjunction with anticholinergic agents to:
   a. Prevent bradyarrhythmia
   b. Prevent dryness of the throat
   c. Prevent nausea and vomiting
   d. None of the above

8. A residual neuromuscular block after general anesthesia can result in:
   a. Impaired pharyngeal function
   b. Increased risk of aspiration
   c. Airway obstruction
   d. All of the above

9. A cyclodextrin compound, Sugammadex, has been developed for the early reversal of neuromuscular blockade by steroidal neuromuscular blocking agents:
   a. It is helpful to reverse the blockade of atracurium early

b. Sugammadex engulfs and envelopes the nondepolarizing neuromuscular blocking agent molecules to prevent them from binding to the receptors
c. Sugammadex is a competitive antagonist of non-depolarizing neuromuscular blocking agents
d. All of the above.

Answers
1. d
2. d
3. d
4. d
5. c
6. b
7. a
8. d
9. b

CHAPTER 7

Central Neuraxial Blockade

Pratibha Jain Shah

Learning Objectives

- Anatomy of subarachnoid and epidural spaces
- Principles for central neuraxial blockade
- Spinal anesthesia
- Epidural anesthesia
- Combined spinal epidural anesthesia
- Methods, complications, post-management after CNB
- Role of CNB in postoperative pain relief
- Adjuvants drugs used in central neuraxial blockade
- Caudal epidural anesthesia in children and adults

INTRODUCTION

Central neuraxial block (CNB) is a blockade of nerve transmission at the level of the spinal cord. In CNB, a local anesthetic (LA) agent is injected around the spinal cord and nerve roots to block sympathetic, sensory, and motor transmission. CNB includes spinal anesthesia (SA), epidural anesthesia (EA), and combined spinal-epidural anesthesia (CSEA). CNB is indicated for regional anesthesia for surgery in the abdomen and lower limb. It is also used for analgesia of the lower part of the body and obstetric anesthesia. CNB can be used for a wide range of conditions.

RELEVANT SPINAL CORD ANATOMY

AS5.2: Describe the correlative anatomy of the subarachnoid and epidural spaces.

Spinal Cord

The spinal cord occupies 2/3 of the vertebral canal. The vertebral canal consists of the spinal cord, CSF, meninges, spinal nerves, and epidural space. The spinal cord extends from the medulla oblongata cranially to the conus medullaris caudally and has five anatomical segments based on their supply area. It ends at the lower border of L1 in adults and L3 in infants (**Fig. 1**). The lumbar and sacral nerves (cauda equina) descend almost vertical beyond the spinal cord to meet their respective foramina. The segmental division of the spinal cord and nerves arising from them are as under:

- Cervical: 8 pairs of nerves
- Thoracic: 12 pairs of nerves
- Lumbar: 5 pairs of nerves
- Sacral: 5 pairs of nerves
- Coccygeal: 1 pair of nerves

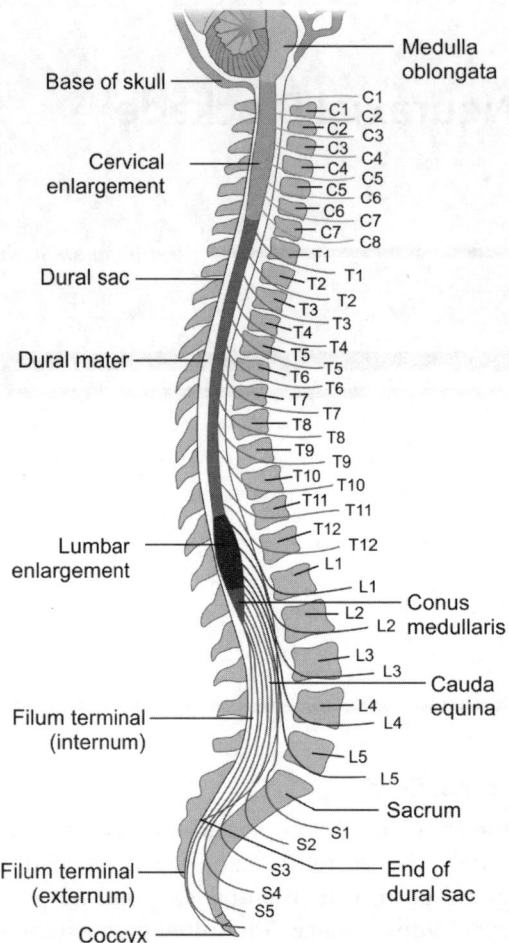

Fig. 1: Spinal cord and spinal nerves.

Meninges

The spinal cord is ensheathed by three meninges (from inside to periphery): the pia mater, the arachnoid mater, and the dura mater (**Fig. 2**). The pia mater is highly vascular and closely invests the spinal cord, which terminates as filum terminale, and connects to the coccyx. The arachnoid mater is a delicate nonvascular layer closely attached to the dura and acts as a principal pharmacological barrier to prevent drug migration into the subdural space. The dura, an outermost layer, merges above with the cranial dura and ends below at the lower border of S2. It comprises longitudinally oriented fibroelastic fibers. Hence the needle's bevel should be kept parallel to these fibers to separate rather than cut them.

Spaces Around the Cord

The potential space between the pia mater and arachnoid mater is the subarachnoid space. It that extends up to S2 and contains CSF, spinal nerves, dentate ligament, and blood vessels. LA is injected here in SA. The space between the arachnoid mater and the dura mater is called subdural space, containing a small amount of serous fluid. The space outside the dura, which extends from the foramen magnum to the sacral hiatus, is called the epidural space. The epidural space is bounded anteriorly by the posterior longitudinal

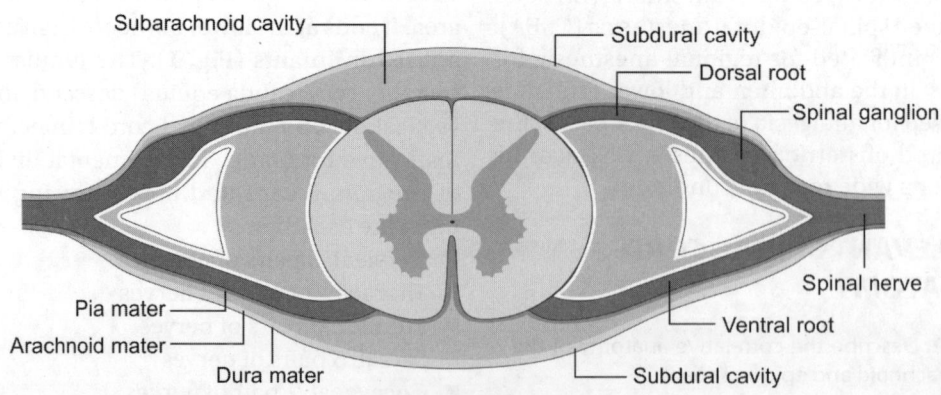

Fig. 2: Meninges.

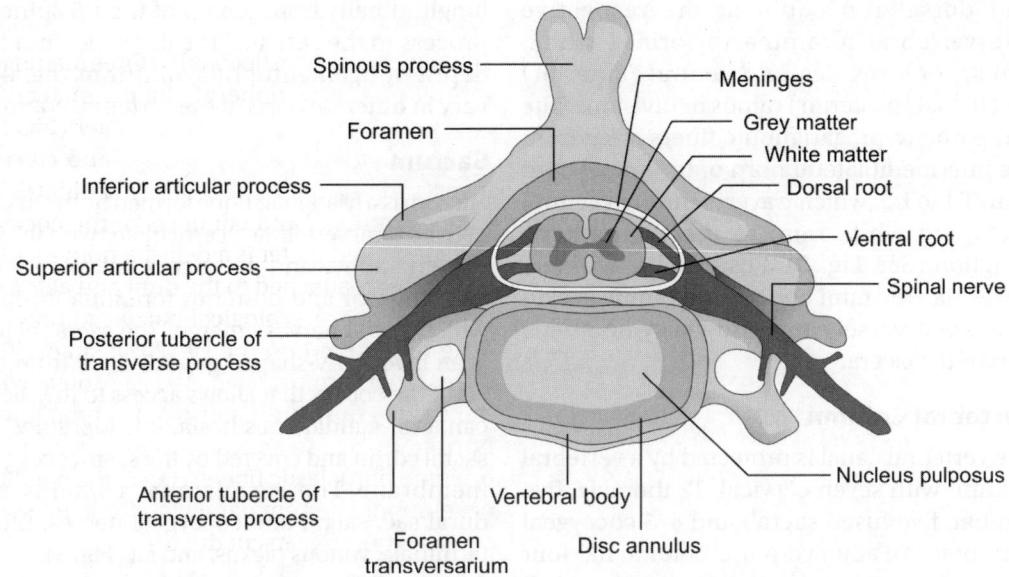

Fig. 3: Cross-section of the vertebral column showing spinal cord, its roots, and division.

ligament and the intervertebral discs, laterally by the pedicles and intervertebral foramina, and posteriorly by the ligamentum flavum and bony laminae (**Figs. 3 and 4**). It contains nerve roots, fat, areolar tissue, blood vessels, and lymphatics.

Spinal Nerves

Spinal nerves have a ventral (anterior) root which is efferent and motor, and a dorsal (posterior), which is afferent and carries various sensory fibers that ascend to the thalamus via different columns. The ventral

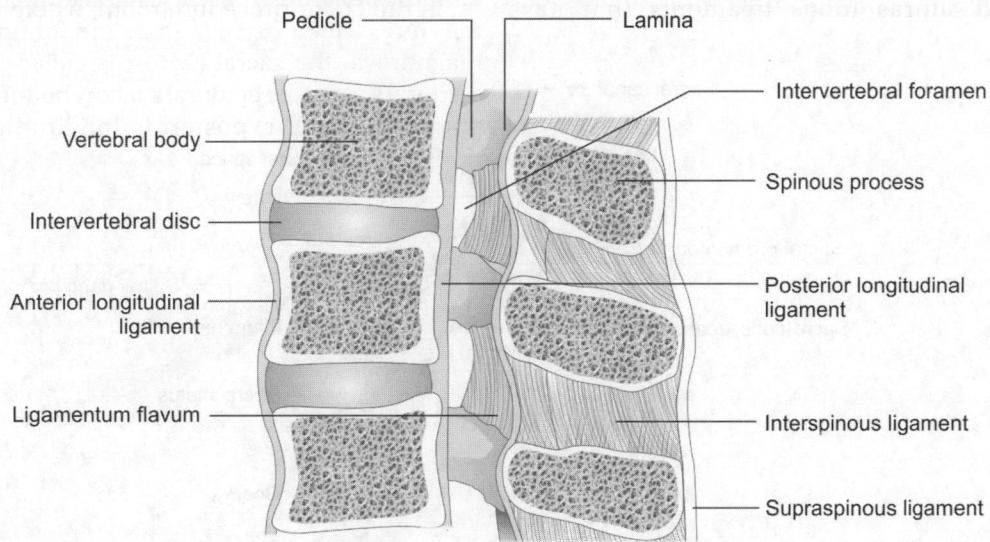

Fig. 4: Various ligaments around the vertebral column.

and dorsal roots join at the respective intervertebral foramina to form a trunk, which soon divides into ventral (anterior) and dorsal (posterior) ramus or divisions. The sympathetic preganglionic fibers arise from the intermediolateral horn of the spinal cord from T 1 to L 2, which traverse through ventral roots and white rami to the sympathetic ganglion (See **Fig. 3**). Postganglionic fibers travel via grey rami and ventral ramus to skin and blood vessels and also via sympathetic nerves to viscera.

Vertebral Column

The vertebral canal is protected by a vertebral column with seven cervical, 12 thoracic, five lumbar, five fused sacral, and 4/5 coccygeal vertebrae. An adult vertebral column has four curvatures: cervical, thoracic, lumbar, and sacrococcygeal curves. Vertebrae at different levels vary in size and shape. The vertebral column is stabilized by the anterior and posterior longitudinal ligaments between the adjacent vertebral bodies; Ligamentum flavum (yellow ligament) between the adjacent lamina; interspinous ligaments between adjoining spinous processes, and supraspinous ligaments that pass longitudinally from the tip of the C5 spinous process to the sacrum. The thickness and the depth of ligamentum flavum from the skin vary in different parts of the vertebral column.

Sacrum

Sacrum is a triangular bone formed by the fusion of five sacral vertebrae. It articulates with the L 5 vertebra above and the coccyx below and has four anterior and posterior foramina through which sacral nerves emerge. The sacral hiatus is an inverted V-shaped gap 3.5–5 cm from the tip of the coccyx that allows access to the sacral canal for caudal anesthesia. It is identified by sacral cornu and covered by the sacrococcygeal membrane The sacral canal contains the dural sac, sacral and coccygeal nerves, filum terminale, venous plexus, and fat (**Fig. 5**).

TECHNIQUE OF PERFORMING CNB

AS5.1: Enumerate the indications for and describe the principles of regional anesthesia (including spinal, epidural and combined).

The four basic steps to perform CNB are:
1. **Preparation:** CNB should be performed in the OT or procedure room, where any

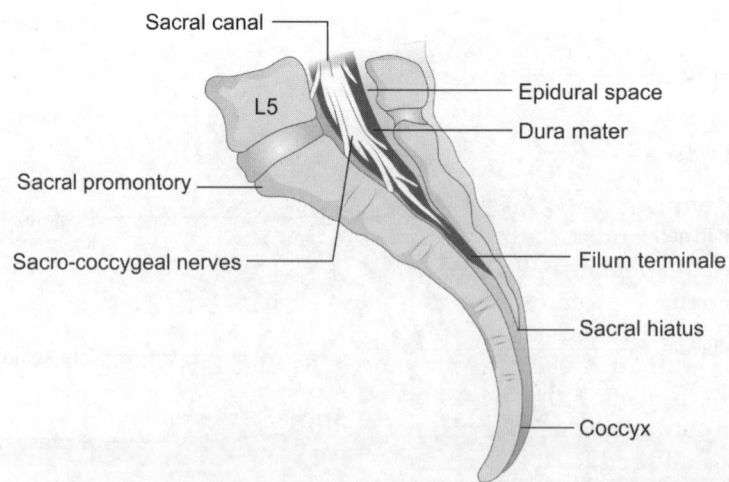

Fig. 5: Sacrum and the sacral canal.

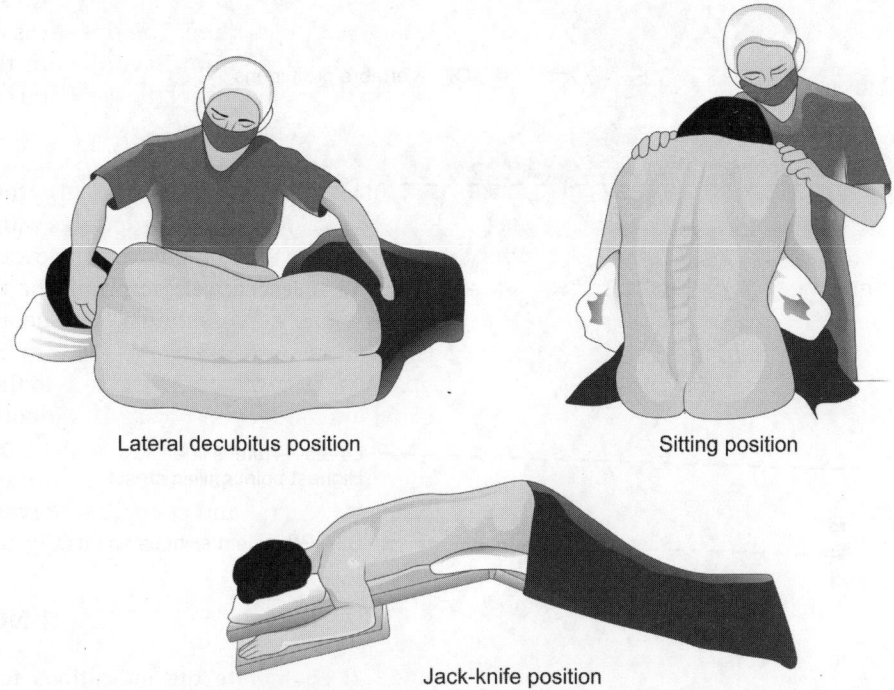

Fig. 6: Different patient positions for administrating CNB.

emergency can be addressed successfully. Both the patient and the OT must be prepared before doing CNB. All safety equipment must be available. Basic monitors (SpO$_2$, NIBP, and ECG) must be attached first. Establish intravenous access and start an infusion. Choose the appropriately sized needle or epidural set.

2. **Position:** CNB is usually performed in lateral decubitus or sitting positions (**Fig. 6**). The sitting position is preferred whenever midline landmarks are difficult to appreciate, especially in obese and pregnant women.
3. **Projection:** The skin at the site of injection is disinfected with an antiseptic solution (chlorhexidine in alcohol), first at the injection site, then outward in a circular manner. The alcohol is allowed to dry completely (to minimize the risk of meningitis), and a sterile drape is applied. The injection site is identified by palpating the spine (**Fig. 7**). The Tuffier's line (between the two iliac crests) is the key reference point to determine the level of L3-L4 interspace. Subarachnoid blocks are usually given at L2-L3 and L3-L4 interspaces in adults.
4. **Puncture:** CNB can be performed via a midline or paramedian approach. A midline approach is preferred in the lumbar area. However, owing to the steep downward slope of the spinous processes and the relatively fixed thoracic spine, the paramedian approach is favored in the thoracic area.

TYPES OF CNB

Spinal Anesthesia

For spinal anesthesia, after local anesthetic infiltration, a fine gauge spinal needle is introduced in the center of the interspinous

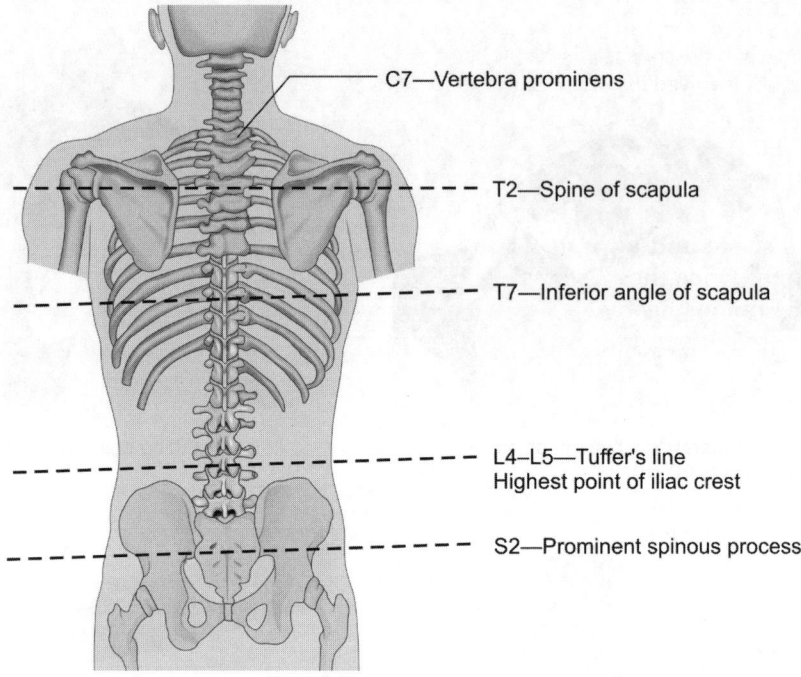

Fig. 7: Various body landmarks with the corresponding spinous process tip.

space and advanced towards the spinal cord. Various structures are punctured as the needle advances (**Fig. 8**). On removal of the stylet, if a free flow of cerebrospinal fluid (CSF) is present, the LA is injected into the CSF. The drug acts directly on the spinal; nerve roots emerging from the spinal cord. The drug floats to spinal segments levels above and below based on the baricity of the formulation.

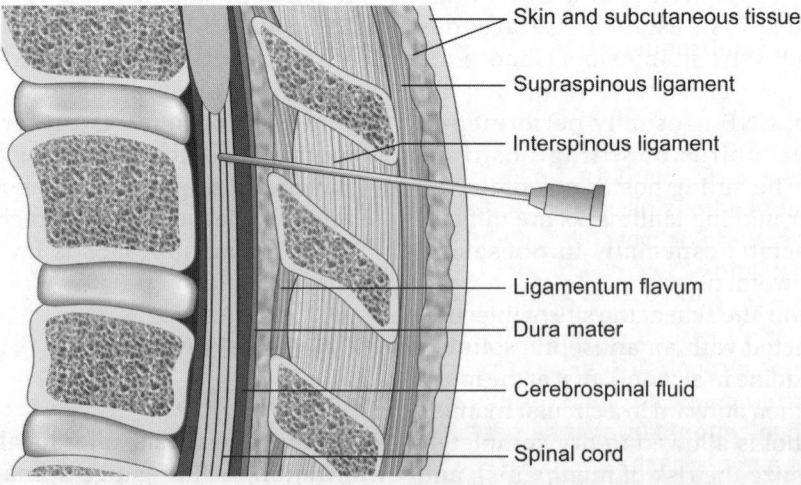

Fig. 8: Structures pierced in midline approach (sagittal section).

Epidural Anesthesia

AS5.5: Observe and describe the principles and steps/techniques involved in caudal epidural in adults and children.

For epidural injection, a large gauge Touhy needle is introduced in the center of the interspinous space and advanced towards the spinal cord. Once the needle gets fixed into the interspinous ligament, the stylet is removed. A loss of resistance (LOR) syringe loaded with either air/saline is attached for epidural space identification. The needle is advanced while applying intermittent pressure to the syringe plunger. On crossing the ligamentum flavum, a giveaway is felt, and a loss of resistance is felt on the syringe plunger as the epidural space has negative pressure. The LA can be injected into the epidural space. An epidural catheter can be inserted for repeat doses of the LA and long-term continuous infusion. The height of the sensory block achieved is determined by testing for sensation at different dermatome levels.

Combined Spinal-epidural Anesthesia

In the combined spinal-epidural (CSE) technique, an initial subarachnoid injection is administered, followed by epidural catheter placement for subsequent administration of epidural medications. The block is administered using a needle-in-needle technique. The epidural space is identified with a Touchy needle, and then a long fine-gauge spinal needle is passed through it to pierce the dura and deliver the drug into the cerebrospinal fluid.

This allows for rapid induction of regional anesthesia, and subsequent administration of medications through the epidural catheter is used to prolong anesthesia. Postoperative analgesic medication can also be delivered for extended periods via the epidural catheter. The CSE technique provides excellent surgical conditions and offers benefits of both spinal and epidural anesthesia. CSE is widely used for labor analgesia as it offers rapid-onset analgesia with minimal risk of toxicity or motor block.

Caudal Anesthesia

Caudal epidural anesthesia is the most widely used regional method in newborns and infants. The epidural space is accessed through the sacrococcygeal ligament. As the block is limited to sacral and lumbar nerves, it has a minimal impact on cardiovascular, respiratory, and bowel function and a limited motor blockade in the legs, and autonomic dysfunction in the bladder and anorectal sphincter. The patient is either lateral or prone, with one or both hips flexed. The sacral hiatus is a groove or notch between two sacral cornua above the coccyx. A needle is advanced at a 45° cephalad to the sacrum through sacral hiatus. A decrease in resistance to needle insertion is appreciated. The angle of the needle's angle is then flattened, and it is advanced 1-2 cm into the sacral canal. The drug is injected slowly into the space (**Fig. 9**).

Indications of Central Neuraxial Blockade

It is indicated for procedures that can be performed with a sensory level of anesthesia below the thorax, such as a lower limb, lower abdominal and perineal surgeries.

Contraindications of Central Neuraxial Blockade

The absolute and relative contraindications for CNB are listed in **Table 1**.

PRINCIPLE OF CENTRAL NEURAXIAL BLOCKADE

Local anesthetic disrupts nerve transmission by blocking voltage-sensitive Na^+ channels primarily on nerve roots emerging from the cord and spinal cord. LA injected into subarachnoid or epidural space raises the

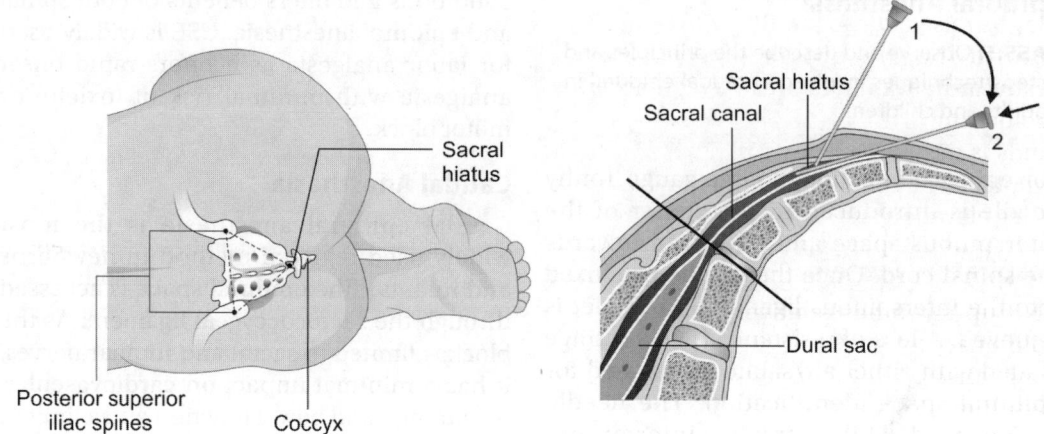

Fig. 9: Caudal anesthesia: The sacral hiatus is present at the apex of the equilateral triangle formed by the two posterior superior iliac spines and coccyx. Angles of the needle during caudal puncture: (1) first stage and (2) second stage.

threshold of channel opening, blocking Na$^+$ entry and thereby depolarization. The blockade of nerve conduction in the posterior nerve root interrupts afferent somatic and visceral sensation, whereas the blockade of anterior nerve root conduction interrupts efferent motor and autonomic outflow. The sensitivity of nerve fibers to LA depends on the axonal diameter, myelination, nerve length in contact with LA, and concentration. The smaller unmyelinated autonomic fibers are more sensitive to LA than sensory fibers, which are more sensitive than motor fibers.

Drug molecules are eliminated from subarachnoid space by absorption into blood vessels in the pia mater and by uptake in the cord substance. The epidural veins remove drugs from the epidural space. The molecular weight, molecular structure, lipo-solubility, and degree of ionization influence drug transport.

PHYSIOLOGICAL EFFECTS OF CENTRAL NEURAXIAL BLOCK

Cardiovascular System

Central neuraxial block causes a drop in blood pressure (BP) and heart rate (HR) that depends on the block height and sympathetic blockade. The BP falls primarily due to blood vessel dilation caused by sympathetic fibers blockade from T5 to L1. The vascular dilatation causes blood pooling and thus reduces venous return and stroke volume. The systemic vascular resistance reduces by 15–18% in the young and may decrease by over 25% in the elderly. The reduction in HR is due to lower right atrial pressure (Brainbridge reflex) and blockade of sympathetic T1-T4 cardio-accelerator fibers

Table 1: Absolute and relative contraindications of central neuraxial blockade.

Absolute contraindications	Relative contraindications
• Patient refusal • Uncooperative patient • Infection at injection site • Raised ICP • Allergy • Suspected spontaneous subarachnoid hemorrhage • Uncorrected severe hypovolemia	• Coagulopathy • Sepsis • Fixed cardiac output • Severe toxemia • Deformity of the spine • Pre-existing neurological disorder • Huge abdominal mass or ascites • Inexperienced anesthesiologist

ICP: increased intracranial pressure

with unopposed parasympathetic activity. HR may be raised due to low BP, which stimulates carotid baroreceptors (Marey's law). Bradycardia should be treated with atropine. Preloading with 10–15 mL/kg intravenous fluids is traditionally used to prevent or treat hypotension. The BP may also be normalized by leg elevation and vasopressor use.

Respiratory System

CNB up to T6 has relatively little effect on pulmonary functions. Thoracic level of block may cause chest tightness and dyspnea. A high block above T6 may affect intercostal and accessory muscles, impede effective breathing and the ability to cough, and induce distress and respiratory failure. A very high block may stop breathing due to medullary hypoperfusion and is referred to as 'total spinal.' Total spinal generally occurs due to massive epidural spread or accidental subdural injection.

Gastrointestinal System

CNB-induced blockade of preganglionic sympathetic fibers from T5 to L1 causes unopposed vagal stimulation and a loss of sympathetic inhibitory effect on the gut, resulting in relaxation of sphincters, increased peristalsis, and secretion. The contracted bowel facilitates abdominopelvic surgeries and early return of bowel function. CNB may induce nausea and vomiting in 20% of patients, primarily related to hyperperistalsis of the gut.

Endocrine System

CNB suppresses stress responses following surgery, such as hyperglycemia and a rise in antidiuretic hormone by blocking afferent impulses.

Genitourinary System

Renal function is well preserved despite a fall in renal blood flow following CNB. Autoregulation of renal blood flow is disrupted when mean arterial pressure goes below 50 mm Hg. CNB blocks both sympathetic and parasympathetic control of the bladder and may result in post-spinal urinary retention. The blockade of the nervi erigentes (S2-S3) results in an engorged flaccid penis.

Temperature Homeostasis

CNB induces hypothermia because of central thermoregulation inhibition, vasodilation-induced heat loss, reduced heat production from reduced catecholamine secretion, and limited heat conservation as shivering is limited to the parts of the body above the block level. The infusion of warm fluid and forced-air warming help limit the temperature drop.

MANAGEMENT AFTER CNB

Shivering should be prevented and aggressively managed with radiant heat and blankets. Nausea and vomiting are primarily managed by correcting BP. Patients should be shifted from recovery once the block has receded successfully (at least four segments regression), hemodynamically stable, and comfortable. Outpatients can be discharged once able to ambulate without orthostatic hypotension and void.

Differential blockade: The sensitivity of nerve fibers to different concentrations of LA varies. This results in different levels of nerve blockade of specific types of fibers. Following spinal injection of LA, sympathetic blockade is two-six segments more cephalad than the sensory block, and the sensory blockade is two or more segments more cephalad than the motor block.

Return of sensibility or reversal of blockade: The sensation of nerve fibers at recovery is restored in an order which is reverse of that during the onset of the blockade. However, the activity of sympathetic fibers returns before that of sensory fibers.

Drugs Used in CNB

Local Anesthetics

LA preparations used in spinal anesthesia can be hyperbaric, isobaric, or hypobaric compared to CSF. For spinal anesthesia, LA is made hyperbaric by adding dextrose. Isobaric LA is used for epidural anesthesia. The common drugs used are:
- 2-chloroprocaine
- Lignocaine
- Mepivacaine
- Bupivacaine
- Levobupivacaine
- Ropivacaine

Adjuvants Drugs

Adjuvants are administered with LA either intensify or prolong the duration of anesthesia.
- Vasoconstrictors (epinephrine) to limit systemic absorption of the drug
- α-2 agonists (clonidine or dexmedetomidine) to enhance sensory and motor block
- Opioids (fentanyl, morphine) bind to opioid receptors and enhance sensory block
- Acetylcholinesterase inhibitors (neostigmine) to prevent the breakdown of acetylcholine
- Alkalinization (sodium bicarbonate) to increase the non-ionized form of LA.

COMPLICATIONS OF CNB

Complications of CNB are related to adverse or exaggerated physiological responses, needle/catheter placement, or drug toxicity. Hypotension and post-dural puncture headache are the most common complication of spinal anesthesia. Young age, female gender, large-bore needle, pregnancy, multiple punctures, and needle bevel perpendicular to the long axis of the spinal cord increase the risk of PDPH. The complications of CNB are listed in **Table 2**.

Table 2: Complications associated with central neuraxial blockade.

Adverse or exaggerated physiological response	Related to technique (needle or catheter placement)	Related to drug toxicity
• Severe hypotension • Nausea-vomiting • Shivering • Dyspnea • Transient hearing loss • Urinary retention • Failed spinal • High spinal (above T4) • Total spinal (intracranial spread) • Cardiac arrest • Anterior spinal artery syndrome • Horner's syndrome	• PDPH • Diplopia (6th cranial nerve palsy) and tinnitus • Backache • Direct nerve injury leading to spinal cord or nerve root damage and cauda equina syndrome • Broken needle or catheter • Epidural or intraspinal hematoma • Inadvertent subdural, subarachnoid or intravascular injection • Infection leading to meningitis or epidural abscess	• Systemic LA toxicity • Transient neurological symptoms • Radiculitis • Arachnoiditis • Ascending myelitis • Cauda equina syndrome

CHAPTER 7 ♦ Central Neuraxial Blockade

MULTIPLE CHOICE QUESTIONS

1. The segmental division of the spinal cord and nerves arising from them are as under *except*:
   a. Cervical: 7 pairs of nerves
   b. Thoracic: 12 pairs of nerves
   c. Lumbar: 5 pairs of nerves
   d. Sacral: 5 pairs of nerves

2. The Tuffier's line (highest point of the iliac crest) corresponds to:
   a. L2 – L3
   b. L3 – L4
   c. L4 – L5
   d. L5 – S1

3. In spinal anesthesia:
   a. The local anesthetic agent acts directly on the spinal cord
   b. The local anesthetic agent acts on the dorsal horn cells
   c. The local anesthetic agent acts on nerve roots emerging from the spinal cord
   d. The local anesthetic agent acts on the ventral horn cells

4. For epidural anesthesia, the epidural space is identified by:
   a. Using an endoscope
   b. By the feel of the needle touching the vertebral body
   c. By loss of resistance syringe loaded with either air/saline
   d. By the free flow of CSF through the needle.

5. Caudal epidural anesthesia is administered by:
   a. Approaching the caudal epidural space between L5 – S1 with the patient in a sitting position
   b. Approaching the caudal epidural space through the sacral hiatus
   c. Approaching the caudal epidural space through L4 – L5 with the needle hub pointed downwards
   d. None of the above

6. Central neuraxial blockade causes a drop in blood pressure and heart rate:
   a. Due to blood vessel dilation caused by sympathetic fibers blockade from T5 to L1
   b. Due to the effect on the vasomotor center in the brain
   c. Due to the systemic effect of the local anesthetic agent
   d. All the above

7. Differential blockade in central neuraxial blockade is related to which of the following:
   a. The sensitivity of nerve fibers to different concentrations of LA varies
   b. Results in different levels of nerve blockade of specific types of fibers
   c. The sympathetic blockade is two-six segments more cephalad than the sensory block
   d. All the above

8. For spinal anesthesia, dextrose is added to the local anesthetic:
   a. To make the pH alkaline
   b. To improve the drug binding to the nerves
   c. To make the drug hyperbaric and restrict the spread of the drug
   d. To provide substrate for uptake of the local anesthetic drug

9. All the below mentioned are complications of spinal anesthesia *except*:
   a. Post-dural puncture headache
   b. Diplopia
   c. Abdominal cramps
   d. Horner's Syndrome

Answers
1. a
2. c
3. c
4. c
5. b
6. a
7. d
8. c
9. c

CHAPTER 8

Regional Anesthesia

Shaloo Garg

Learning Objectives

- Common regional blocks
- Agents used for regional anesthesia
- Pharmacology of local anesthetic agents and adjuvant agents
- Modes of administration including ultrasound and peripheral nerve stimulation for blocks
- Potential complications of regional anesthesia
- Continuous regional anesthesia
- Anatomy of brachial plexus

REGIONAL ANESTHESIA

Regional anesthesia (RA) is a method where a peripheral nerve is blocked with local anesthetic (LA) agents to cause anesthesia or prevent pain. It can be local infiltration, nerve or nerve plexus block, or neuraxial block (Spinal or Epidural).

RA does not affect the consciousness of the patient and has many advantages as compared to general anesthesia (GA). It also helps in early post-procedure recovery, pain relief, and rehabilitation. RA can be given alone or synergistically with GA, sedation, or a post-procedure technique for pain relief in acute or chronic pain.

History

The slow progress of discoveries has defined RA. Harvey Cushing is credited with coining the term RA for his method of blocking a nerve plexus under direct vision during GA. In 1900, it was demonstrated that 50–60% of cases could be done without narcosis. Blocking of nerve trunks at the exit point of the cranial foramina made possible thyroid, larynx, and other head and neck surgeries. Similarly, by blocking the respective nerve plexus, amputations of the extremities, resection of joints, and pelvic surgeries were performed.

Sir Benjamin Ward Richardson worked with many agents for the alleviation of pain. Effects of cold in numbing were used by Napoleon's surgeon. He used ether spray for local freezing, which gave way to ethyl chloride.

Cocaine soon found utility for topical applications, and Parke-Davis advertised that it could "make the coward brave, the silent eloquent, and render the sufferer insensitive to pain." Due to its undesirable effects, physicians soon started to look for alternative anesthetic agents.

Lignocaine, an amide, was a major discovery in 1940. It did not have the allergic potential of ester drugs and was soon followed by bupivacaine, prilocaine, and later ropivacaine.

The spread of RA in the United States was greatly facilitated by the work of Gaston

Labat, who published his influential textbook, 'Regional Anesthesia.' Most currently used techniques of RA were devised during the first decade of the twentieth century.

For a successful regional block, certain prerequites have to be met. These are a drug, syringe, and needle, along with other factors like detailed knowledge of the physiology of pain, anatomy of the nerves and ability to localize them, and monitoring administration of drugs.

PHYSIOLOGY OF PAIN

Plato and Aristotle opined that pain is an emotion and not a sensation, much like pleasure, which is a passion of the soul. With the advent of science and a better understanding of physiology, the religious interpretation of pain took a backseat.

Pain is a sensory perception by specific pain receptors and nerve endings. This is transmitted through specific nerve fibers to the spinal cord and well-defined pathways to higher centers (Fig. 1). Any intervention utilizing drugs or trauma can modulate or interrupt this transmission, leading to analgesia or altered pain perception. The physiology of pain is described in detail in chapter 17.

LOCAL ANESTHETICS

AS5.4: Describe the pharmacology of commonly used drugs and adjuvant agents in regional anesthesia.

Mechanism of Action

Local anesthetics consist of a lipophilic and a hydrophilic portion separated by a connecting hydrocarbon chain. Hydrophilic tertiary amines act by binding to the Na^+ channel, thereby blocking the depolarization-induced influx of Na^+ and blocking the propagation of nerve impulses. Differential blockade of nerve types depends on myelination, diameter, etc. Sensitivity is more for autonomic, sensory, and motor fibers in that order.

Classification

Local anesthetic agents have a lipophilic benzene ring linked to an amine group by a hydrocarbon chain of amide or ester linkage **(Tables 1 and 2)**.

Pharmacodynamics

Local anesthetics exist in free equilibrium in both charged (ionized) and neutral (nonionized) forms. The ionized form

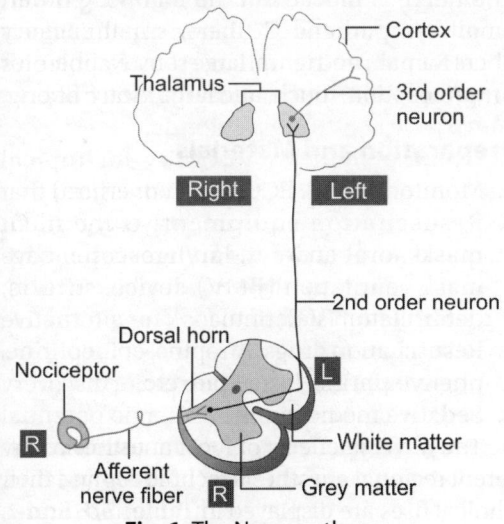

Fig. 1: The Nerve pathway.

Table 1: Classification of local anesthetic agents based on chemical linkage.	
Ester	**Amide**
Ester linkage	Amide linkage, stable in solution
Rapidly hydrolyzed by plasma pseudocholinesterases (avoid in patients with deficiency)	Metabolized by hepatic microsomal P450 enzymes
A significant metabolite, para-amino benzoic acid (PABA), is a known allergen	Rare allergic reactions may be from multidose vials containing a methylparaben preservative (structure similar to PABA)

Table 2: Classification of local anesthetic agents based on the duration of action.

Short-Acting (15–30 min)	Intermediate-acting (1–3 h)	Long-acting (2–4h)
Procaine	Lignocaine	Bupivacaine
Chlorprocaine	Prilocaine	Ropivacaine
	Mepivacaine	Dibucaine

Table 3: Comparative pharmacology of local anesthetic agents.

Classification	Potency	Onset	Duration of action (mins)	Max single dose (mg)	Toxic plasma concentration (mcg/mL)	pK	Protein binding (%)
Ester							
Chlorprocaine	1	Rapid	30–45	600		8.7	
Amide							
Lignocaine	1	Rapid	60–120	300	> 5	7.9	70
Prilocaine	1	Slow	60–120	400	> 5	7.9	55
Bupivacaine	4	Slow	240–480	175	> 3	8.1	95
Levo bupivacaine	4	Slow	240–480	175		8.1	> 97
Ropivacaine	4	Slow	240–480	200	> 4	8.1	94

binds to the receptor and exerts the drug's action, and the nonionized, lipid-soluble form allows the drug to penetrate the nerve membrane. Protein binding directly correlates with the duration of action (**Table 3**).

Adjuvants to Local Anesthetics

Peripheral nerve blocks provide significant anesthetic and analgesic benefits for our patients. Analgesic adjuvants such as opioids, α_2-agonists, NMDA receptor antagonists, and other agents can be added to LAs both to facilitate onset and to prolong anesthetic and analgesic effects by mechanisms existing in the peripheral nervous system (PNS). Several agents are effective when administered in the perineuronal or intra-articular space and when given in intravenous regional anesthesia (IVRA) or local infiltration (**Table 4**).

Tissue vascularity and drug absorption based on the vascularity of the tissue, the greatest degree of absorption is seen with intercostal, followed by caudal, epidural, brachial plexus, and subcutaneous injections.

Peripheral Nerve blocks

AS5.3: Describe the principles and steps/techniques involved in peripheral nerve blocks.

Local anesthetics are injected around specific nerves or nerve bundles to prevent the transmission of impulses along those nerves. The nerve is blocked in the following order: Small sympathetic C fibers, small sensory fibers for pain and temp, large sensory fibers for proprioception/touch, and large motor fibers.

Preparation and Materials

1. Monitors (SpO$_2$, ECG, blood pressure)
2. Resuscitation equipment: Oxygen, O$_2$ masks, oral airways, laryngoscope, bag-mask ventilation (BMV) device, suction, defibrillator, IV Cannula
3. Resuscitation drugs: Atropine, epinephrine, phenylephrine, intra lipid, etc.
4. Sedative medications

The adverse effects of local anesthesia, different regional anesthesia techniques and their clinical uses are displayed in **Tables 5, 6 and 7**, respectively.

Table 4: Additives to local anesthetics.

Class	Drug	Dose	Action	Side Effects
Vasoconstrictors	Epinephrine	5 mcg/mL (commonly used)	Vasoconstriction, ↑ duration, and ↑ intensity of the block	Tachycardia, hypertension, arrhythmias
Opioids	Morphine	150–3000 mcg	↑ Duration of neuraxial block, ↑ quality of surgical anesthesia, and postoperative analgesia	Nausea, itching, respiratory depression, sedation
	Fentanyl	20–50 mcg		
	Buprenorphine	0.3 mg		
Alpha 2 agonists	Clonidine	15–30 mcg	↑ duration of sensory and motor block	Bradycardia, hypotension
Bicarbonate	Soda bicarbonate	8.4%	↑ membrane penetration, ↓ onset time, reduces pain during infiltration	
Steroid	Dexamethasone	4–10 mg	↑ duration of sensory and motor block	

Table 5: Adverse effects of local anesthesia.

	Clinical features	Prevention	Treatment
Allergic reaction (Rare—less than 1%. Usually due to additive)	Rash, urticaria, and laryngeal edema, with or without hypotension and bronchospasm	Cross sensitivity not seen. Intradermal testing	Symptomatic treatment
LAST (Local anesthetic systemic toxicity)	• CNS: Lightheadedness, circumoral numbness, facial tingling, slurred speech, seizures, unconsciousness, respiratory arrest • CVS: cardiovascular depression, circulatory arrest, dysrhythmias (especially with bupivacaine) • ECG: ↑PR, ↑QRS, ↑QT intervals	• Incremental injection • Use of vasoconstrictors • "Test dose" of local with epinephrine can indicate likely IV injection if associated with a significant and rapid ↑HR, ↑BP, or T-wave inversion. • Avoid hypercarbia and acidosis • Reduce dose in Renal and Hepatic disease and CHF.	Stop injecting LA, get help; maintain airway (intubate if necessary); give 100% oxygen and consider hyperventilation in the presence of metabolic acidosis; Treat seizures CPR/ modified ALCS (Reduce individual doses of epinephrine (<1 mcg/kg/ dose) Avoid β and calcium channel blockers, vasopressin) Treat arrhythmias. Initiate lipid therapy. Consider ECMO

Contd...

Contd...

	Clinical features	Prevention	Treatment
Methemoglobinemia (Benzocaine, Prilocaine)	Dyspnea, cyanosis loss of consciousness >50% met-Hb dysrhythmias, seizures, coma and death Blood—"chocolate-brown" color ABG—normal pO_2 +/– metabolic acidosis Co-oximetry—met-Hb level		Supplemental O_2, 1% methylene blue 1–2 mg/kg IV (restores iron in Hb to its normal reduced O_2-carrying state), hyperbaric O_2.
Neural tissue toxicity	Patchy groin numbness an persistent isolated myotomal weakness to cauda equina syndrome		

Table 6: Different regional anesthesia techniques.

Technique	Example	Indication
Topical or Surface	• Spray • Pledget • Skin surface application • Nebulization • EMLA patch	• SSG • IV cannulation • Awake fibre-optic laryngoscopy/bronchoscopy • Mucous membrane of nose, mouth, genito-urinary tract
Local infiltration	• Subcutaneous injection	• IV cannulation • Wound infiltration for anesthesia and analgesia
Peripheral nerve block	• Brachial plexus • Lumbar plexus • Nerve blocks • TAP block	• Anesthesia for procedure • Postoperative analgesia • Acute or chronic pain management
Intravenous regional anesthesia (Bier's Block)	• Lignocaine is the most commonly used drug	• Upper limb surgery • Lower limb surgery

5. Barrier equipment: Cap, mask, sterile gloves, sterile gown
6. Block needle: Short bevel (blunt), echogenic, or insulated needle
7. Infusion catheter (if performing continuous nerve block)
8. Local anesthetic (LA) drug in appropriate dose and concentration
9. Method of nerve localization: Nerve stimulator, ultrasound machine
10. Documentation: Consent, site of procedure, allergy

Nerve localization techniques

Ultrasound-guided: Ultrasound (US) imaging is based on a transducer emitting sound waves (produced by the piezoelectric crystal) in the range of 4–17 MHz into the tissues and receiving sound reflected or scattered back to the receiver. Tissues have different acoustic impedance causing attenuation, reflection, refraction, and scattering. Anechoic structures (e.g., blood vessels) appear black because US waves are transmitted through these structures with no reflection. Hypo-echoic

Table 7: Clinical uses of local anesthetics.

Drug	Clinical Use	Concentration (%)	Onset	Duration (min)	Recommended maximum single dose (mg)
Lignocaine	Topical	4	Fast	30–60	300
	Infiltration	0.5–1	Fast	60–240	300/500 with epinephrine
	IVRA	0.25–0.5	Fast	30–60	300/500 with epinephrine
	PNB	1–1.5	Fast	60–180	300/500 with epinephrine
Prilocaine	Infiltration	0.5–1	Fast	60–120	600
	IVRA	0.25–0.5	Fast	30–60	600
	PNB	1.5–2	Fast	90–180	600
Bupivacaine	Infiltration	0.25	Fast	120–480	175/225 with epinephrine
	PNB	0.25–0.5	Slow	240–960	175/225 with epinephrine
Levo-Bupivacaine	Infiltration	0.25	Fast	120–480	150
	PNB	0.25–0.5	Slow	840–1020	150
Ropivacaine	Infiltration	0.2–0.5	Fast	120–360	200
	PNB	0.5–1	Slow	300–480	250
Chlorprocaine	Infiltration	1	Fast	30–60	800/1000 with epinephrine
	PNB	2	Fast	30–60	800/1000 with epinephrine
EMLA (eutectic mixture of LA)	Topical	(Lignocaine 2.5% + Prilocaine 2.5%)	Slow	120	2500 -10000 2 g (about half a 5 g tube) or approx. 1.5 g/10 cm² for 1-5 h for minor procedures

structures (proximal nerves, adipose tissue) appear dark/near black because US waves are transmitted through these structures with little reflection. Hyper-echoic structures (e.g., bone, tendons) appear bright because transmission of US waves is blocked, and the strong signal returned to the transducer gives these structures a white appearance.

Nerve locators: Nerve stimulation, as seen in **Figure 2**, is used to confirm the identity of the targeted nerve. The peripheral nerve stimulators help identify nerves by stimulating the nerves with low-intensity electric current. This stimulation results in a motor response or evokes a patient response to sensation. It is also used to ensure the needle is not intraneural with no stimulation at a low current. Peripheral nerve stimulators allow measurement of stimulus amplitude, pulse width, frequency, and electrical impedance.

Anatomical landmarks: Adequate knowledge of anatomy is a must. Patient positioning and monitoring equipment and slow incremental injection of the drug after repeated aspiration for blood or CSF should be done. Accept only low injection pressures (<20 psi) to avoid intraneural injections. Epinephrine can

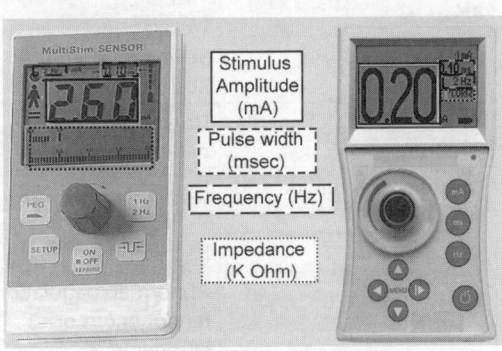

Fig. 2: Peripheral nerve locators.

be added to LA as a vascular marker (e.g., 1:500,000 [2.5 mcg/mL]).

Potential Complications of Regional Anesthesia

Peripheral nerve blocks are relatively safe and associated with very few complications. The complications noted are sensory deficit, motor deficit, toxicity from local anesthetics, and nausea/vomiting. The neurological deficits are related to nerve trauma, while nausea and vomiting result from drug effects post systemic absorption. Permanent neurologic complications are rare but probably underreported. The contra indications of regional anesthesia is discussed in **Table 8**.

Continuous Regional Anesthesia

Continuous perineural infusions of LAs are a safe and effective method for postoperative analgesia and reducing opioid analgesic medications. A continuous peripheral nerve block can be administered by inserting a catheter percutaneously with its tip adjacent to a target nerve/plexus. The catheter placement is usually guided by ultrasound or a peripheral nerve stimulator. A LA can be administered as a continuous infusion through this catheter to provide a prolonged block that may be titrated to the desired effect. The LA can be administered using a syringe infusion pump or disposable volumetric pump. Several disposable infusion pumps are currently available that allow adjusting basal rates, bolus volume, and lockout times.

Similarly, continuous regional anesthesia can be administered through epidural and spinal catheters in case of central neuraxial blocks.

BRACHIAL PLEXUS BLOCK

AS5.2: Describe the correlative anatomy of the brachial plexus.

The brachial plexus innervates bones, joints, muscles, and the skin of the upper extremity. It is formed by ventral rami of C5 to T1 (**Fig. 3 and Table 9**).

Approaches to the Brachial Plexus

The brachial plexus has four common approaches (**Fig. 4 and Table 10**).

Interscalene Block

AS5.6: Observe and describe the principles and steps/techniques involved in common blocks used in surgery (including brachial plexus blocks).

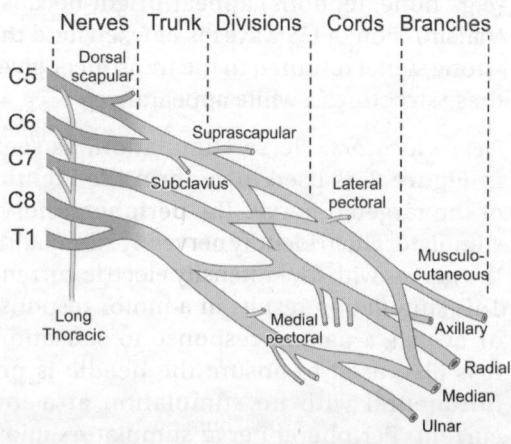

Fig. 3: Organization and distribution of the brachial plexus nerves.

Table 8: Contraindications to regional anesthesia	
Contraindications	
Absolute	Relative
Patient refusal	Severe anatomic abnormalities
Infection at site of needle puncture	Un-cooperative patient
True allergy to amide and ester LA	Neurologic disease or nerve injury
	Bacteremia
	Abnormal coagulation (endogenous or iatrogenic)

Table 9: Distribution of the nerves in brachial plexus.

Nerve	Dermatome	Muscle Innervated
Nerves to subclavius	C4 to C6	Subclavius muscle
Dorsal scapular nerve	C5	Rhomboid and levator scapulae muscle
Long thoracic nerve	C5 to C7	Serratus anterior muscle
Suprascapular nerve	C5, C6	Supraspinatus and infraspinatus muscles
Pectoralis nerve (median and lateral)	C5 to T1	Pectoralis muscles
Subscapular nerves	C5, C6	Subscapularis and teres major muscles
Thoracodorsal nerve	C6 to C8	Latissimus dorsi muscle
Axillary nerve	C5, C6	Deltoid and teres minor muscles; skin of shoulder
Radial nerve	C5 to T1	Extensor muscle of the arm and forearm (triceps brachii, extensor carpi radialis, supinator and anconeus muscles, and extensor carpi ulnaris muscles) and brachioradialis muscle; digital extensors and abductor pollicis muscle; skin over the posterolateral surface of the arm
Musculocutaneous nerve	C5 to C7	Flexor muscles on the arm (biceps brachii, brachialis, and coracobrachialis muscles); skin over lateral surface of forearm
Median nerve	C6 to T1	Flexor muscles on the forearm (flexor carpi radialis and palmaris longus muscles); pronator quadratus and pronator teres muscles; digital flexors (through the palmar interosseous nerve); skin over anterolateral surface of the hand
Ulnar nerve	C8, T1	Flexor carpi ulnaris muscle, adductor pollicis muscle, and small digital muscles; medial part of flexor digitorum profundus muscle; skin over medial surface of the hand

Table 10: Brachial plexus—approaches for brachial plexus block.

Brachial plexus block	Interscalene block	Supraclavicular block	Infraclavicular block	Axillary block
Anatomy	Roots and trunks	Trunks or divisions	Cords	Branches
Landmark	At the level of the C6 vertebral body (Chassaignac's tubercle) between the anterior and middle scalene muscles, i.e. interscalene groove	Interscalene groove, about 1 cm superior to the clavicle and lateral to the subclavian artery	In delto-pectoral groove, 1 cm below the clavicle.	Just superior to the pulsation of the axillary artery at the lateral border of the pectoralis major muscle
Coverage	Muscles of the shoulder. Lateral 2/3 of clavicle Shoulder Proximal humerus	Entire arm and hand	Hand, forearm, elbow, and lower arm. At this level, musculocutaneous nerve has not divided and will be blocked	Distal to elbow. Axillary artery can be thought of as the hub of a wheel with 4 spokes: • Superior anterior: Median nerve

Contd...

Contd...

Brachial Plexus Block	Interscalene Block	Supraclavicular block	Infraclavicular block	Axillary block
				• Inferior-anterior: Ulnar nerve • Inferior-posterior: Radial nerve • Superior-posterior: Musculocutaenous nerve (in coracobrachialis
Distributions missed:	**Cephalad cutaneous shoulder** (above the clavicle): innervated by the supraclavicular nerves Due to the vertical distribution of the roots at the point of injection, the C8-T1 roots are often missed. **Hand and forearm**: lower trunk is often inadequately blocked			Since, the musculocutaneous nerve has already divided at this level, it must be anesthetized separately
Problems	Horner's syndrome Hoarseness hemidiaphragm paresis Severe hypotension and bradycardia due to Bezold-Jarisch reflex. Pneumothorax, Epidural or subarachnoid injection and Accidental vertebral artery injection	Highest incidence of pneumothorax, Phrenic nerve palsy	Intravascular injections	Intravascular injections
Advantage			No change in pulmonary function. Minimal risk of pneumothorax	Least complications
Patient position	Head up at 30° allow shoulder to drop inferiorly head turned away	Head up at 30°; head turned away	Supine or semi-sitting; head turned away	Supine; arm abducted 90° at shoulder; +/− flexed at elbow

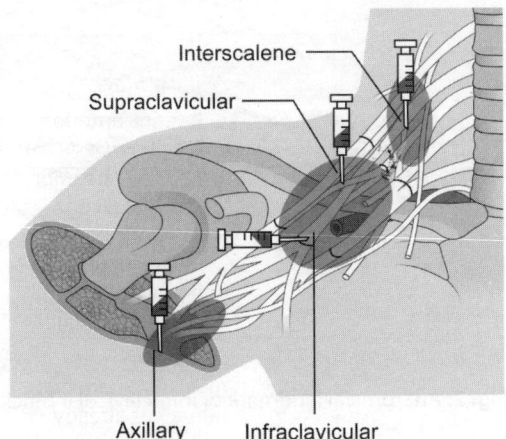

Fig 4: Approaches to brachial plexus block.

The interscalene approach to the brachial plexus should ideally be performed in awake patients. The upper arm and shoulder are reliably blocked. The key landmark shown in **Figure 5** is the interscalene groove between the anterior and middle scalenus muscle. It is palpated at the level of the cricoid cartilage (C6) and the lateral border of the sternocleidomastoid muscle. The external jugular vein often crosses this point, but this is not a reliable landmark. The position of the needle is in the interscalene groove. It is important to use a short regional block needle (maximum 50 mm) and maintain a caudad direction angle. When a nerve stimulator is used, a motor response is most often observed in the C5-6 distribution of the superior trunk, but sometimes middle trunk (C7) stimulation is seen. Stimulation of the diaphragm via the phrenic nerve occurs when the needle position is too anterior. When the needle tip is too posterior, shoulder elevation (dorsal scapular nerve) is seen. A posterior approach to the interscalene block was described in 1912 but was largely forgotten until it was reintroduced in 1990 using a peripheral nerve stimulator. The dermatomes blocked by the interscalene block are seen in **Figure 9**.

Supraclavicular Block

The supraclavicular approach to the brachial plexus provides the most reliable anesthesia for the entire arm. The anatomical landmarks are shown in **Figure 6**, and the most common technique is the subclavian perivascular approach. The interscalene groove is palpated and followed distally until the pulsation of the subclavian artery is felt. This should be

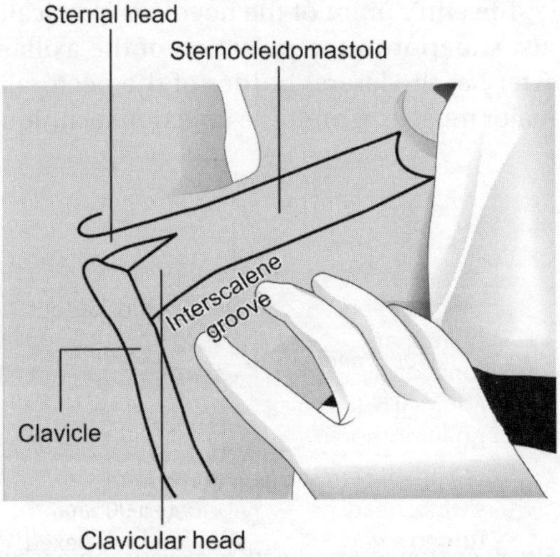

Fig. 5: Anatomical landmarks of interscalene block.

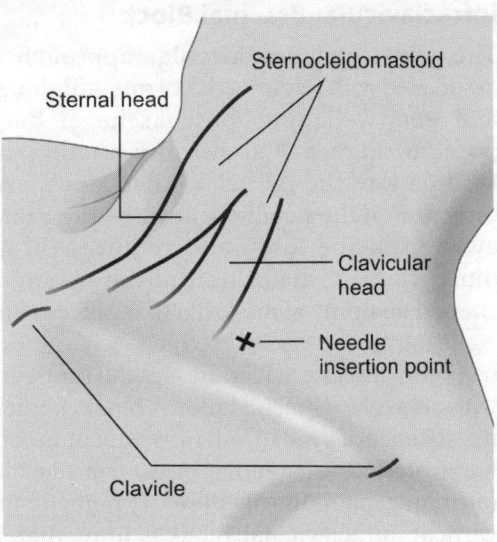

Fig. 6: Anatomical landmark of supraclavicular block.

at the midpoint of the clavicle, about 1 cm posterior to it. It is important to note that the cupola of the lung is medial to the insertion point of the needle, which is shown in **Figure 9**. Entry to the sheath can be identified by a 'click' as the needle pierces the tough fascia, by paresthesia, or by an appropriate motor response when a nerve stimulator is used. The subclavian artery runs within the fascia, just anterior and inferior to the brachial plexus. If the needle punctures the artery, it should be withdrawn a few milimeter carefully until it lies outside the artery but still within the sheath. The 'plumb-bob' technique is another supraclavicular approach.

The needle entry site is immediately superior to the clavicle, just lateral to the point where the sternocleidomastoid is attached to the clavicle. The angle of needle entry is 90° to the table. **Figure 9** shows the dermatomes targeted in this technique. The injection is made at the level of the trunks or the proximal divisions, where the fascial sheath is at its most compact. This could explain the reliability of the block and its relatively short onset of action.

Infraclavicular Brachial Block

The classical infraclavicular approach is associated with minimal risk of pneumothorax and good reliability but has never been popular. **Figure 7** shows the anatomical landmark of the infraclavicular block. The direction of the needle is towards the axilla, away from the lung, and requires three-dimensional visualization of the pyramid-shaped anatomy of the axilla to be successful.

Recently, the vertical infraclavicular block has been described. It addresses the problems with an axillary brachial plexus block, namely the absence of a radial and musculocutaneous nerve block. The latter may be used to alleviate tourniquet pain. The needle entry point for the vertical infraclavicular block is immediately below the clavicle at a point midway between the sternal notch and the acromion. The needle

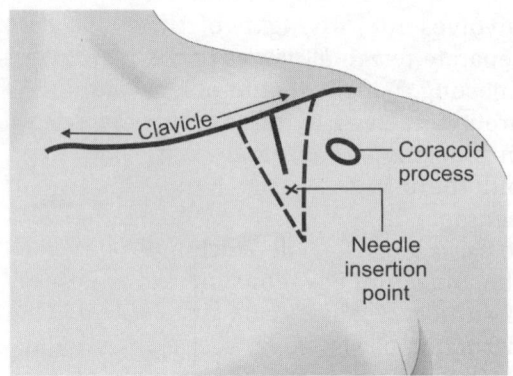

Fig. 7: Anatomical landmark of infraclavicular block.

must be advanced in a vertical direction to a maximum depth of 4 cm. **Figure 9** shows the dermatomal distribution of this block.

Axillary Approach to Brachial Block

The axillary approach is most suitable for surgery on the forearm, wrist, and hand, though the radial side of the forearm is sometimes missed. The anatomical landmarks are seen in **Figure 8**. The shoulder and the elbow should be in 90° abduction and flexion, respectively. A deliberate transarterial technique has been described, but the main complication from this block remains hematoma formation as a result of arterial puncture.

The entry point of the needle is classically just superior to the pulsation of the axillary artery at the lateral border of the pectoralis major muscle. A multiple injection technique

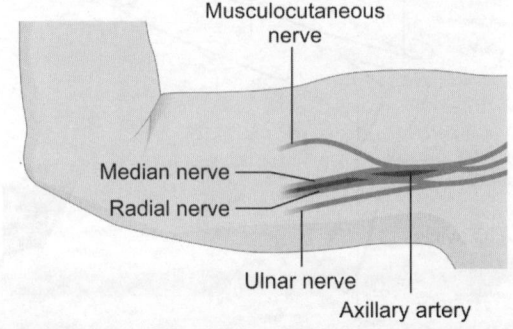

Fig. 8: Anatomical landmark of axillary approach to brachial block.

involves identifying two, three, or four separate terminal nerves in the plexus and injecting a small amount of local anesthetic around each. It increases the success rate in blocking the musculocutaneous nerve, but there is a slightly higher chance of neuropraxia after the block. An alternative is to use a single injection technique and block the musculocutaneous nerve separately if surgery occurs in its distribution. The dermatomal distribution is seen in **Figure 9**. The musculocutaneous nerve is blocked separately by injecting local anesthetic in the belly of the coracobrachialis muscle, just superior to the pulsation of the axillary artery and at 90° to the skin. Because the injection is made at the level of the terminal branches, the missed segment(s) show a nerve territory distribution and not a dermatomal pattern, as is the case when the injection is placed at the level of the roots.

About 25–40 mL volume of local anesthetic in prescribed concentration (**Table 7**) is injected in the desired areas depending upon the approach. Individual nerve blocks can be performed distally for selective blockade or as rescue blocks (inject 3–5 mL of LA).

Distal Blocks of Peripheral Nerves of Upper Extremity

Radial, ulnar, median, musculocutaneous, or digital nerves can be blocked depending upon the indication.

LOWER-EXTREMITY BLOCKS

The lumbosacral plexus innervates the muscles, joints, skin, and peritoneal lining of the abdominopelvic wall (**Figs. 10 and 11**). It also innervates the inferior extremities. It is formed by the ventral rami of L1 to S5. The lower extremity is innervated by the lumbar (L1–4) and lumbosacral plexuses (L4–S3). The lumbar plexus gives rise to the femoral, obturator, and lateral femoral cutaneous nerves. It also gives rise to iliohypogastric, ilioinguinal, and genitofemoral nerves.

In the lower extremity, individual nerve blocks are commonly performed by infiltration

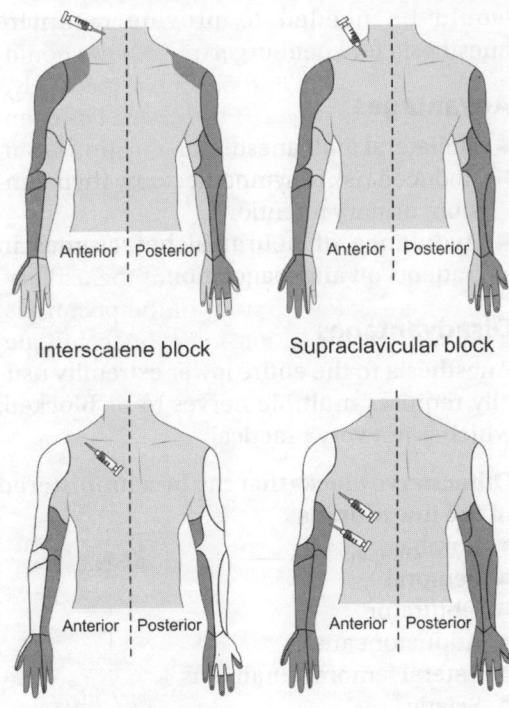

Fig. 9: Dermatomal distribution of various approaches to brachial block.

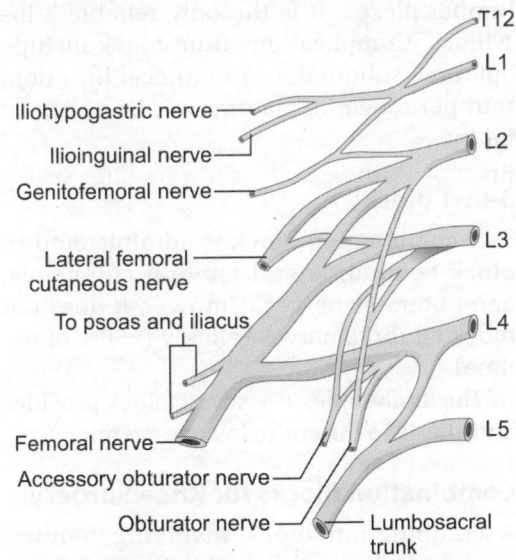

Fig. 10: Lumbar plexus nerve distribution.

CHAPTER 8 ♦ Regional Anesthesia

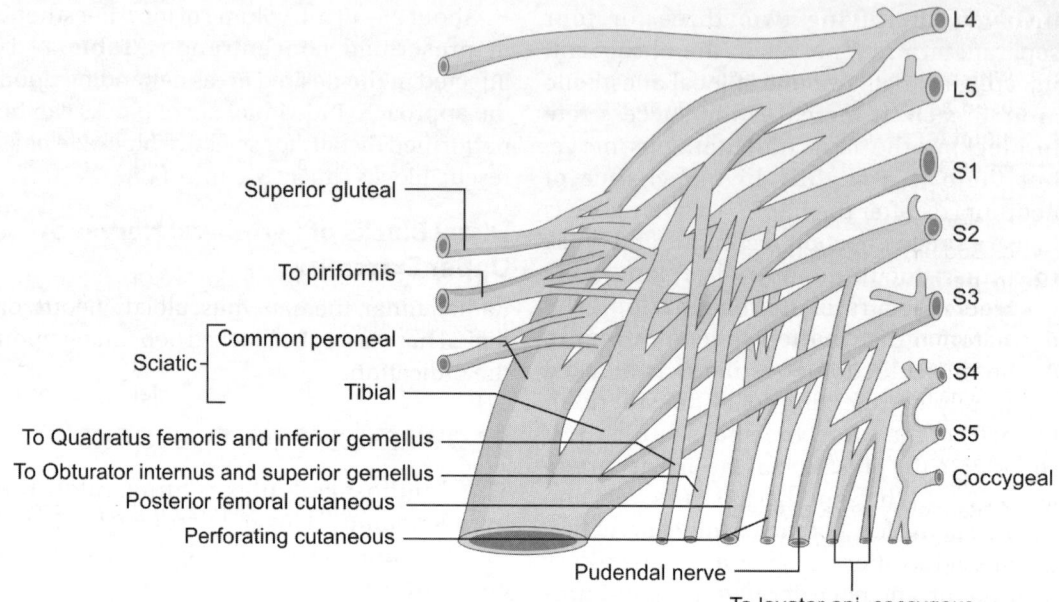

Fig. 11: Lumbosacral plexus nerve distribution.

without nerve stimulation, the femoral nerve is the only exception.

Combination Blocks

The psoas compartment/lumbar plexus block—achieves blockade of the entire lumbar plexus. It is the only reliable 3-in-1 block. Complications from block include epidural, subdural, or intrathecal injection, retroperitoneal hematoma, and/or visceral injury.

3-in-1 Block

This combination block is administered to block femoral, lateral femoral cutaneous, and obturator nerves. However, it does not block all three nerves reliably (<50% of the time).

The lumbar plexus + sciatic block provides anesthesia to the entire lower extremity.

Combination Blocks for Knee Surgery

A combination block involving femoral [anterior], obturator [medial], lateral femoral cutaneous [lateral], and sciatic [posterior] would be needed to provide complete anesthesia for knee surgery.

Advantages
- Unilateral limb anesthesia
- Reduced risk of sympathectomy (hypotension, urinary retention)
- Avoidance of neuraxial hematomas in patients on anticoagulation.

Disadvantages
Anesthesia to the entire lower extremity usually requires multiple nerves to be blocked, which is not very practical.

Other nerve blocks that can be administered in the lower limbs
- Lumbar
- Femoral
- Obturator
- Adductor canal
- Lateral femoral cutaneous
- Sciatic
- Popliteal
- Saphenous
- Ankle

CHAPTER 8 ♦ Regional Anesthesia

MULTIPLE CHOICE QUESTIONS

1. Which of the following agent is commonly used as an adjuvant to a local anesthetic agent for peripheral nerve blocks:
   a. Ketamine
   b. Ketorolac
   c. Magnesium sulfate
   d. Sodium bicarbonate

2. In peripheral nerve block, the nerve is blocked in the following order:
   a. Motor fibers > large sensory fibers > small sensory fibers.
   b. Small sensory fibers > large sensory fibers > Motor fibers.
   c. Large sensory fibers > small sensory fibers > Motor fibers.
   d. Randomly block all fibers.

3. Ultrasound helps identify nerves for blockade:
   a. As nerves appear hyperechoic
   b. As nerves appear hypoechoic
   c. Nerves travel adjacent to blood vessels, so a local anesthetic is injected adjacent to vessels.
   d. None of the above

4. The supraclavicular brachial plexus block is administered:
   a. At the level of the C6 vertebral body between the anterior and middle scalene muscles
   b. In the deltopectoral groove, 1 cm below the clavicle
   c. In the Interscalene groove, about 1 cm superior to the clavicle and lateral to the subclavian artery
   d. At the apex of the triangle formed by the two heads of the sternocleidomastoid muscle and the clavicle

5. Regards the axillary approach to the brachial plexus:
   a. Most suitable for surgery on the forearm, wrist, and hand
   b. The radial side of the forearm is sometimes missed
   c. Multiple injections with small amounts of the local anesthetic after identifying two, three, or four terminal nerves provide an excellent block
   d. All the above

Answers
1. d   2. b   3. b   4. c   5. d

9. Monitoring of a Patient Under Anesthesia

DV Bhargava

Learning Objectives

- Minimum monitoring standards
- Monitoring oxygen saturation
- End-tidal carbon dioxide
- Monitoring ECG and temperature
- Monitoring noninvasive blood pressure and arterial blood pressure
- Monitoring central venous pressure
- Brain function and neurological monitoring
- Cardiac output
- Fluid status monitoring
- Neuromuscular monitoring
- Respiratory gas monitoring
- Intraoperative echocardiography
- Intraoperative record keeping

INTRODUCTION

AS4.5: Observe and describe the principles and the steps/techniques in monitoring patients during anesthesia.

The dictionary meaning of 'monitoring' applies best to the fundamental job description of a vigilant anesthesiologist caring for a patient under anesthesia. Monitoring a patient under anesthesia constitutes 'a watch' on the patient by constantly observing the variations in various physiological parameters through the use of clinical signs and employment of various invasive or noninvasive devices and occasional blood sample analysis to preserve normal homeostasis.

Monitoring a patient under anesthesia reduces the adverse events and accidents during the period by providing a warning about the clinical deterioration of the patient. Monitoring helps the anesthesiologist take vital proactive measures for prevention, early detection, treatment of the cause, and minimizing the adverse effects of any abnormal deviations. These deviations in physiological parameters detected during such monitoring are interpreted in the context of the specific patient's clinical situation. The importance of monitoring a patient under anesthesia undergoing an operation or a diagnostic or therapeutic procedure cannot be overstated.

Monitoring in a Hospital

A patient admitted to a hospital is constantly under varying levels of monitoring depending on the clinical condition. It may vary from intermittent/periodic recording of vital parameters [pulse, blood pressure (BP), and oxygen saturation (SpO_2) checked intermittently by the nursing staff] or continual determination of vital parameters by an automated bedside monitor or the constant monitoring of a critically ill patient while being connected to a bedside monitor with a real-time display.

Need for Monitoring Under Anesthesia

Monitoring a patient while undergoing an invasive procedure or surgery in the operation theatre is completely different when compared to monitoring a patient in other sections of the hospital. A patient under general anesthesia, especially when paralyzed and under invasive mechanical ventilation, cannot report any pain, discomfort, or distress. Similarly, a patient under sedation while undergoing a procedure may not reliably report pain, difficult breathing, or any discomfort in any part of the body. To ensure organ preservation, monitoring of the patient is essential.

Clinical Signs Monitored

Monitoring of the physiological status of the patient can be performed only by the use of clinical signs. The responsibility for monitoring these signs while the surgeon performs the procedure lies primarily with the anesthesiologist. These signs may include direct physical observation of changes in skin color, temperature, sweating, shivering, movement, breathing, secretions, eye signs and variations in pulse characteristics, and deviations in BP. The detection of clinical signs, intuitively, constitutes one of the primary methods of monitoring a patient under anesthesia.

Limitations Encountered while Monitoring Under Anesthesia

Patients undergoing surgery are cleaned and draped almost completely, constituting one of the various aseptic precautions to prevent surgical infection. This limits the accessibility to look for various signs and measure certain physiological parameters under the surgical drapes. In addition, the clinical condition of a patient undergoing surgery is dynamic due to the effects of anesthetic medications, ongoing surgical intervention, and patient positioning in certain surgical procedures. Hence, the information about the clinical condition must be available reliably and continuously.

Physiological Parameters Monitored

Apart from drug administration to maintain the anesthetic state and record keeping during the entire duration of the surgery, an anesthesiologist is overwhelmed with repeatedly monitoring various clinical signs, like pulse and BP. With these limitations, intermittent automatic measurements of certain parameters can be done by applying monitors over the patients. These vary from the simple intermittent measurement of pulse rate, intermittent BP measurement, and SpO_2 to the advanced methods like invasive measurement and continuous display of various hemodynamic parameters, pressure waveform analysis, continuous cardiac output determination, monitors for inhaled anesthetic administration, depth of neuromuscular blockade, and determining of the depth of anesthesia.

STANDARDS FOR MONITORING UNDER ANESTHESIA

In 1982, ABC Television aired a program titled "Deep Sleep: 6,000 will die or suffer brain damage," where the adverse events due to mishaps during the administration of anesthesia were highlighted with various patient accounts. The program concluded that anesthesia was 1000 times more dangerous than traveling in an airplane 30,000 feet in the sky. Dr. Ellison C Pierce Jr was triggered by the thought that adverse events under anesthesia could be prevented by early detection of clinical deterioration by standard monitoring. He worked with other like-minded anesthesiologists around the globe to highlight the importance of standard monitoring of a patient under anesthesia.

Institution of Minimum Monitoring Standards

The Anesthesia Patient Safety Foundation (APSF), with the vision 'that no one shall be harmed by anesthesia care,' was founded in 1985 (www.apsf.org). A set of standards for minimum monitoring of patients under anesthesia (The Harvard Standards) were adopted in 1985 and were published in August 1986 by an independent risk management committee from the Harvard Medical School. On 21 October 1986, The American Society of Anesthesiologists (ASA) introduced the first medical standard of care for basic intraoperative monitoring. Amendments to the original standards are periodically incorporated to suit contemporary practice.

Several professional anesthesiology societies worldwide also have defined the standards for monitoring a patient under anesthesia. The Indian Society of Anaesthesiologists (ISA) promulgated monitoring standards as 'basic' and 'desirable' for monitoring patients under anesthesia. The ISA enshrines 'Eternal Vigilance' in its emblem to highlight the primary responsibility of the anesthesiologist to a patient under anesthesia.

Minimum Monitoring Standards

The foremost monitoring standard states that the presence of a qualified anesthesiologist is mandatory for any intervention in a patient under anesthesia or monitored anesthesia care. It is vital to understand that the minimum standard of anesthetic monitoring should not be altered even for a seemingly 'fit' patient without co-morbidities. All standards for monitoring patients under anesthesia uniformly prescribe the following basic parameters:

- *ECG*: Continuous monitoring of ECG during all types of anesthetics
- *SpO_2*: Continuous monitoring of SpO_2 during all types of anesthetics with audible variable pitch pulse tone for oxygen saturation
- *Blood pressure*: Continual BP determination (at least every 5 min) and evaluation of blood pressure and heart rate during all types of anesthetics
- *End-tidal carbon dioxide*: Monitoring of end-tidal carbon dioxide readings and breathing circuit disconnection audible alarms in all patients undergoing mechanical ventilation
- Body temperature (for procedures lasting more than 30 min)

American Society of Anesthesiologists (ASA) Minimum Monitoring Standards

The American Society of Anesthesiologists (ASA) minimum monitoring standards are followed globally (**Table 1**). The ASA standards apply to all anesthesia care, i.e., general anesthetics, regional anesthetics, and monitored anesthesia care. The objective of the ASA standards is to encourage quality patient care, but they do not guarantee a patient outcome.

Additional Standards

The Association of Anesthetists (UK) guidelines published in 2019 recommends the addition of the following monitoring:
1. Quantitative neuromuscular monitoring - whenever neuromuscular blocking drugs are administered.

Table 1: Features of the American Society of Anesthesiologists (ASA) standards for basic anesthesia monitoring.

Personnel-related	Qualified anesthesia personnel shall be present throughout all types of anesthesia care.
Parameter-related	During an anesthetic, ventilation, circulation, and temperature will be continually monitored.
Oxygenation	Patient will be adequately exposed and illumination adequate to assess color. a. An oxygen analyzer with a limit alarm will monitor inspired oxygen. b. Blood oxygenation will be quantitatively assessed with a pulse oximeter with variable pitch pulse tone and audible alarm.
Ventilation	a. The following qualitative clinical signs will be verified: chest excursion, reservoir breathing bag movements, auscultation of breath sounds, and correct positioning of the endotracheal tube or supraglottic airway device. b. Continual end-tidal carbon dioxide analysis shall be performed using a quantitative method such as capnography with audible alarms. c. During regional anesthesia or monitored anesthesia care, the adequacy of ventilation will be evaluated by qualitative clinical signs.
Circulation	a. Arterial blood pressure and heart rate will be determined at least every five minutes. b. Electrocardiogram will be continuously displayed. c. Circulation will be evaluated, in addition, by at least one of the following: palpable pulse, heart sounds auscultation, tracing of intra-arterial pressure, or pulse plethysmography or oximetry.
Body temperature	Will be monitored when clinically significant changes in body temperature are expected or suspected

2. Processed electroencephalogram monitoring—when total intravenous anesthesia is administered along with neuromuscular blocking drugs.
3. Capillary blood glucose and ketone monitoring are immediately accessible in every location.
4. An anesthetic record should be made with an accurate summary of the information provided by all monitoring devices (electronic preferable with integration to the hospital electronic health record system).

Advanced Monitoring

Advanced methods of monitoring can be employed on per case-to-case basis depending on the patient's clinical situation and the complexity of the surgery planned.

Equipment for Monitoring

Monitoring a patient under anesthesia, notwithstanding the presence of a qualified anesthesiologist, often becomes synonymous with electronic equipment and instrumentation that the patient is often connected to during the surgery. To overcome the limitations of reliably detecting clinical signs in a patient undergoing surgery under anesthesia, various patient monitoring methods are often utilized for intraoperative decision-making. The clinical information available with the gainful employment of various monitoring equipment is amazing. **Figure 1** shows some parameters that are displayed by a 'multipara monitor' employed for the perioperative monitoring of a patient. The range of basic and advanced monitoring techniques available for patient monitoring in

CHAPTER 9 ♦ Monitoring of a Patient Under Anesthesia

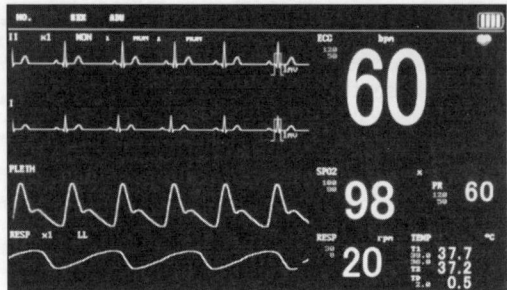

Fig. 1: 'Multipara monitor' continuously displays various physiological parameters. It shows a continuous running display of electrocardiographic leads, heart rate, pulse oximeter plethysmograph, oxygen saturation, blood pressure, respiratory waveform, respiratory rate, and temperature.

an operation theatre has been summarized in **Table 2** and **Figure 2**.

ECG Monitoring

Continuous display of ECG waveform during the entire period of surgery under anesthesia is essential. Intraoperative ECG monitoring is noninvasive, continuous, has a minimal recurrent cost, is simple to operate, and has no adverse effects on the patient. It is the standard of care for a patient under any anesthesia. The extent of intraoperative ECG monitoring depends on the patient's preoperative condition and the complexity of the surgical intervention.

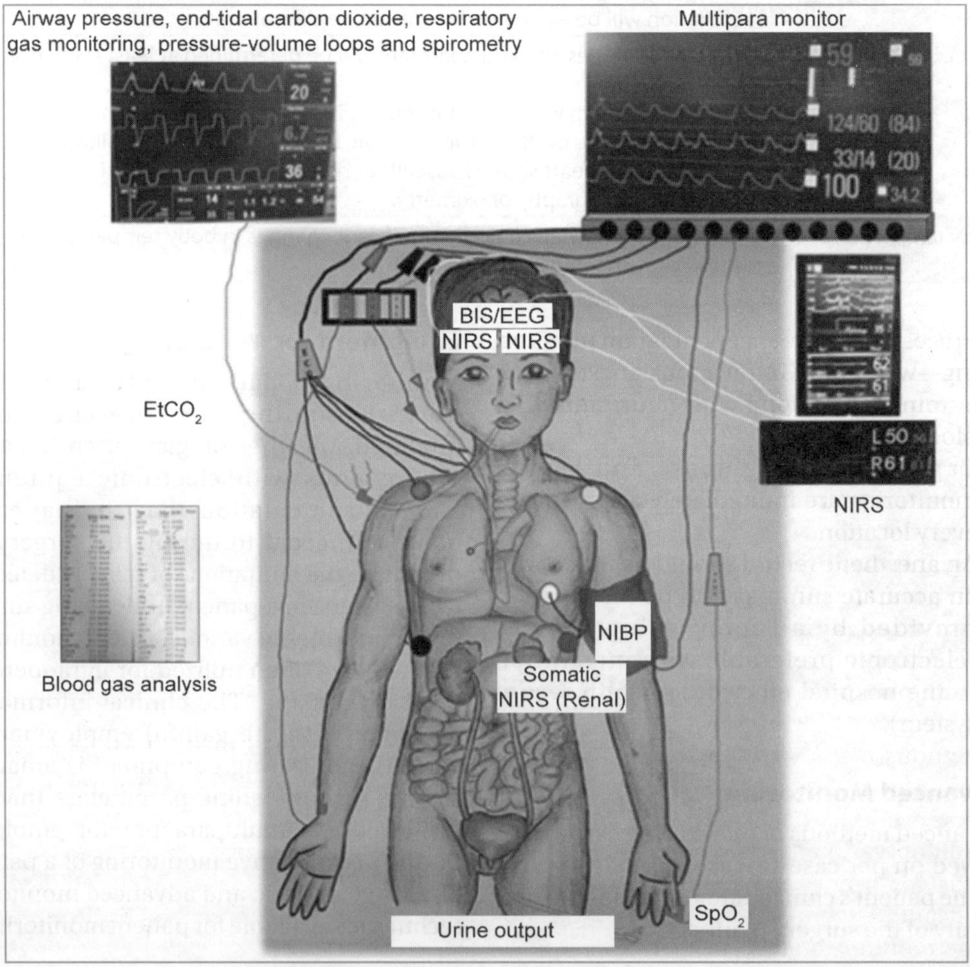

Fig.2: Schematic diagram of monitoring under anesthesia.

Table 2: Different modes of monitoring under anesthesia

Cardiovascular	**Clinical** • Heart rate • Pulse rate • Capillary refill • Mentation	**Equipment based** • Continuous electrocardiogram • Non-invasive blood pressure • Invasive arterial blood pressure • Central venous pressure • Pressure plethysmography • Pulmonary artery catheter/PCWP • Non-invasive continuous arterial pressure	**Cardiac output** • Pulmonary artery catheter based • Pulse contour analysis • Esophageal Doppler • Bioimpedance • Bioreactance • Echocardiography (TEE and TTE)
Respiratory	**Clinical** • Chest excursions • Breathing pattern	**Equipment based** • SpO_2 • Capnography • Respiratory gas • Thoracic impedance	**Ventilator based** • Disconnection • Hypoxia • Airway pressures • Flow volume loops
Temperature	**Blood temperature** Pulmonary artery catheter	**Core temperature** • Swan Ganz catheter • Distal esophagus • Nasopharynx	**Shell temperature** • Skin temperature • Rectal
Others	**Blood gas analysis** • Lactate trends • Electrolyes • Acidosis/Alkalosis	**Neuromuscular** • TOF • Single twitch • Tetany • Double burst stimulation	**Renal** Urine output monitoring

Electrode Placement

ECG electrode placement in the intraoperative period may need modifications due to the planned surgical incision and electromagnetic interference. Intraoperative ECG electrodes can be placed as per various systems. Commonly, three and four-electrode systems are monitored during anesthesia for elective non-cardiac surgery. Five-electrode system is usually employed for patients with significant cardiac illness undergoing cardiac surgery under anesthesia. More ECG electrodes facilitate the simultaneous continuous display of more ECG leads on the monitor and facilitate early detection of adverse events like ischemia and arrhythmia. In addition, various types of visual and audible alarms for bradycardia, tachycardia, and significant ST-segment changes can be set up on the monitor to alert the anesthesiologist early.

ECG Display Modes

The ECG monitor display utilized for patient monitoring under anesthesia caters to a variety of adjustable selections in terms of the number of ECG leads simultaneously displayed on the monitor, size alterations, and alternative display modes (filter, monitor, and diagnostic mode) to minimize artifacts and noise, detection of pacing spikes and options to automatically detect arrhythmias and ST-segment changes in multiple leads. Usually, two ECG channels, Lead II and Lead V, are employed for continuous display during the intraoperative period as this combination has a high sensitivity for the detection of perioperative ischemic events. Some alternate methods, using only one display channel, for the three-electrode system to facilitate ischemia and arrhythmia monitoring are tabulated in **Table 3**.

Table 3: Three-electrode system modifications.

3-electrode system	RA	LA	LL	Lead selected
MCL_1	Ground	Left clavicle	V_1	III
CS_5	Right clavicle	V_5	Ground	I
CM_5	Manubrium	V_5	Ground	I
CB_5	Right scapula	V_5	Ground	I
CC_5	Right anterior axillary line	V_5	Ground	I

Benefits of ECG Monitoring

Patients with pre-existing coronary artery disease require close monitoring of the ST segment changes for early detection of perioperative myocardial ischemia and infarction. ST-segment depressions are more commonly encountered than ST-segment elevations during the perioperative period. They occur due to an imbalance in the oxygen supply/demand mismatch during the procedure. Continuous ECG monitoring with ST-segment monitoring provides a lead time for the anesthesiologist to correct this imbalance. Similarly, arrhythmias during the intraoperative period are promptly detected by continuous ECG monitoring.

ECG Artifacts

Artifacts on ECG display may occur due to initial poor skin contact, altered skin contact due to blood/antiseptic solutions, sweating, interference due to electrocautery or other electromagnetic interference, and damaged cables.

Pulse Oximetry

Pulse oximetry is considered the most useful technological advancement in the monitoring and safety of patients during anesthesia, recovery, and critical care. The blood oxygen saturation in capillaries is measured non-invasively with a pulse oximeter. The device utilizes an electronic processor and a pair of small light-emitting diodes facing a photodiode through a translucent part of the patient's body, usually a fingertip or an earlobe. The percentage of oxygen saturation of the hemoglobin in blood is shown by this monitor by the use of a simple, non-invasive probe. It is a precalibrated, non-invasive, inexpensive, easy-to-use monitor of the oxygen saturation of a patient. Takuo Aoyago, a Japanese bioengineer, invented the prototype of a pulse oximeter and patented it in 1972. Initially developed as an ear-piece oximeter, the present-day pulse oximeters are self-contained battery-operated models commonly applied over the fingertip.

Principle

Light absorbance of oxygenated blood is different from that of deoxygenated blood. Reduced hemoglobin absorbs light in the red range (660 nm) more than oxygenated hemoglobin. Further, oxygenated hemoglobin absorbs light in the near-infrared range (940 nm) more than deoxygenated hemoglobin. Two wavelengths of light, 660 nm and 940 nm, are emitted by a light source across the tissue. At the same time, the probe is clipped to the fingertip, and the absorption of each component of emitted light in the tissue is detected by a photodetector. Using the principle of Beer-Lambart Law, the concentration of a given solute (oxygenated or deoxygenated hemoglobin) is determined by the amount of each wavelength of light absorbed.

Derivation of Oxygen Saturation

The pulsatile component of the total tissue due to the arterial pulse is determined by deducting the non-pulsatile component

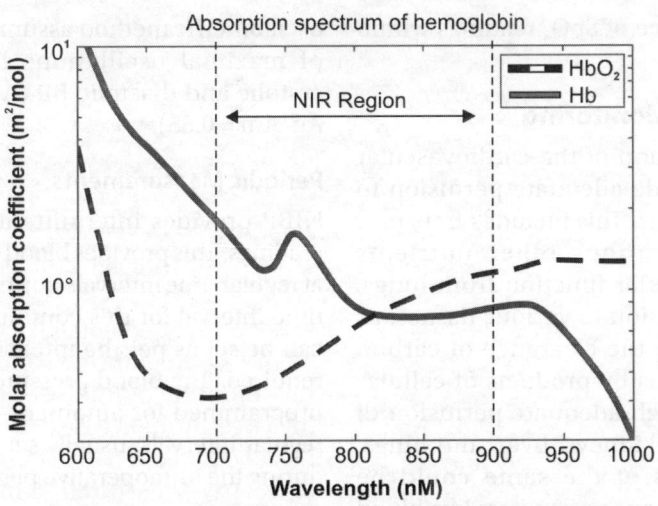

Fig. 3: Oxygen absorption spectrum of hemoglobin.

(bone, muscle, tissue) from the total absorbed light. The ratio of differential light absorption in pulsatile to the non-pulsatile component is input into a nomogram. This nomogram has been derived from healthy volunteers breathing progressive hypoxic mixtures. The oxygen saturation in the pulsatile component of the tissue (SpO_2) derived from this nomogram is displayed by the pulse oximeter. Pulse oximetry thus utilizes these two physical principles of differential light absorption and deduction of non-pulsatile components of tissue to detect the percentage of oxygenated hemoglobin in the pulsatile arterial blood (**Fig. 3**).

Pulse Plethysmography

An essential benefit of a pulse oximeter is a plethysmograph display. The variation of plethysmograph amplitude indicates volumetric changes associated with pulsatile arterial blood flow (**Fig. 4**). Newer monitors use the plethysmograph wave area to estimate the cardiac output and blood volume.

Limitations of Pulse Oximetry

Abnormal forms like methemoglobin and carboxyhemoglobin affect its accuracy. Ambient fluorescent light, nail polish, electrical interference, and patient motion commonly interfere with the functioning of the oximeter. In addition, poor perfusion, cold extremities, arrhythmias, and peripheral vascular disease may also affect the SpO_2 readings. Failure to detect hypoventilation and subsequent hypercarbia without a fall in oxygen saturation is possible when supplemental oxygen is administered under anesthesia. Other patient monitoring methods, like capnography and clinical vigilance, thus remain important

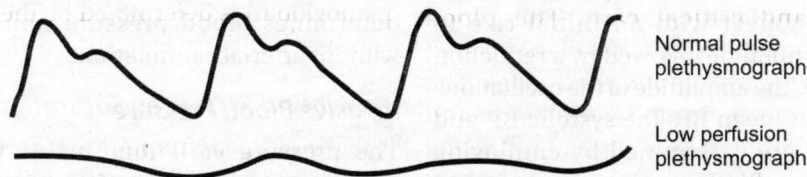

Fig. 4: Normal pulse plethysmograph and pulse plethysmograph in low perfusion state.

even in the presence of SpO_2 readings within normal limits.

Blood Pressure Monitoring

The primary function of the cardiovascular system is to provide adequate perfusion to various body tissues. This includes transport of oxygen and various other nutrients necessary for cellular function from lungs, splanchnic circulation to various tissues, as well as facilitating the clearance of carbon dioxide and various by-products of cellular metabolism through adequate perfusion of organs, including kidneys, liver, and lungs. The effectiveness of the same could be determined by various parameters like blood pressure, pulse rate, cardiac output, oxygen saturation in blood, partial pressure of oxygen and carbon dioxide, and blood levels of various electrolytes and metabolites. A vital physiological parameter that determines this function is arterial blood pressure.

Noninvasive Blood Pressure

Arterial blood pressure in the operation theatre can be determined by a noninvasive method using a cuff, usually over the arm (brachial arterial pressure) by an automatic oscillometric method. This is denoted as noninvasive blood pressure (NIBP). The cuff is inflated around the arm and deflated while the pressure inside the cuff is monitored. The oscillations within the cuff occur due to arterial pulsations.

Working Principle of NIBP

The cuff is inflated beyond the systolic pressure where no blood supply occurs. As cuff deflation occurs, the oscillometric waveforms appear with an initial rise in oscillation amplitude followed by a reduction in amplitude. The amplitude of the oscillations is maximal at mean BP. The systolic BP and diastolic BP are determined by employing algorithms, which vary with different machine manufacturers. The conventional oscillometric method assumes fixed fractions of maximal oscillations for determining systolic and diastolic BP (As/Am = 0.55 and Ad/Am = 0.85).

Periodic Measurements

NIBP provides intermittent blood pressure readings. This provides blood pressure readings at regular time intervals during the surgery. The time interval for this continual measurement can be set as per the intensity of monitoring required. The blood pressure monitor can be programmed for automatic measurement at regular intervals, usually set at 3 or 5 minutes during the intraoperative period.

Limitations of NIBP

Critically ill patients who are expected to have major fluctuations in blood pressure during surgery may not be suitable for NIBP monitoring. The measurements may differ from those obtained by the auscultatory method in pregnant and obese patients. The accuracy of NIBP is unreliable in patients with arrhythmias, in severe shock or vasodilated states, as the changes in oscillations with variations in cuff pressure are small and non-uniform.

Continuous Noninvasive Arterial Pressure (CNAP)

Continuous noninvasive arterial pressure (CNAP) provides a continuous estimation of blood pressure and employs photoplethysmography and vascular unloading techniques, using counter-pressure to maintain constant finger volume. A counter-pressure is applied to the finger during arterial pulsation to maintain constant blood volume, as photoplethysmography estimates. This method determines blood pressure noninvasively without arterial cannulation.

Invasive Blood Pressure

The pressure variations inside the artery resulting from each cardiac contraction is measured by inserting a cannula into the lumen of an artery. Arterial access is usually obtained via radial, femoral, or dorsalis pedis arteries. It provides a continuous measure of the arterial pressure along with the display of the arterial pulse waveform. The pressure waveforms derived directly from the cannula inside the lumen are transmitted via a non-compressible fluid-filled tube into a transducer.

Working Principle of Pressure Transducer

The transducer has a flexible diaphragm attached to a Wheatstone bridge via a strain gauge. Mechanical energy from arterial waveforms displaces the diaphragm, and this energy is converted into electrical signals. The resistance of the wire or silicone in the strain gauge increases with increasing stretch. A Wheatstone Bridge is employed to determine the unknown change in resistance with each transmitted arterial pulsation. This information is computed and transmitted as multiple sine waves. Fourier analysis of the multiple sine waves resulting from an arterial waveform results in the display of a simple continuous arterial waveform on the monitor (**Fig. 5**).

Transducer Zeroing

The transducer is fixed at the level of the heart (mid-axillary line in the fourth intercostal space) for leveling. It is zeroed to atmospheric pressure for accurate readings before it starts measuring the pressures. In addition, optimal damping of the transducer system is assessed for the correct blood pressure assessment.

Limitations and Risks

Although it gives a continuous beat-to-beat reading of the blood pressure, invasive blood pressure monitoring is associated with risks related to arterial cannulation like injury, hematoma, and peripheral ischemia.

Additional Uses

Arterial waveform analysis by systolic pressure variation (SPV), and pulse pressure variation (PPV) is utilized to determine the volume status of a patient and predict the

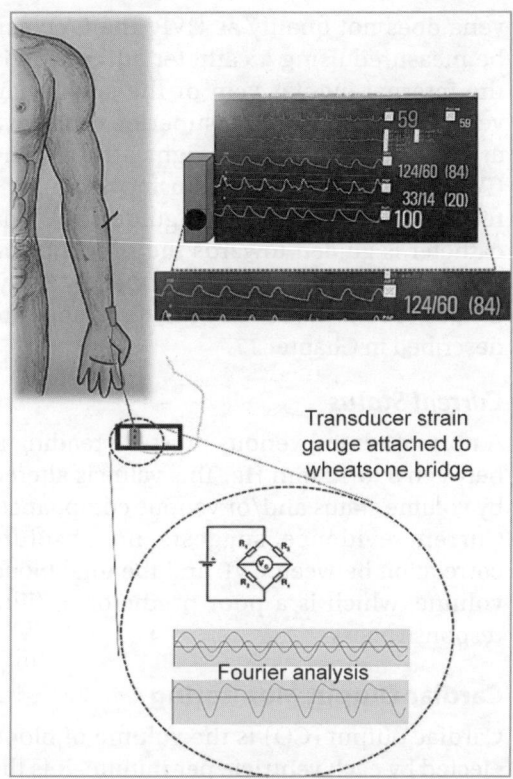

Fig. 5: Pressure transducer system showing various components. Intra-arterial cannula, connected to a transducer via non-compressible fluid-filled tubing, and then to the monitor for display. The transducer contains a diaphragm connected to a strain gauge and a Wheatstone bridge.

requirement of fluid resuscitation in patients with hemodynamic shock. Arterial waveform analysis is also used to calculate cardiac output using pooled algorithms.

Central Venous Pressure Monitoring

Central venous pressure (CVP) is a measure of pressure in the superior vena cava. It is a surrogate method of estimation of preload and right atrial pressure. It is often used as an assessment of hemodynamic status.

Measurement of CVP

The point of measurement of the central venous pressure must be intrathoracic. Thus measurement of pressure in inferior vena does not qualify as CVP. The CVP can be measured using a catheter advanced via the internal jugular vein or the subclavian veins and placed in the superior vena cava at its junction with the right atrium. The CVP catheter is introduced using Seldinger's technique (catheter over a guidewire). The catheter is guided towards the right atrium. The correct placement is confirmed by X-ray. Details of central venous catheterizations are described in Chapter 17.

Current Status

A normal central venous pressure reading is between 8 to 12 mm Hg. This value is altered by volume status and/or venous compliance. Current evidence suggests no absolute correlation between CVP and the total blood volume, which is a poor predictor of fluid responsiveness.

Cardiac Output Monitoring

Cardiac output (CO) is the volume of blood ejected by each ventricle per minute. It is the product of stroke volume and heart rate. CO varies with heart rate or rhythm, preload, contractility, and afterload. CO monitoring is essential to determine tissue perfusion and oxygen delivery. Cardiac output (CO) monitoring is an important tool in high-risk, critically ill, hemodynamically unstable patients and in whom large fluid shifts are expected.

Thermodilution Cardiac Output

The thermodilution method, using a pulmonary artery catheter (PAC) or Swan Ganz catheter), is considered the gold standard for monitoring CO. The method works on the principle of measuring the rate of change of temperature of a cold saline injectate as it traverses from the right atrium to the pulmonary artery. The CO is calculated using the Stewart Hamilton equation. The PAC is introduced through the right internal jugular vein and traverses the right atrium and ventricle to reach the pulmonary artery. The passage of the PAC along the blood flow is facilitated by balloon floatation.

Newer Cardiac Output Monitoring Methods

Complications associated with PAC led to the development of newer minimally or non-invasive methods. The newer monitors are based on the Ficks principle, thermodilution, Doppler, pulse contour analysis, ultrasound, and bioimpedance. Each method has its limitations and advantages. None of these monitors can accurately measure CO, so they are used mainly to estimate trends.

Fluid Status Monitoring

The estimation of total body blood volume is difficult. Till recently, CVP was considered a guide to fluid status, but of late, its utility and accuracy have been challenged.

Central Venous Pressure

Central venous pressure has traditionally been used to determine the adequacy of fluid preload. However, it is unreliable in assessing volume status or left ventricular function. Care must be taken when interpreting CVP in patients during mechanical ventilation, particularly when positive end-expiratory pressure (PEEP) levels exceeding 10 cm water are being used or during respiratory distress when pleural pressures fluctuate widely.

Fluid Responsiveness

The emergence of the concept of fluid responsiveness and its impact on patient outcomes has changed the way fluid status is estimated. Initially, this concept was used to deliver a 'fluid challenge' with a bolus of fluid intravenous and look for a resultant change in the blood pressure. Adequacy of circulatory volume status can be determined by the response of filling pressures to fluids. A rise in

CVP by 3 mm Hg indicates no volume deficit. The result of this test can also be assessed by noting changes in cardiac output in case it is being monitored. If the hemodynamics improved after the administration of fluids, the patient was considered fluid deficient, and more fluid was administered.

Static and Dynamic Indicators of Preload

Technology to determine static and dynamic parameters that indicate cardiac preload is available. These parameters determine the volume status more accurately.

- Pulse pressure and volume variation are commonly used to determine hypovolemia. Greater than 10% variation in the pulse trace dimension with respiratory cycle changes during mechanical ventilation indicates volume deficit. Pulse plethysmograph monitors which quantify variation in pulse pressure are available for clinical use today.
- Ultrasonography of the inferior vena cava and right ventricle can provide information on circulating volume status and overall cardiac function. However, interpretation of the images is highly user-dependent and may be complicated by the presence of valvular dysfunction and positive pressure ventilation.
- Non- and semi-invasive cardiac output monitors that record beat-by-beat stroke volume and display stroke volume variation. Currently, these monitors are considered the gold standard for estimating circulatory volume status.

Goal-directed Therapy

Intravascular volume management has currently shifted to 'Goal-directed Therapy.' The changes in parameters recorded by the new cardiac output monitors help assess the fluid response. Most monitors use variations in pulse pressure or volume to estimate fluid status. Variations of more than 10% in the area under the pulse curve are considered a fluid deficit state. The patient is administered fluids to attain a preset hemodynamic goal of cardiac output.

Temperature Monitoring

Anesthetic medications may impair the normal response to hypothermia. A fall in peripheral temperature can cause a redistribution of central heat to the periphery, causing a drop in core temperature. The operating room temperature is usually maintained at around 20–22°C. The patient under anesthesia is thus at risk of hypothermia. Hypothermia can lead to various adverse physiological effects, including shivering and increased oxygen consumption which can be detrimental during the surgery.

Therapeutic Hypothermia

Certain surgeries (open-heart surgeries) require the cooling of the patient for myocardial preservation and to reduce metabolic requirements. Therapeutic hypothermia facilitates better surgical outcomes. Cooling and re-warming of the patient must be done carefully, and continuously monitor the body temperature.

Sites for Temperature Monitoring

Core temperature can be measured using temperature probes. Probes in the pulmonary artery catheter, nasopharynx, distal esophagus, tympanic membrane, and urinary bladder catheter denote core temperature. Skin temperature can be measured by direct application of a probe over the skin or by application of infrared thermometers. The increased gradient between core temperatures denotes reduced peripheral perfusion, as seen in patients in shock with cold peripheries.

End-tidal Carbon Dioxide Monitoring

The amount of carbon dioxide in the exhaled gas can be continuously analyzed by sampling the exhaled gas from the anesthetic circuit. The

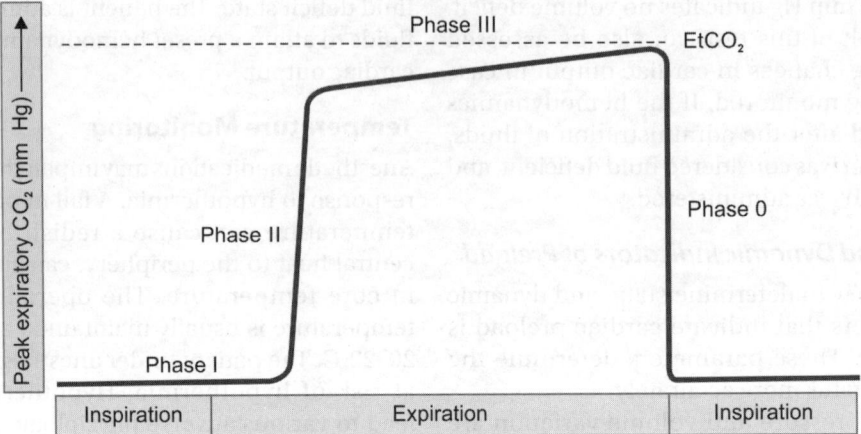

Fig. 6: Phases of a capnography.

gas sample must be collected at the patient end of the breathing circuit. The sampled gas is continuously drawn for infrared analysis. The CO_2 levels measured at the end of expiration constitute $EtCO_2$ (end-tidal CO_2). In healthy patients, $EtCO_2$ values are usually 3–5 mm Hg less than the PCO_2 in the blood. The absence of an $EtCO_2$ waveform after intubation should raise suspicion of esophageal intubation. This requires immediate repositioning the endotracheal tube into the trachea from the esophagus. The $EtCO_2$ waveform provides valuable information about CO_2 production and clearance (ventilation).

Phases of Capnography

There are four phases of capnography (**Fig. 6**).
a. Phase 0 (inspiratory phase): Inspiration ($PECO_2 = 0$ mm Hg).
b. Phase I (latency phase): From the beginning of expiration (represents anatomical dead space of the respiratory tract) and is not different from the inspiratory phase graph before it ($PECO_2 = 0$ mm Hg),
c. Phase II: A rapid increase in $PECO_2$ (represents exhalation of mixed air).
d. Phase III (Plateau phase): a small increase in $PECO_2$, which happens at the peak at the end of tidal expiration ($EtCO_2$) (represents the alveolar expiratory flow). $PECO_2$ is close to alveolar carbon dioxide tension (P_ACO_2).

Types of $EtCO_2$ Monitors

Two commonly used $EtCO_2$ monitors are the side-stream monitors and the main-stream monitors. Side-stream monitors aspirate the gas sample from the exhaled gas (taken from the T-adapter of the ventilator tubing) and analyze it. In the main-stream monitors, a sampling window is inserted directly in line with the ventilator circuit for CO_2 measurement.

Neurological Monitoring

Monitoring of the central nervous system includes assessment of various aspects of cerebral function. The central nervous function can be assessed using the following modes:
a. *Processed EEG monitoring:* It is commonly monitored using the bispectral index (BIS) and entropy. Analysis of changes in processed EEG waveforms derived by applying one or two electrodes over the forehead to estimate the depth of anesthesia to prevent awareness. Examples of such processed EEG algorithms include BIS and Entropy.
b. *Intracranial pressure monitoring:* It is commonly monitored by pressure transduction

from catheters placed in the subarachnoid space.

c. *Cerebral oxygenation:* It is commonly monitored by estimation of the jugular venous oxygen saturation ($SjvO_2$) and using near-infra-red spectroscopy (NIRS) monitoring. NIRS uses the principle of reflectance oximetry to assess the cerebral oxygenation status.

d. *Blood supply and emboli to the brain:* Transcranial Doppler of various intracranial blood vessels, like the middle cerebral artery, is used to assess cerebral blood flow. In addition, it is used to detect embolic events in the brain.

e. *Evoked potentials:* Evoked potential monitoring is done in procedures with a risk of mechanical injury or ischemia of neural structures due to the surgical procedure. This may occur in surgeries of the spine (mechanical trauma) and aortic aneurysms (interruption of blood supply to the spinal cord). SSEP (Somatosensory EP) and MEP (Motor EP) are the most commonly used evoked potentials where a stimulating electrode and a sensing electrode are used to continuously assess the function of the neural track at risk (sensory/motor).

Neuromuscular Monitoring

Hypnosis, analgesia, and immobility achieved with homeostasis and physiological stability are the cornerstones of anesthetic practice. Immobility, along with hypnosis under general anesthesia, is mandatory for certain types of surgery. Neuromuscular paralysis is achieved using muscle relaxants that act at the neuromuscular junction.

Train of Four Monitoring

The most common method for monitoring neuromuscular paralysis is applying a train-of-four (TOF) count. The TOF monitor generates four successive supramaximal stimuli at 0.5-second intervals (**Fig. 7**). Deep neuromuscular blockade results in no response to all four stimuli. As the blockade recovers, the response to the stimulus is counted initially as the number of responses out of four. The ratio of the last twitch height to the first is called the TOF ratio. TOF ratio of >0.9 is essential before tracheal extubation to prevent various airway-related complications. The monitors work on the principles of either mechanomyography, electromyography, or acceleromyography. The new neuromuscular monitors usually use acceleromyography technology. Apart from TOF count, other methods used are post-tetanic stimulation, post-tetanic count, and double burst stimulation.

Respiratory Gas Monitoring and Spirometry

Airway pressures, lung compliance, and inspired oxygen levels are monitored in patients under anesthesia with mechanical ventilation (**Fig. 8**). Spirometry and pressure-volume loops are inbuilt into the anesthesia workstations. In addition, levels of inhalation anesthetics like sevoflurane, isoflurane, and desflurane in the inhaled breathing gas mixture

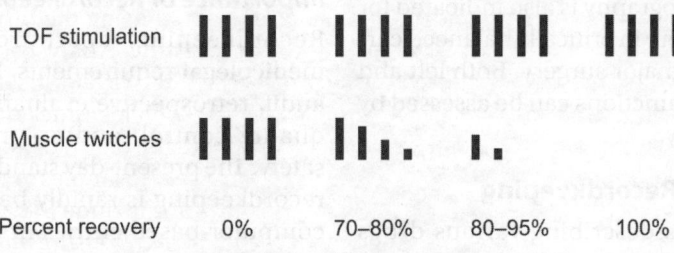

Fig. 7: Train of four response.

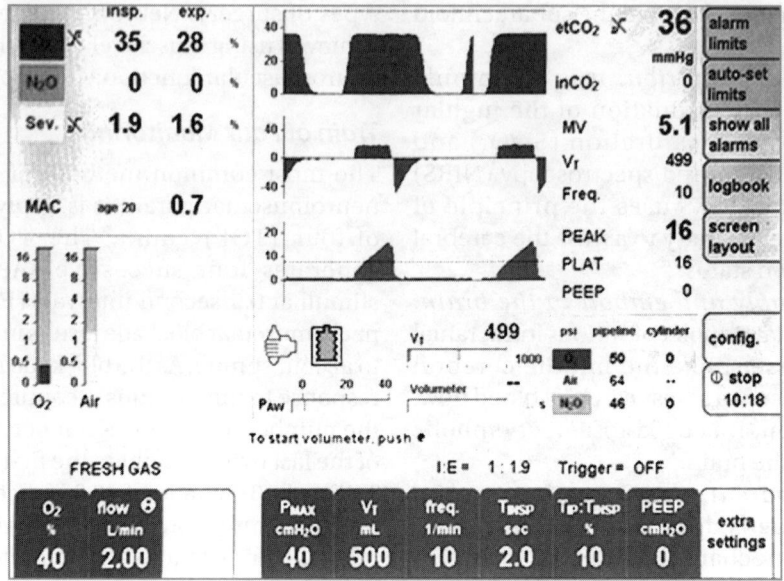

Fig. 8: Respiratory gas monitoring and spirometry under anesthesia.

are monitored to maintain adequate depth of anesthesia.

Intraoperative Echocardiography

Intraoperative transesophageal echocardiography is a critical component of contemporary heart surgery. It plays a key role in surgical planning, determining cardiac chamber filling and function, and assessing surgical interventions. It is also used for the early detection of cardiac complications such as cardiac tamponade. It plays a vital role in trans catheter device closure of cardiac shunts (such as ventricular septal defect, atrial septal defect, etc.) to help identify the shunt and place the occluder device optimally. Intraoperative echocardiography is also indicated for non-cardiac surgery in critically balanced cardiac patients for major surgery. Both left and right ventricular functions can be assessed by echocardiography.

Intraoperative Recordkeeping

Anesthetic charts describing various drugs and fluids administered, intraoperative events like intubation, central venous cannulation, and arterial cannulation, along with hemodynamic variations of heart rate, BP, SpO_2, etc., on a timeline are mandatory for each case administered an anesthetic. These anesthetic charts form part of medical documents for the patient. Meticulous recordkeeping and documentation are necessary for all cases.

History

The initial history of record keeping, by Harvey Cushing and Ernest Codman, using carefully written charts was improvised to an auditable format by Nosworthy. Most institutions have their unique way of anesthetic recordkeeping.

Importance of Recordkeeping

Recordkeeping, apart from catering to medicolegal requirements, helps in internal audit, retrospective evaluation for research, quality control, and assurance of patient safety. The present-day standard of anesthetic recordkeeping is rapidly being upgraded to computer-based entries in real-time, which are either stored on a local database or a cloud network. This facilitates rapid access and helps to build large databases suitable for developing artificial intelligence algorithms. Maintaining medical record archives is a legal requirement.

MULTIPLE CHOICE QUESTIONS

1. **The Minimum Monitoring Standard recommended under anesthesia includes all *except*:**
   a. Neuromuscular transmission
   b. Electrocardiogram
   c. End-tidal carbon dioxide
   d. Body temperature

2. **The foremost monitoring standard states that the presence of:**
   a. A qualified anesthesiologist is desirable for any intervention in a patient under any kind of anesthesia
   b. A qualified anesthesiologist is mandatory for any intervention in a patient only under general anesthesia
   c. A qualified anesthesiologist is mandatory for any intervention in a patient under anesthesia or monitored anesthesia care
   d. A qualified anesthesiologist is desirable for every intervention in a patient under general anesthesia

3. **About a pulse oximeter:**
   a. Works on the principle that light absorbance of oxygenated blood differs from that of deoxygenated blood
   b. Reduced hemoglobin absorbs light in the red range (660 nm) more than oxygenated hemoglobin
   c. The pulsatile component of the total tissue with the arterial pulse is determined by deducting the non-pulsatile component
   d. All of the above

4. **Pulse oximeter readings may be erroneous in all *except*:**
   a. Patients with anemia
   b. Patients with nail polish
   c. Patients with severe jaundice
   d. Patients with poor peripheral perfusion

5. **For the correct measurement of central venous pressure, the cannula tip must be:**
   a. In the superior or inferior vena cava
   b. In the right atrium
   c. Intrathoracic
   d. All of the above

6. **Fluid deficit is indicated by:**
   a. A greater than 10% variation in the pulse pressure or volume
   b. A greater than 5% variation in the pulse pressure or volume
   c. Pulsus alternans
   d. Central venous pressure < 6 mm Hg

7. **End-tidal carbon dioxide is the:**
   a. Estimated average carbon dioxide level
   b. Carbon dioxide level at the mid-point of the capnograph
   c. Carbon dioxide level measured at the end of expiration
   d. Same as the arterial carbon dioxide tension

8. **Which of the following is a neurological function monitor?**
   a. Entropy
   b. Bispectral index
   c. Near-infra-red spectroscopy
   d. All of the above

9. **Regarding intraoperative medical record-keeping:**
   a. It is a medicolegal requirement
   b. Helps administration calculate drug usage
   c. It helps determine the patient's hemodynamics
   d. None of the above

Answers
1. a
2. c
3. d
4. a
5. c
6. a
7. c
8. d
9. a

CHAPTER 10

Ensuring Homeostasis Under Anesthesia

Mukul Chandra Kapoor

Learning Objectives

- Arterial blood pressure control
- Carriage of respiratory gases
- Hemoglobin oxygen dissociation curve
- Preservation of cellular respiration
- Acid-base balance and its relevance
- Maintenance of body temperature
- Interventions to maintain homeostasis

INTRODUCTION

AS4.4: Observe and describe the principles and the steps/techniques in maintenance of vital organ functions in patients undergoing surgical procedures.

The loss of consciousness and loss of voluntary control over breathing due to suppression of the brain and muscle function makes a patient susceptible to multi-organ damage. With the induction of anesthesia, the body homeostasis is disturbed, particularly in terms of oxygenation, expiration of carbon dioxide, maintenance of body temperature, fluid homeostasis, and cardiac/respiratory function. The relative complexity of general anesthesia makes the intervention and monitoring requirement to maintain organ function more intense.

ARTERIAL BLOOD PRESSURE CONTROL

The baroreceptor reflex, antidiuretic hormone, and renin-angiotensin system have a significant role in cardiovascular homeostasis. In addition, local mechanisms like myogenic vascular response and the endothelial nitric oxide system also influence cardiovascular homeostasis. These mechanisms directly or indirectly affect arterial blood pressure to maintain homeostasis. Hypertension, atherosclerosis, cardiac disease, kidney disease, and central nervous system disease alter cardiovascular function.

Arterial baroreceptors are present in the aortic arch and the carotid bodies. Baroreceptors are mechanoreceptors activated by the stretching of the vessel. This sensory input from them to the central nervous system triggers a response to influence the peripheral vascular resistance and cardiac output. These receptors transmit the action potentials to the solitary nucleus, which signals the autonomic neurons to secrete hormones to affect the cardiovascular tone and heart rate.

Arterial pressure reflects the cardiac output, arterial elasticity, and peripheral vascular resistance. Blood pressure is by many activities and anesthesia. Maintaining blood pressure within normal limits is essential to prevent damage to the heart and other systems. The arterial pressure is maintained at a high enough pressure for proper tissue perfusion but not so high as to cause harm. In the case of acute hypotension, the baroreceptors attempt to raise arterial pressure to allow adequate tissue perfusion.

Most anesthetic agents have cardiac depression properties and can potentially cause hypotension. In addition, some anesthetic agents, both inhaled and intravenous, vasodilate the vascular tree to reduce peripheral resistance and cause hypotension. On the other hand, inadequate depth of anesthesia may cause the hormonal release to cause hypertension. Judicious maintenance of acceptable blood pressure levels is essential during anesthesia.

OXYGEN CARRIAGE

Oxygen is the fundamental elements required for cellular metabolism and is essential for the survival of living cells. Oxygen is the electron transport chain's terminal electron acceptor in the synthesis of adenosine triphosphate (ATP) by oxidative phosphorylation within the mitochondria. ATP is the coenzyme that supplies energy for all metabolic processes in the cells. The primary objective of organ preservation under anesthesia is to ensure adequate oxygen delivery to the tissues. To understand this fundamental objective, one should recollect the mode of oxygen transport in the blood and its delivery to the tissues and the factors determining efficient oxygen carriage.

Uptake and Transport of Oxygen

Ventilation of the lungs help to transport oxygen from the atmosphere to the alveolus. Deoxygenated venous blood gets oxygenated in the pulmonary capillaries after oxygen diffusion across the alveolar-capillary membrane. The transport of oxygen is fundamental to facilitating aerobic respiration. Oxygen transport within the human body occurs through both convection and diffusion. One hemoglobin molecule binds up to four oxygen molecules in the pulmonary capillaries. Global oxygen delivery describes the total amount of oxygen delivered to the tissues each minute and is a product of the cardiac output and arterial oxygen content. The systemic capillaries release oxygen to the tissues.

A partial pressure gradient transfers oxygen from the atmosphere to the alveoli and from the arteries and capillaries to tissues and mitochondria. Oxygen moves passively across membranes due to a partial pressure gradient. Fick's law of diffusion governs the flow of oxygen and carbon dioxide across the blood-gas barrier of the alveolar wall, interstitial fluid, and pulmonary capillary endothelium. The diffusion of gases depends on the area and thickness of the membrane, the partial pressure difference of the gas across the membrane, and the diffusion constant of the individual gases (depending on the solubility of gas and its molecular weight).

Oxygen Cascade

The oxygen cascade (**Fig. 1**) describes the sequential falls in oxygen partial pressure from the atmosphere to cellular mitochondria. The partial pressure of oxygen reduces from 160 mm Hg (in atmospheric air) to 105 mm Hg (in alveoli - PAO_2) to 95 mm Hg (in the blood - PaO_2) to 40 mm Hg (capillaries) to 25 mm Hg (cell) to 4–22 mm Hg (mitochondria). The

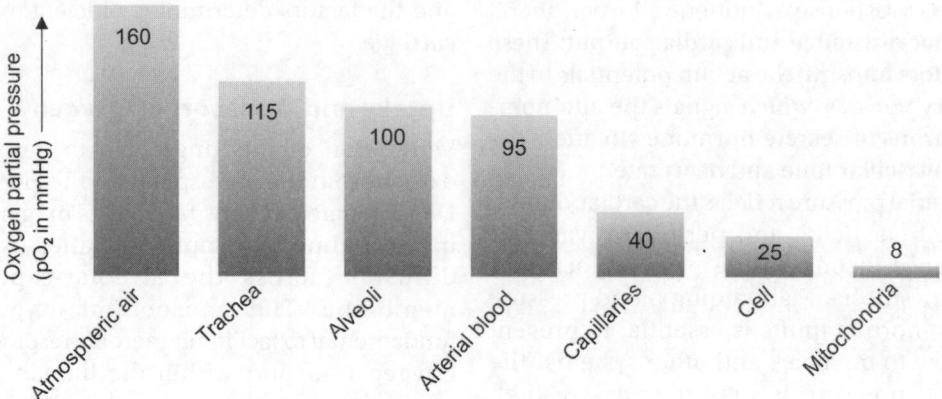

Fig. 1: Oxygen cascade.

oxygen partial pressures at different cascade levels may vary depending on the magnitude of the ventilation-perfusion mismatch, diffusion defects, venous oxygen tension, and metabolic activity.

The partial pressure of oxygen in the venous blood is about 40 mm Hg. The pressure gradient for oxygen is from the alveolar PAO_2 of 105 mm Hg down to the venous PvO_2 of 40 mm Hg (a partial pressure difference of 65 mm Hg). An oxygen gradient of 65 mm Hg is associated with the diffusion of 250 mL of oxygen each minute (average O_2 consumption per minute). The extraction ratio (ratio of oxygen consumption to oxygen delivery expressed as a percentage) is about 25% but can double if tissue demand increases.

Role of Hemoglobin in Oxygen Carriage

Hemoglobin is the primary oxygen carrier in the blood to meet the tissue oxygen demand. Typically, hemoglobin carries 98% of the oxygen in the blood. Oxygen cooperatively binds reversibly to hemoglobin, forming oxyhemoglobin after diffusion across the alveolar membrane. Up to four oxygen molecules can be carried simultaneously by one hemoglobin molecule. Hemoglobin binds reversibly to oxygen and carries it in the blood from the lungs to the tissues for aerobic metabolism in the mitochondria. Adequate levels of hemoglobin are thus crucial for oxygen carriage.

Role of Hemoglobin in Carbon Dioxide Carriage

Hemoglobin, as carbaminohemoglobin, is also responsible for carbon dioxide carriage from the tissues to the lungs. Carbon dioxide is also transported in the plasma (dissolved) and as bicarbonate. Deoxygenated blood has a greater carbon dioxide affinity than oxygenated blood (known as the Haldane effect). Adequate levels of hemoglobin are thus crucial for carbon dioxide carriage and elimination.

Oxygen Content

The maximum hemoglobin oxygen-carrying capacity in the adult blood is 1.39 mL/g. This value of oxygen, carried by each gram of hemoglobin when fully saturated, is known as Huffner's constant. In addition to hemoglobin, oxygen is also carried dissolved in plasma. The oxygen content of blood is the volume of oxygen carried in every 100 mL of blood. Oxygen content is calculated by:

Oxygen Content = (O_2 carried by Hb) + (O_2 in plasma) = ($1.31 \times Hb \times SpO_2 \times 0.01$) + ($0.023 \times PaO_2$)

[Where: Hb - Hemoglobin (g/dL); 1.31 - Huffner's constant (reduced from maximum binding capacity of 1.39 mL/g Hb due to the presence of abnormal hemoglobins); SpO_2 - Arterial oxygen saturation (%); PaO_2 - partial pressure of arterial oxygen]

The maximum oxygen capacity is 20.85 mL O_2/100 mL of blood at a hemoglobin level of 15 g/100 mL. Under normal conditions, arterial blood has a PaO_2 of 100 mm Hg and is almost 100% oxygen saturation. The hemoglobin of 100 mL of blood carries approximately 20 mL of oxygen. 5 mL of oxygen is extracted from every 100 mL of blood in the capillaries. Venous blood has 15 mL of oxygen per 100 mL of blood, at a PO_2 of 40 mm Hg, and is 75% saturated with oxygen.

Hemoglobin-oxygen Binding Kinetics

When a molecule of oxygen binds to heme, the shape of the globin chain is altered, leading to an overall change in the quaternary structure of hemoglobin. Subsequent oxygen molecules bind with greater affinity. The reaction of each of the four subunits of hemoglobin with oxygen occurs sequentially, with each sub-unit facilitating the next. This change in the shape of subunits facilitating substrate binding to other subunits is called positive cooperativity. The kinetics of the binding of the fourth unit is faster than the previous reactions so that oxygen continues to combine with hemoglobin, despite the hemoglobin molecule having fewer available binding sites.

Hemoglobin-oxygen Dissociation Curve

Hemoglobin exists in 2 forms: taut (with a low oxygen affinity) and relaxed (with a high oxygen affinity). The taut form predominates in the tissues (high carbon dioxide, acidic pH), promoting oxygen release. In contrast, the relaxed form predominates in areas of alkaline pH, low carbon dioxide, and high partial pressures of oxygen (in the alveoli). This relationship between hemoglobin, oxygen binding, carbon dioxide tension, and pH is known as the Bohr effect. The sigmoid-shaped hemoglobin-oxygen dissociation curve best describes this relationship (**Fig. 2**).

The Shift of Hemoglobin-oxygen Dissociation Curve

Various chemical and physiological factors may cause a shift of the hemoglobin-oxygen

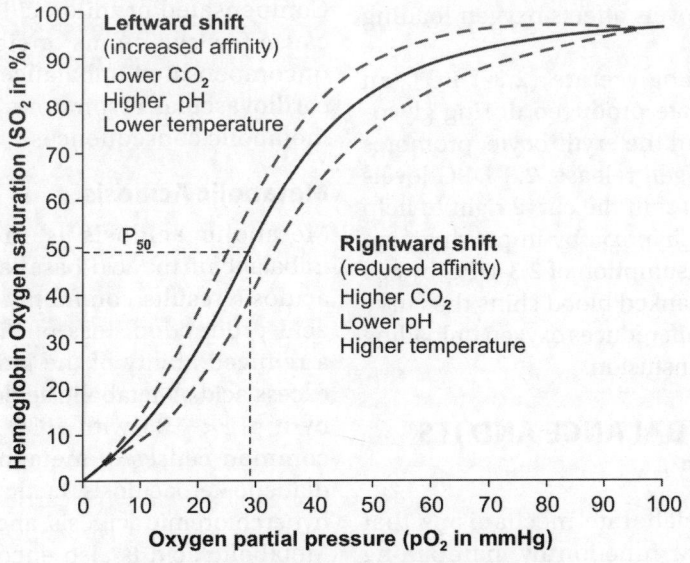

Fig. 2: Hemoglobin-oxygen dissociation curve.

Table 1: Factors causing a shift in the hemoglobin-oxygen dissociation curve.

Leftward shift (↓P_{50})	Rightward shift (↑P_{50})
↑ pH (↓H⁺)	↓ pH (↑H⁺)
↓ $PaCO_2$	↑ $PaCO_2$
↓ 2,3-diphospho-glycerate	↑ 2,3-diphospho-glycerate
↓ Temperature	↑Temperature
Fetal hemoglobin	Adult hemoglobin
Carbon monoxide poisoning	
Methemoglobinemia	

dissociation curve to the right or left. The partial pressure of oxygen at which hemoglobin is 50% saturated (P_{50}) is the reference point used to determine changes in the position of the curve. P_{50} is a marker of hemoglobin's oxygen affinity. A shift to the right reduces the affinity of hemoglobin for oxygen, causing better tissue oxygen delivery despite low oxygen content. On the other hand, a shift to the left increases affinity for oxygen, and there is reduced oxygen delivery to the tissue despite high oxygen content. **Table 1** lists the various factors and their effects on the curve. Change in these factor levels affects oxygen loading and unloading.

2,3-Diphosphoglycerate (2,3-DPG), an organic phosphate produced during glycolysis and found in the erythrocyte, promotes hemoglobin oxygen release. 2,3-DPG levels rise in anemia to shift the curve right to help minimize tissue hypoxia by improving oxygen release. Consumption of 2,3-DPG by cell metabolism in banked blood shifts the curve to the left. This shift reduces oxygen unloading to tissue after transfusion.

ACID-BASE BALANCE AND ITS RELEVANCE

The body has elaborate mechanisms that maintain cellular function by maintaining blood H⁺ concentration within a narrow pH range of 7.43 to 7.37 (with an ideal pH of 7.40). The tissue enzyme systems malfunction at abnormal pH and disturbance of these mechanisms can have serious clinical consequences. Acid-base equilibrium is also related to fluid metabolism and electrolyte balance. Acid-base balance is maintained by intracellular/bicarbonate buffering, pulmonary compensation, and renal compensation.

The pH indicates acidosis or alkalosis in a patient, although pH moves toward the normal range with compensation. Acidosis is an abnormally acidic (pH < 7.35) while alkalosis is an abnormally basic pH (pH > 7.45). Acid-base imbalances are classified as *metabolic* if the change in pH is primarily due to an alteration in serum bicarbonate and *respiratory* if the change is primarily due to a change in pCO_2 (increase or decrease in ventilation). The body's homeostatic mechanisms compensate for the acid-base imbalances to normalize the pH. Metabolic acid-base disorders result in respiratory compensation (change in pCO_2), while respiratory acid-base disorders result in metabolic compensation (change in HCO_3). Compensated or mild acid-base disorders cause few symptoms or signs. Severe and uncompensated imbalances have multiple cardiovascular, respiratory, neurologic, and metabolic consequences.

Metabolic Acidosis

Metabolic acidosis is indicative of an imbalance in the acid-base balance. Metabolic acidosis results commonly from increased acid production, loss of bicarbonate, and a reduced ability of the kidneys to excrete excess acids. Metabolic acidosis is suggested by a pH < 7.35 with HCO_3 <22 mEq. The common causes of metabolic acidosis are diabetic ketoacidosis, lactic acidosis, shock, hyperchloremic acidosis, and kidney disease. Metabolic acid is also encountered during surgery after restoring circulation following tourniquet and arterial clamp release.

Respiratory Acidosis

Respiratory acidosis occurs when the lungs cannot adequately remove the carbon dioxide produced. Carbon dioxide accumulation causes body fluids, especially the blood, to become too acidic. A rise in pCO_2 to > 40 mm Hg is suggestive of respiratory acidosis. An increase in HCO_3 by 3 to 4 mEq/L can compensate for a 10 mm Hg rise in pCO_2 sustained for 4–12 h. A more significant rise in HCO_3 indicates a primary metabolic alkalosis, while a lesser increase suggests inadequate compensation or coexisting primary metabolic acidosis. The common causes of respiratory acidosis are respiratory disease, skeletal/metabolic disorders restricting diaphragm/chest movements, and respiratory depressant drugs.

Metabolic Alkalosis

Metabolic alkalosis results from decreased hydrogen ion concentration leading to increased bicarbonate concentrations. A rise in HCO_3 to >28 mEq/L is suggestive of metabolic alkalosis. Each mEq/L increase in HCO_3 can be compensated by increasing pCO_2 by 0.6 to 0.75 mm Hg. A more significant increase implies concomitant respiratory acidosis, and a lesser increase indicates respiratory alkalosis. Common causes are gastric acid and chloride loss due to recurrent vomiting or nasogastric suction and diuretic use.

Respiratory Alkalosis

Respiratory alkalosis results from a low-level of carbon dioxide due to hyperventilation. A fall in pCO_2 to < 38 mm Hg suggests respiratory alkalosis. In about 4–12 hours, HCO_3 compensates by decreasing 4–5 mEq/L for every 10 mm Hg decrease in pCO_2. A significant decrease suggests a primary metabolic acidosis. A less significant decrease implies inadequate compensation or a concomitant primary metabolic alkalosis. Common causes of respiratory alkalosis include anxiety, panic, and fever.

BODY TEMPERATURE

Body temperature is tightly regulated for normal physiological functioning. The mean core temperature in healthy humans is 36.5°C–37.3°C. Inadvertent changes in the body temperature are common during surgery due to exposure of the patient to the cold ambient temperature, cold fluids, and exposure of body cavities. The incidence of inadvertent hypothermia is quite high. Temperature changes adversely affect the body's physiological processes and patient outcomes. Exposure to vasodilating anesthetic agents also promotes heat loss in the body. Under anesthetic conditions, the body cannot restrict heat loss by its protective mechanisms. In the postoperative period, patients who develop hypothermia may shiver as a protective mechanism to gain heat. Shivering is, however, associated with a rise in oxygen consumption and discomfort. It is thus paramount to ensure thermal homeostasis under anesthesia.

INTERVENTION TO MAINTAIN HOMEOSTASIS BASED ON MONITORING

To ensure organ preservation, monitoring of the patient is essential. Details of monitoring and the standards prescribed are described in Chapter 9.

Heart Rate

Heart rate is maintained within 10% of the basal line rate of the patient. Tachycardia is controlled with analgesics or enhancing the depth of anesthesia, as assessed by the attending anesthesiologist. Beta-blockers can be administered if adequate analgesia and anesthetic fail to treat tachycardia. Bradycardia is treated as per cause determined, e.g., anticholinergics treat vagal preponderance.

Blood Pressure

Blood pressure is maintained within 10% of the basal value of the patient. Hypertension is controlled with analgesics or enhanced anesthesia depth, as assessed by the attending anesthesiologist. Vasoactive drug therapy may be resorted to control hypertension. Fluids are used initially for hypotension. Vasopressor therapy is resorted to if there is no response to volume infusion.

Oxygen Saturation

The oxygen saturation of blood in capillaries is measured non-invasively with a pulse oximeter. Reduced oxygen saturation is treated as per the assessment of cause by the attending anesthesiologist. Correct placement of the airway device is confirmed. Saturation may be improved by increasing the percentage of oxygen in the inspired breathing gas or improving ventilation dynamics (positive end-expiratory pressure application, changing breathing gas delivery pattern, etc.).

End-tidal Carbon Dioxide

Respiratory rate and ventilation pattern are manipulated to maintain normocarbia. Hypercarbia can lead to hypertension apart from the ill effects of retained carbon dioxide on various organs. Hypocarbia can reduce oxygen delivery to tissues by promoting vasoconstriction and shifting the hemoglobin-oxygen curve to the left.

Temperature

Covering the exposed areas of the patients, convective or surface warming, infusing warm fluids, and other measures help prevent hypothermia.

MULTIPLE CHOICE QUESTIONS

1. The following mechanisms play a role in maintaining blood pressure *except*:
   a. Pituitary-hypophyseal axis
   b. Baroreceptors
   c. Renin-angiotensin system
   d. Antidiuretic hormone
2. Most inhaled anesthetic agents in clinical doses have the following effects on the cardiovascular system *except*:
   a. Decrease systemic vascular resistance
   b. Decrease pulmonary vascular resistance
   c. Cause myocardial depression
   d. Cause baroreceptor depression
3. Fick's law of diffusion governs the flow of respiratory gases:
   a. In the upper airway
   b. In the anesthesia machine
   c. Across the blood-gas barrier of the pulmonary capillary endothelium
   d. In resuscitation
4. If the partial pressure of oxygen in the alveoli is about 100 mm Hg, the partial pressure of oxygen delivered to a cell would be about:
   a. 95 mm Hg
   b. 40 mm Hg
   c. 25 mm Hg
   d. 08 mm Hg
5. Each molecule of hemoglobin can carry four molecules of oxygen. The amount of oxygen carried by 100 mL of the blood of an average person is about:
   a. 18 mL
   b. 20 mL
   c. 30 mL
   d. 40 mL
6. P_{50} is a marker of hemoglobin's oxygen affinity. Which of the following is correct about P_{50}?
   a. A rise in pH shifts the P_{50} left
   b. A rise in temperature shifts the P_{50} left
   c. A rise in 2,3-Diphosphoglycerate levels shifts the P_{50} left
   d. A rise in arterial carbon dioxide levels shifts the P_{50} left
7. A patient undergoing surgery may get hypothermic due to:
   a. Exposure of the patient to the cold ambient temperature
   b. Exposure to body cavities
   c. Heat loss due to vasodilatation by anesthesia agents
   d. All of the above

OSCE

A patient is admitted to the ICU with severe respiratory distress. An emergent arterial blood gas analysis (ABG) is done to determine the cause of his distress.

8. If the ABG shows the following result pH 7.1; pO_2 53.5 mm Hg; pCO_2 90 mm Hg; HCO_3 25 mmol. It indicates that the patient is in:
   a. Metabolic acidosis
   b. Metabolic alkalosis
   c. Respiratory acidosis
   d. Respiratory alkalosis

9. If the ABG shows the following result pH 7.3; pO_2 53.5 mm Hg; pCO_2 85 mm Hg; HCO_3 30 mmol. It indicates that the patient is in:
   a. Respiratory acidosis
   b. Metabolic acidosis
   c. Partially compensated respiratory acidosis
   d. None of the above

10. If the ABG shows the following result pH 7.6; pO_2 53.5 mm Hg; pCO_2 45 mm Hg; HCO_3 28 mmol. It indicates that the patient is in:
    a. Respiratory alkalosis
    b. Metabolic alkalosis
    c. Mixed respiratory and metabolic alkalosis
    d. None of the above

11. If the ABG shows the following result pH 7.5; pO_2 65.1 mm Hg; pCO_2 25 mm Hg; HCO_3 23 mmol. It indicates that the patient is in:
    a. Metabolic alkalosis
    b. Respiratory alkalosis
    c. Normal ABG with hypoxemia
    d. None of the above

Answers
1. a
2. d
3. c
4. c
5. b
6. a
7. d
8. c
9. c
10. b
11. b

11. Organ Protection During Anesthesia

Mukul Chandra Kapoor

Learning Objectives

- Central nervous system protection
- Cardiovascular system protection
- Respiratory system protection
- Kidney protection
- Gastrointestinal tract and liver protection
- Protection of other organs

INTRODUCTION

The loss of consciousness and loss of voluntary control over breathing due to suppression of the brain and muscle function makes a patient susceptible to multi-organ damage. With the induction of anesthesia, the body homeostasis is disturbed, particularly in terms of oxygenation, expiration of carbon dioxide, maintenance of body temperature, fluid homeostasis, and cardiac/respiratory function. Organ Preservation under these altered circumstances is a primary goal of the administration of anesthesia. In addition to these alterations, anesthetic agents exert organ toxicity.

The basic principles of organ preservation are similar to general anesthesia, regional anesthesia, and monitored anesthesia care. The relative complexity of general anesthesia makes the intervention and monitoring requirement to maintain organ function more intense.

General anesthesia protects against both ischemic myocardial and brain reperfusion injuries. Anesthetic preconditioning is one of the useful ways to diverse the organ protective effects. Preconditioning inhibits the mitochondrial permeability transition that leads to either apoptosis or necrosis of myocardium and neuronal cell.

CENTRAL NERVOUS SYSTEM PROTECTION

The brain is the most important vital organ to protect under anesthesia. It needs a continuous delivery of oxygen and nutrients. To sustain consciousness, satisfactory perfusion and adequate oxygen delivery are vital. It is essential to maintain a constant supply of glucose, too, as the brain has virtually no glucose stores. Within seconds of ischemia resulting from a reduction in cerebral blood flow (CBF), loss of consciousness ensues. Permanent brain damage occurs with just 3–8 min of insufficient blood supply. The brain has a high blood flow to meet its high metabolic requirements. Although the brain constitutes only 2% of body mass (1400 g), it receives a disproportionate 12–15% of the resting cardiac output in the adult. Under anesthesia, the brain metabolism has to be maintained by ensuring good perfusion and oxygenation.

Glucose as a Substrate

Glucose is the main energy substrate for the brain and is also a precursor of neurotransmitters, such as γ-aminobutyric acid, glutamate, and acetylcholine. To maintain a constant substrate supply, it is essential to maintain a constant CBF. The brain's basal oxygen consumption at rest is ~50 mL min^{-1}, which is used almost completely by the oxygen-dependent metabolism of glucose for energy production. Under aerobic conditions, oxidative phosphorylation produces 38 molecules of ATP for every glucose molecule.

Anaerobic Metabolism in the Brain

The brain has a limited capacity for anaerobic metabolism. In anaerobic metabolism, glycolysis produces only two molecules of ATP from one molecule of glucose. Under hypoxic conditions, the anaerobically-produced lactate is utilized to carry out the fundamental processes essential for cell structure maintenance. Unless perfusion is re-established immediately to restore aerobic metabolism, permanent cell death occurs in hypoxia. The cerebral metabolic rate (CMR) is the rate at which the brain utilizes metabolic substrates. Similarly, CMR followed a suffix such as oxygen, glucose or lactate denotes the consumption of the said substrate.

Autoregulation

Autoregulation is a physiological process of maintaining near-constant CBF, regardless of changes in systemic blood pressure. It depends on the capacity of the cerebral circulation to adjust its vascular resistance. Autoregulation is almost instant (occurs within 1–10 s of change in pressure) in the mean arterial pressures (MAP) range of 50–150 mm Hg. CBF is dependent on the MAP, above and below the autoregulation range. The changes in vascular resistance are mediated primarily by the endothelium-derived relaxing factor and nitric oxide. In chronic arterial hypertensives, the upper and lower limits of autoregulation are both reset to higher levels. Preservation of autoregulation by maintaining the MAP in the optimal range is an essential goal of anesthesia.

Regional Autoregulation in the Brain

CBF is variable across the brain and largely dependent on neuronal activity. An increase in activity, either regional or general, causes an increase in the CMR, resulting in proportional increases in blood flow. This method of matching oxygen or glucose delivery to metabolic requirements is termed flow-metabolism coupling. The change occurs within seconds of increased functional cerebral activity. N**itric oxide** of neuronal origin seems to be the most likely cause of the metabolism-associated vasodilatation. However, many chemical mediators, such as H$^+$, carbon dioxide, adenosine, glycolytic intermediates, K$^+$, and phospholipid metabolites, have been implicated.

Effect of Volatile Anesthetics on Brain Metabolism

Most anesthetic agents reduce the metabolism of brain tissue and thus are cerebro-protective. Volatile anesthetics are intrinsic vasodilators. They also decrease Cerebral Metabolic Rate of Oxygen (CMRO$_2$) in a dose-dependent manner. In the presence of intact flow-metabolism coupling, volatile anesthetics cause a coupled decrease in both CMRO$_2$ and CBF. Intravenous anesthetic agents, such as thiopentone and propofol decrease CMRO$_2$.

Factors Influencing Cerebral Oxygen Delivery

- *Partial pressure of carbon dioxide:*
  - An increase in $PaCO_2$ causes vasodilatation and increases CBF.
  - A decrease in $PaCO_2$ causes vasoconstriction and decreases CBF.
- *Mean arterial pressure*: CBF directly depends on the mean arterial pressure and helps maintain cerebral oxygen delivery.
- *Cardiac output*: Depends on the heart rate and stroke volume, which are influenced by preload, afterload, and contractility.
- *Hemoglobin level*: Hemoglobin carries oxygen to cerebral tissue and indicates oxygen-carrying capacity in the blood.
- *Arterial oxygen saturation*: Determines the amount of O_2 in the blood available for delivery to tissues. It can be measured using pulse oximetry or through arterial blood gas monitoring.

Factors Influencing Cerebral Oxygen Consumption

- *Temperature*: Hyperthermia increases consumption while hypothermia decreases consumption.
- *Pain*: Analgesia decreases consumption while pain increases consumption.
- *Mental state*: Anxiety increases consumption while sedation/anesthesia decreases consumption.

Situations Needing Special Attention to Cerebral Oxygenation

- *Cardiac surgeries*: Coronary artery bypass grafting (both off-pump and on-pump); cardiac surgeries on cardiopulmonary bypass; deep hypothermic circulatory arrest.
- *Vascular surgeries*: Carotid endarterectomy, aortic arch surgeries, aneurysm surgeries (cerebral vasoconstriction resulting from clamping and unclamping of the aorta).
- *Neurosurgeries*: Cerebral aneurysm surgery; surgeries in sitting position; pediatric neurosurgeries
- Surgeries in hypotensive anesthesia
- Surgeries in severely hypotensive patients

Monitoring Cerebral Oxygenation

- *Invasive methods*: Brain tissue oxygen tension (direct method); jugular venous oxygen saturation (surrogate method)
- *Non-invasive method*: Near-infrared spectroscopy (transcutaneous cerebral oximetry).

Spinal Cord Protection

The spinal cord receives 75% blood supply from a single anterior spinal artery, formed by the anastomosis of two branches of the contralateral vertebral arteries. The blood supply of the anterior spinal artery is augmented by its anastomosis with the anterior cervical arteries, radicular artery of Adamkiewicz, and posterior intercostal arteries. The flow in spinal arteries depends on collaterals and is often bidirectional. It can be shunted to the rest of the body if perfusion pressures are low.

During surgery, there is a need to ensure good blood pressure to maintain spinal cord perfusion. Spinal cord perfusion during low perfusion states, such as aortic clamping, can be enhanced by lowering cerebrospinal fluid (CSF) pressure by CSF drainage. The metabolic requirements of the spinal cord during ischemia can also be lowered by local cooling of the spinal cord and by the administration of pharmacological neuroprotective adjuncts during surgery.

Protection of Peripheral Nerves

The peripheral nerves can get compressed and injured by odd positioning for surgery. It is important to ensure proper patient positioning and padding of pressure points under anesthesia to prevent nerve compression/injury. Peripheral nerves also need to be protected from injury during the performance of peripheral nerve blocks by using ultrasound image guidance.

CARDIOVASCULAR SYSTEM PROTECTION

Protection of the Heart

The heart pumps blood to the entire body, and its protection is of utmost importance under anesthesia. All effort is made to ensure that the usual preoperative hemodynamics of the patients are maintained under anesthetic conditions. There is a need to maintain the balance between oxygen demand and supply under anesthesia for myocardial protection.

Factors Influencing Oxygen Demand/Supply

- Tachycardia and hypertension increase the metabolic load and oxygen demand of the heart and may precipitate ischemia in patients with compromised coronary anatomies.
- The reduction in blood supply in bradycardia and hypotension may cause ischemia despite lower metabolic demand.
- Maintenance of adequate blood volume (preload) is important for optimal filling of the pumping chambers of the heart and ensuring adequate cardiac output.
- Peripheral vasoconstriction increases the impedance of the blood pumped by the heart (afterload) and increases the oxygen demand of the heart.
- A rise in circulating catecholamines (as in pain and hypothermia) increases the contractility of the heart and increases the oxygen demand.
- Anemia reduces the capacity to carry oxygen and causes tachycardia which increases the oxygen demand of the heart. Hemoglobin levels >10 gm% are recommended to maintain adequate oxygen supply.

Maintaining the Blood Supply of the Coronaries

The heart primarily receives its **blood supply during diastole,** unlike the other organs of the body, which are primarily perfused during systole. For cardiac protection under anesthesia, it is important to maintain a diastolic blood pressure of around 60 mm Hg to maintain coronary supply, especially in patients with coronary artery disease.

Protection of Major Vessels

When major vessels are cannulated to access the central venous system, ultrasound image guidance must be used to avoid injury to the vessels and the adding structures.

Prevention of Coagulopathy

Surgical trauma induces a procoagulable state. Immobilization and temporary suspension of the natural venous pumps under anesthesia promote coagulation. Patients undergoing pelvic surgeries and long-duration surgeries are more prone to develop thromboembolism following this heightened coagulation. Under anesthesia, it is important to protect against thromboembolism by using mechanical devices, like pneumatic stockings, and with pharmacological therapy, intra- and post-operatively.

RESPIRATORY SYSTEM PROTECTION

The respiratory system is responsible for exchanging respiratory gases, and its protection is of utmost importance. Maintenance of the airway is vital for an anesthesiologist, especially during the delivery of general anesthesia.

Protection from Infection

The respiratory track may be invaded, during the process of general anesthesia, by the passage of an endotracheal tube or a supraglottic airway device. It is important to ensure asepsis during airway intervention. The patients are also advised to brush their teeth and perform a chlorhexidine mouthwash preoperatively to reduce micro-organic flora in the oral cavity.

Prevention of Soiling of Trachea and Lungs

Under the influence of sedation and anesthesia, the protective airway reflexes are obtunded, making the patient prone to aspiration of fluids and foreign material in the oral cavity. Regurgitation of gastric contents after losing consciousness exposes the lungs to contamination. The airway thus needs to be secured with a device that provides a barrier between the oral cavity and the trachea, such as a cuffed endotracheal tube. To prevent the adverse effects of aspired gastric contents, patients are advised not to consume solid food (at least 6 hours) and clear fluids (at least 2 hours) before induction of anesthesia. Patients with acid reflux and peptic disorders are advised medication to suppress gastric acid production or to neutralize the acid present. An oral cavity toilet is recommended before tracheal extubation to prevent soiling of the lungs by oral secretions that may have collected.

Lung Protective Ventilation

The ventilation of the lungs under general anesthesia is usually managed by mechanical ventilators. The ventilation mode, tidal volume delivery, and permissible airway pressures need to be set as per the patient's physiology and pathology. Atelectasis and barotrauma are two ends of a spectrum of lung morbidity under anesthesia, and both need to be prevented. To prevent atelectasis, continuous positive pressure is given. To prevent barotrauma, airway inflation pressures are restricted, and low tidal volume ventilation is administered.

Tracheal Protection

The inflation pressure of the endotracheal tube cuff is quantitatively monitored and kept lower than usual capillary perfusion pressures as tissue ischemia promotes fibrosis and consequent tracheal stenosis. Tight-fitting endotracheal tubes are not recommended to prevent tracheal mucosal trauma. Correct endotracheal tube depth of insertion is ensured to prevent trauma to the vocal cords on the expansion of the tube cuff.

KIDNEY PROTECTION

The kidneys receive 15–30% of the cardiac output, i.e., 500–600 mL/min. The blood flows to the cortex first, which extracts 80% of its oxygen content, leaving the balance to the medulla. The limited blood supply of the outer medulla has a low oxygen tension (10 mm Hg), and near-total extraction of oxygen (80%) takes place here. The oxygen demand-supply balance is precariously balanced, and any reduction in renal blood flow or an increase in demand due to solute load can result in tubular ischemia. The ascending limb of the loop of Henle is very vulnerable to hypoxic damage. Renal autoregulation maintains renal blood flow at mean arterial pressures > 70 mm Hg. Anemia increases the risk of kidney injury by impairing oxygen delivery to an already hypoxic renal medulla.

Perioperative Strategies to Prevent Renal Damage

The major perioperative goals to prevent kidney are:
- Maintaining normal hemodynamics
- Maintaining intravascular volume depletion
- Optimize cardiac output
- Avoid intravascular volume depletion
- Adequate hydration and avoiding loop diuretics
- Hematocrit optimization
- Avoid nephrotoxic drugs
- Optimal glucose control.

GASTROINTESTINAL TRACT AND LIVER PROTECTION

Liver Protection

The liver is responsible for all body metabolism as well as that of most drugs. A healthy liver has a substantial functional reserve capacity and can tolerate a lot of insult and injury. Preoperative evaluation of liver impairment is important, as the extent of the perioperative injury is related to pre-existing liver diseases. To protect the liver, hepatotoxic drugs must be avoided. Hypotension must be prevented to prevent liver damage. All volatile anesthetics can potentially impair liver function and must be used cautiously in patients with compromised liver functions. Halothane hepatitis and hepatitis associated with other volatiles have been reported.

Gastrointestinal Tract

In patients undergoing prolonged surgeries and with an acid-peptic disease, pharmacological prophylaxis with drugs to reduce/neutralize stomach acid is recommended to protect against stress-induced peptic ulcerations. Prolonged gut ischemia, as seen in hypotensive states and patients with high doses of vasopressors, leads to disruption of the gut mucosal barrier. Bacterial translocation across this breached barrier may lead to septicemia. Adequate hemodynamics must be maintained during anesthesia to prevent this.

OTHERS

Eye Protection

Eyes must be covered and kept moist during anesthesia to prevent corneal dryness, erosions, and accidental injuries. In prone position surgeries, eyes must be free of pressure and compression. In facial surgeries, eyes may need to be taped to prevent soiling from blood, antiseptics, and tissue debris. In patients with open eye injuries, the eyes must be protected from potential elevations of intraocular pressure by avoiding the use of drugs like succinylcholine.

Pressure Point and limb Protection

The protection of pressure points and limbs are described in Chapter 20.

MULTIPLE CHOICE QUESTIONS

OSCE

A 26-year-old man met with a vehicular accident and sustained a head injury and multiple injuries. He was brought in an unconscious state to the hospital. On arrival at the hospital, he maintained his airway but had shallow respiration. He responded only to painful stimuli. His blood pressure was recorded as 90/60 mm Hg, and his heart rate was 120/min. His oxygen saturation was 88%. The patient's trachea was intubated, and he was placed on mechanical ventilatory support.

1. Considering the above picture, what can be the effects of his injury on the brain?
   a. Cerebral hypoperfusion
   b. Fall in the availability of glucose in the brain
   c. Cerebral hypoxia
   d. All of the above
2. If this man has a cardiac arrest and is not administered cardiopulmonary resuscitation, then:
   a. Permanent brain damage can occur within 10 min
   b. Permanent brain damage occurs within 3–8 min
   c. Permanent brain damage will occur within 15 min
   d. Permanent brain damage will not occur as he is receiving mechanical ventilation
3. The primary substrate for the metabolism of the brain is:

a. Lactate
b. Acetate
c. Glycogen
d. Glucose

4. **In the autoregulation range, factors influencing cerebral oxygenation include all *except*:**
   a. Arterial carbon dioxide level
   b. Arterial blood pressure
   c. Hemoglobin level
   d. Cardiac output

5. **Mechanical ventilatory support helps manage such patients by:**
   a. Preventing cerebral hypoxia
   b. Preventing hypercarbia and thereby an increase in cerebral perfusion
   c. Airway protection
   d. All of the above

6. **Lung protective ventilation was followed to:**
   a. Prevent damage by high airway pressures
   b. Prevent damage by delivery of high tidal volumes
   c. Prevent atelectasis
   d. All of the above

OSCE

A 75-year-old man has suffered an inferior wall myocardial infarction. His current vital parameters are heart rate: 45/min, BP: 90/50 mm Hg, SpO_2: 92%, and respiratory rate: 20/min.

7. **With the current parameters:**
   a. He will suffer further myocardial ischemia
   b. He will improve as the oxygen demand of the heart is low
   c. His condition can improve with the administration of dopamine to increase cardiac output
   d. He will benefit from the use of a vasodilator like nitroglycerine

8. **He should be administered an analgesic like morphine as pain:**
   a. Increases peripheral vascular resistance
   b. Increases heart rate and oxygen demand
   c. Increases catecholamine levels
   d. All of the above

9. **To improve his coronary perfusion:**
   a. We should attempt to increase his systolic blood pressure
   b. We should attempt to increase his diastolic blood pressure
   c. We should attempt to increase his mean blood pressure
   d. None of the above

10. **This patient develops acute renal failure. The cause could be:**
    a. Low renal perfusion
    b. Cardiac-renal syndrome
    c. It cannot be related to the heart dysfunction
    d. Drug-induced

Answers

1. c
2. b
3. d
4. b
5. d
6. d
7. a
8. d
9. b
10. a

CHAPTER 12

Postoperative Care

Pradeep Pendlaya

Learning Objectives

- Post-anesthesia care unit
- Protocols in the Post-anesthesia care unit
- Management of patients in the Post-anesthesia care unit
- Monitoring in the Post-anesthesia care unit
- Post-anesthesia care unit recovery assessment tools
- Resuscitation in the Post-anesthesia care unit
- Special management requirements in the Post-anesthesia care unit

INTRODUCTION

Postoperative care is the care a patient receives after his surgery. The modalities of postoperative care needed depends on the type of surgery as well as health history. It includes pain management, maintenance of body homeostasis, wound care, and physiotherapy. Prompt assessment and treatment of postoperative complications are very important for the comprehensive care of surgical patients. Interventions that are required include prompt pain control, assessment of the surgical site and drainage tubes, monitoring the patency of intravenous access and rate of intravenous fluids, consciousness, hemodynamics, sensory levels, and circulation to ensure patient safety.

POST-ANESTHESIA CARE UNIT (PACU)

AS6.1: Describe the principles of monitoring and resuscitation in the recovery room.

A post-anesthesia care unit (PACU) is an area that provides postoperative care. PACU is the transitional area for intensive observation after surgery before transferring the patient to the ward or home. The primary objective of a PACU is to protect the patient and prevent complications after surgery. It is a well-monitored and intensively staffed area. All patients who have received general anesthesia, regional anesthesia, or monitored anesthesia care are admitted to the PACU till they have recovered well enough to be shifted to the inpatient ward. In the PACU, patients are in the care of an anesthesiologist. The PACU is adjacent to minimize transport for immediate access to anesthesia and operating room (OR) personnel if needed.

PACU Protocols
- A patient transported to the PACU is accompanied by an anesthesiologist who monitors and manages the patient during transportation.
- On arrival at the PACU, the patient is re-evaluated and the anesthesiologist briefs the nurse about the patient regarding the exact nature of the surgery, its duration, and complications if any. At handover, in addition to written notes, all instructions must also be verbally conveyed to the PACU nurse.
- General medical supervision and coordination of patient care in the PACU is usually the responsibility of an anesthesiologist.
- The patient's condition is continually evaluated by the nursing staff and periodically by the assigned anesthesiologist.
- The assigned anesthesiologist is responsible to ensure the fitness of the patient for shifting from the PACU to the hospital ward.
- The nurse charts the following parameters in the PACU:
  - Anesthetic medications used
  - Other medications received
  - Blood loss
  - Fluid replacement
  - Urine output

Positioning in PACU
Many patients are at risk of aspiration as they are brought to the PACU semiconscious and nursed in the supine position. All patients administered general anesthesia must be nursed in the semi-Fowler position, defined as a body position with the head end of the bed elevated at an angle of 30–45° with legs straight or bent. Positioning patients in this semi-recumbent position improves oxygenation and ventilation by permitting better diaphragmatic and chest wall movement. Patients who have undergone oral surgery, like a tonsillectomy, must be nursed in a lateral position, typically called a post-tonsillectomy position.

Temperature Management
Exposure to the cold OR temperature makes the patient hypothermic. To rewarm the body to normothermia, shivering is triggered to generate heat by muscular movement. Oxygen consumption, however, may increase four times during shivering. Oxygen supplementation is thus essential during shivering. The patient is also rewarmed in the PACU with forced air warmers, blankets, and warm fluids. Shivering may also be pharmacologically controlled with systemic low-dose opioids such as pethidine or tramadol.

Pain Management
After surgery, patients may require significant analgesia and/or sedation following significant surgical trauma. Patients may receive ongoing analgesia regimens like intravenous opioid infusion, epidural infusion, regional block infusion, or patient control analgesia infusion. Patients should be monitored and assessed using standard validated pain scores. The visual analog scale (VAS) is commonly used, and the patient is asked to numerically self-quantify pain. Appropriate pharmacological analgesia is given to relieve the patient. In case of severe non-responsive pain, regional blocks may be administered.

Monitoring
During the stay in PACU, the following parameters must be monitored-oxygenation (with pulse oximeter), breathing, circulation (pulse, electrocardiogram, and blood pressure), respiration, level of consciousness, and temperature. Critical patients are observed and monitored by additional methods appropriate to the patient's medical condition.

Circulation Assessment

Postoperative hypertension and tachycardia are very common. The cause of these disturbances must be assessed. The most common cause is inadequate analgesia, and an adequate analgesic supplement must be administered. Hypertension and tachycardia may also be secondary to hypercarbia if the patient is not breathing well. The patient can have hypotension, and the cause must be ascertained. The most common cause of hypotension is intravascular volume depletion due to blood and fluid loss. Adequate fluids/blood must be administered. Bradycardia, if present, must be corrected urgently by administration of atropine after ensuring that the cause is not hypoxia.

Respiratory Assessment

Respiratory complications are the most common major problem in the immediate postoperative period. Appropriate monitoring, early diagnosis, and early management are critical to preventing respiratory compromise. Unexplained tachycardia and tachypnea are indicators of compromised respiration. Incomplete reversal of neuromuscular blockade is the commonest cause of inadequate breathing. The patient may also not be able to maintain airway patency in case of delayed recovery due to the residual effects of inhaled and intravenous general anesthetic agents. In case of upper airway obstruction due to falling back of the tongue, an oro-/nasopharyngeal airway may be placed to clear the obstruction. Less commonly, delayed recovery may be attributed to electrolyte imbalance, acid-base abnormalities, hypoglycemia, or cerebrovascular accidents.

Oxygenation

The use of pulse oximetry helps identify hypoxemic patients and the need for oxygen therapy. Oxygen is administered with the help of a face mask or nasal prong if the oxygen saturation falls below 94%. Obese and critically ill patients are particularly at risk of desaturation. Treatment includes administering 100% oxygen, suctioning of secretions, jaw-thrust maneuver to maintain airway, and insertion of an oral or nasal airway. If none of these interventions are successful, then endotracheal intubation, cricothyroidotomy, or tracheostomy may be necessary. Uncommonly, obese patients and patients with obstructive sleep apnea may require noninvasive ventilation support. In patients with chronic obstructive pulmonary disease, oxygen should be carefully titrated because too high an oxygen concentration can abolish the hypoxic ventilatory drive and precipitate ventilatory failure with high carbon dioxide levels.

POSTOPERATIVE NAUSEA AND VOMITING

Nausea, vomiting, and/or retching are commonly experienced by patients in the PACU. Postoperative nausea and vomiting (PONV) affect about 10% of the population after exposure to general anesthesia. Serotonin antagonists (ondansetron and granisetron) are the primary drugs used to treat PONV. Dexamethasone is also very effective in treating PONV.

MENTAL CARE

Patients, especially the elderly and critically ill, may develop delirium, have delayed emergence, display anxiety, or have postoperative cognitive dysfunction (POCD). Patients with neurological dysfunction may require counseling, pharmacological control, and physical restrain. In case delirium occurs, oxygen saturation should be checked. All nonessential drugs should be stopped.

PACU RECOVERY ASSESSMENT

To safely discharge patients from the PACU, a scoring system was described by a Mexican

Table 1: Modified Aldrete recovery score.	
Criteria	Score
Consciousness	
Fully awake, in full contact	2
Arousable on calling	1
Not responding	0
Mobility	
Able to move 4 extremities on command	2
Able to move 2 extremities on command	1
Unable to move extremities	0
Breathing	
Able to breathe deeply and cough freely	2
Dyspnea or limited breathing	1
Apnea	0
Circulation	
BP ± 20% of preanesthetic level	2
BP ± 20-49% of preanesthetic level	1
BP ± 50% of preanesthetic level	0
Oxygen saturation	
Saturation >90% on room air	2
Needs supplementation maintain >90%	1
Saturation <90% despite supplementation	0

anesthesiologist, Jorge Antonio Aldrete, in 1970. The objective of this scoring was to determine the return of protective reflexes and motor function after discontinuation of anesthesia. A score of 9 or 10 indicates readiness for transfer or discharge to the next phase of recovery. Currently, most hospitals use a modified version of the Aldrete scoring system (**Table 1**) to determine fitness for discharge from the PACU.

CRASH CART

> **AS6.2:** Observe and enumerate the contents of the crash cart and describe the equipment used in the recovery room.

A PACU has to cater to all possible postoperative emergencies. A crash cart should be available to cater to such emergencies. The contents of the crash cart vary with institutions and need to be designed to meet the requirements of the institution. A typical crash cart has all

Table 2: Resuscitation equipment and medications in a typical crash cart.	
Equipment and Disposable	Drugs
• Monitor with defibrillator or AED with leads • Airway (oral and nasal) all sizes • McGill forceps, large and small • Laryngoscope and endotracheal tubes • Bag valve mask (adult and pediatric) • Nasal cannula (adult and pediatric) • Non-rebreather oxygen face masks (3 sizes) • IV start packs • Ringers Lactate & Normal saline solution • IV sets with extension • Angiocaths (various sizes) • Syringes (all sizes) • Gauze • Alcohol preps • Adhesive plaster • Syringe nasal adaptor • Nebulizer • Salbutamol Inhaler • Backup Suction device • Nasogastric tubes (all sizes) • Tongue depressor	• Tablet Aspirin • Tablet Nitroglycerin sublingual • Inj Dextrose 50% and 25% Inj Naloxone Inj Epinephrine Inj Adenosine Inj Noradrenaline Inj Dopamine Inj Vasopressin Inj Diltiazem Inj Atropine sulfate Inj Neostigmine Inj Amiodarone Inj Hydrocortisone Inj Phenaramine Inj Procainamide Inj Lidocaine Inj Calcium Inj Dexamethasone Inj Frusemide Inj Diazepam Inj Midazolam Inj Sodium bicarbonate Inj Magnesium sulphate

resuscitation equipment and medications (**Table 2**).

COMMON COMPLICATIONS IN THE RECOVERY ROOM

> **AS6.3:** Describe the common complications encountered by patients in the recovery room, their recognition and principles of management.

Wound Care

Sterile dressing placed in the OR is generally left intact for 24 to 48 hours unless there are signs of infection (pain, redness, heavy drainage). If there are signs of infection, wound re-exploration may be needed along with up-gradation of systemic antibiotics. A drain tube, if present, is monitored for the quantity and quality of the drainage. Drain tubes must be removed as soon as drainage falls because they serve as a nidus for infection. Sutures, skin staples, and other wound closures are usually kept in place for a week or longer, depending on the surgical intervention.

Deep Venous Thrombosis Prophylaxis

The consequences of deep venous thrombosis (DVT) are severe, and prophylaxis is often warranted. Surgical intervention increases coagulability, and after surgery, the patient may be kept immobile for a prolonged duration which makes the patient prone to DVT. Depending on the estimated DVT risk, prophylaxis should begin in the OR or earlier. DVT prophylaxis in the postoperative period may be administered using compressive stockings, pneumatic calf compression devices, or systemic low molecular heparin. Early ambulation or physiotherapy must be attempted as soon as it is safe to prevent DVT.

Fever

Postoperative fever is common because of an inflammatory or metabolic response to surgery. Fever may also be due to pneumonia, urinary tract infection, wound infections, DVT, drug-induced, and infections of implantable devices. Optimal and timely ambulation, removal of urinary catheters, and meticulous wound and drain care can reduce the risk of complications, as mentioned above. Incentive spirometry, steam nebulization, and chest physiotherapy can help decrease the risk of respiratory morbidity. The common causes of postoperative fever have been enumerated as "six Ws":

- Wound infections
- Water (UTIs)
- Wind (atelectasis, pneumonia)
- Walking (DVTs)
- Wonder drugs (drug-induced fever)
- Widgets (implantable devices, drains)

Urinary Care

Urinary retention is common after surgery. The causes include anticholinergics, opioids, immobility, decreased oral intake, and residual effects of central neuraxial blockade. Urine output must be monitored. Bladder catheterization is indicated in patients with distended bladder and those who have not urinated for 6 to 8 hours after surgery. Applying suprapubic pressure during voiding (Credé maneuver) and simulating micturition (by the sound of a running tap) help relieve the retention. Sometimes an indwelling bladder catheter is needed after prolonged surgery, especially if patients have a history of retention. Care must be taken to prevent catheter-related urinary tract infection (CAUTI) by following recommended protocols. An indwelling catheter must be removed as soon as possible to decrease the risk of infection.

Bowel Care

Patients should be fasting for four hours after anesthesia whenever muscle relaxants have been used (two hours in other cases). The fasting period may be optimally increased if the intestines have been extensively handled or operated upon. During the postoperative period, nausea/vomiting, abdominal distension, postoperative ileus, delayed gastric emptying, and hiccups are common, especially in patients undergoing abdominal surgeries. In such cases, intestinal distension by pooling gastric and intestinal juices is avoided by retaining the nasogastric tube postoperatively to allow drainage of these fluids. Oral intake must be started as soon as bowel sounds are heard.

Constipation, secondary to anesthetic drugs, bowel surgery, postoperative immobility, and opioids, is also commonly seen.

Constipation is treated by avoiding opioid use and early postoperative ambulation. Patients without gastrointestinal surgery can be given laxatives (bisacodyl, senna, cascara). An enema is the last resort.

Glycemic Control

Surgery is associated with the release of stress hormones and catabolism. The release of these hormones disturbs glucose homeostasis. Hyperglycemia is common after surgery and may become uncontrolled after major surgery in patients suffering from diabetes mellitus. Hyperglycemia also hinders wound healing. Good glycemic control is vital in the postoperative period to avoid complications of hyperglycemia. Parenteral insulin is usually needed to control blood sugar levels.

Nutrition

Loss of muscle mass and strength occur in patients after major surgery. It is estimated that with complete bed rest, young patients lose about 1 % of muscle mass per day, while older patients lose up to 5 % per day. For optimal recovery, patients should be ambulated early, and they must exercise as much as permissible. Oral intake should be encouraged. In case oral feeding is not possible, enteral nutrition must to administered. Parenteral nutrition must be restricted to those patients who cannot be administered enteral nutrition.

MULTIPLE CHOICE QUESTIONS

1. **The objectives of a post-anesthesia care unit (PACU) include:**
   a. To protect the patient and prevent complications after surgery
   b. Transit for transfer of the patient to the ward after surgery
   c. To intensively monitor the patient after surgery
   d. All of the above

2. **All patients administered general anesthesia must be nursed:**
   a. With the head end of the bed elevated at an angle of 30-45° with legs straight or bent
   b. In a supine position with oxygen supplementation
   c. In lateral position with head turned to the side to prevent aspiration
   d. In a sitting position for airway protection

3. **Postoperative shivering:**
   a. Increases oxygen consumption
   b. May promote hypoxia
   c. It is related to exposure to low operating room temperatures
   d. All of the above

4. **Postoperative nausea and vomiting can be controlled with all *except*:**
   a. Dexamethasone
   b. Serotonin antagonists
   c. Ranitidine
   d. Domperidone

5. **The following are assessed in the Modified Aldrete Recovery score *except*:**
   a. Circulation
   b. Breathing
   c. Consciousness
   d. End-tidal carbon dioxide

6. **The following may be used in the PACU for deep venous thrombosis (DVT) prophylaxis:**
   a. Compressive stockings
   a. Pneumatic calf compression devices
   b. Physiotherapy
   c. All the above

7. **A common cause of urinary retention in the PACU is:**
   a. Prostate hypertrophy
   b. Excessive intravenous fluids
   c. Residual effects of neuraxial blockade
   d. Residual effects of neuromuscular blockade

Answers
1. d
2. a
3. d
4. c
5. d
6. d
7. c

13

Intensive Care

Ram Murti Sharma, Manish Bharti

Learning Objectives

- Structure and function of ICU
- Admission/Discharge criteria
- Management of unconscious patient
- Mechanical ventilation
- Hemodynamic management and vasoactive drug therapy
- Monitoring
- Prevention and treatment of infections
- Nutrition
- General supportive and nursing care

INTRODUCTION

AS7.1: Visit, enumerate and describe the functions of an intensive care unit.

The intensive care unit (ICU) is a distinct organizational and geographic entity for clinical activity and care in a hospital. The ICU provides an integrated service to the hospital in cooperation with other hospital departments. The ICU of any hospital is considered a *'hospital within a hospital.'* It is where the sickest of the patients are cared for, such as patients requiring life support for organ failure, serious infections, poisonings, life-threatening injuries, and patients after major surgeries. ICU is considered an "economic arrangement for the treatment of grave illness."

In the present standards, the ICUs now serve as a necessity rather than an option. Modern ICUs are equipment intensive and have well-structured and sophisticated equipment for monitoring and providing life support. ICU patients are prone to develop life-threatening complications, including infections, because of the serious nature of the illness and various lifesaving interventions. The traditional arrangement for working in intensive care has now evolved into a specialized branch. ICUs are further categorized into Medical ICU, Surgical ICU, Neuro ICU, etc., depending upon the specific purpose and degree of the dependency of the patient.

STRUCTURE AND FUNCTION OF INTENSIVE CARE UNIT

Functions

ICUs primarily provide supportive care to sustain life till the underlying disease process is partly or completely cured. The basic ICU arrangement comprises the infrastructure and equipment to support the airway, oxygenation, ventilation, and circulation. Often, patients are admitted to ICU for an appropriate level of monitoring and prevention of any unexpected complications, especially after major surgical procedures. Patients are admitted to an ICU with a working diagnosis, and once the life-threatening issues are treated, they are transferred back to the medical or surgical ward for further care. Rarely patients are discharged home from ICU on some form of life support therapy like domiciliary bi-level positive airway pressure (BiPAP) and domiciliary oxygen therapy.

The Basic Structure

Most ICUs may have 10 to 12 beds or 10% of total hospital beds in a C-shape or U-shape with a central nursing station. Beds may be separated by curtains or removable wood or aluminum partitions. ICU should have isolation rooms including positive and negative pressure chambers to provide a protective environment for the patients at risk for infections and health-care staff, respectively. The ICU is located such that it is adjacent or close to an elevator to move patients to and from the emergency department, operating rooms, high dependency units, and radiology.

Criteria for Admission and Discharge

> **AS7.2:** Enumerate and describe the criteria for admission and discharge of a patient to an ICU.

Patients with potentially reversible conditions benefitting from ICU care should only be admitted.

Who Qualifies for ICU Care?

Patients requiring advanced respiratory or hemodynamic support are admitted to ICU. Patients with acute onset organ failure (acute kidney injury), altered sensorium, multiple injuries, following major surgeries requiring intensive monitoring, patients resuscitated after cardiac arrest, and poisonings qualify for admission to ICU. Patients with a reasonable chance of a meaningful functional recovery only should be admitted.

Patients not Appropriate for ICU Care

Patients with no hope of recovering to an acceptable quality of life should not be admitted. Age should not be a barrier to admission to intensive care. Still, doctors should recognize that increasing age is associated with diminishing physiological reserve and an increasing chance of serious coexisting disease. It is important to respect patient autonomy. Patients should not be admitted to intensive care if they have a written desire not to receive intensive care, for example, in an advanced directive. The patients who are "too well to benefit" and "too sick to benefit" from critical care services should not be admitted to ICU.

Discharge from the ICU

Discharge from the ICU should be considered for the patient if the primary condition that necessitated ICU admission has been resolved. Stable vitals, including the minimal need for oxygen support and hemodynamic parameters, support and no longer required intensive monitoring, can be safely transferred back to the wards.

MANAGEMENT OF AN UNCONSCIOUS PATIENT

> **AS7.3:** Observe and describe the management of an unconscious patient.

Three main causes of coma in ICU patients are brain injuries, cerebrovascular accidents, and toxic metabolic encephalopathies. While managing the underlying cause of coma, these patients are prone to develop complications such as airway obstruction, aspiration, pressure ulcers, and pulmonary thromboembolism. Preventing these complications is one of the biggest challenges for critical care specialists. Fall in GCS ≤8 needs securing airway with tracheal intubation. Pressure ulcers are better prevented by turning patients every 2 hours in bed and are one of the important nursing quality indicators. Regular physiotherapy prevents the development of contractures.

MECHANICAL VENTILATION

AS7.4: Observe and describe the basic setup process of a ventilator.

Setting up a Ventilator

Almost 40% to 50 % of patients in ICU may require ventilator support during their stay in ICU. The common reason for initiating ventilator support in ICU patients is either hypoxemic or hypercapnic respiratory failure. Patients presenting with shortness of breath and having clinical signs of respiratory distress are potential candidates for mechanical ventilation. The decision for tracheal intubation and mechanical ventilation is based on the conglomeration of clinical assessment supported by ABG and various standard indices.

Placing Patients on Mechanical Ventilation

Placing patients on ventilators demands high-level expertise and constant nursing care. One needs to safely secure the airway by tracheal intubation and setting up a ventilator per the disease physiology, ensuring patients' safety under all considerations. Tracheal intubation in ICU patients must be performed by an expert as these patients often have significantly deranged physiology due to underlying hypoxia, hypotension, and acidosis. Various standard techniques are described to facilitate safe endotracheal intubation, including rapid sequence and modified rapid sequence induction and intubation.

Managing Mechanical Ventilation

At the beginning of the illness, patients often have marked respiratory distress, including highly variable tidal volumes and minute ventilation. These predispose the patients at risk for respiratory exhaustion and hence respiratory failure. At times, distressing pleural pressure swings predispose the patients at risk for self-inflicted lung injury (SILI), which, if left unattended, can be dangerous and life-threatening. As a standard of care, initial ventilation settings are controlled, which allow and facilitate complete rest to the patient's deranged physiology.

Modes of Controlled Ventilation

Traditionally, the initial mode is conventional mechanical ventilation (CMV) [volume-controlled CMV (V-CMV) or pressure-controlled CMV (P-CMV)]. V-CMV requires the user to set the desired tidal volume, and the respiratory rate, in addition to universal settings like a fraction of inspired oxygen, peak-end-expiratory pressure (PEEP), flow rate, and inspiratory:expiratory (I:E) ratio. In the P-CMV mode, the desired peak pressure to ventilate is set in place of tidal volume. All patients receive 100% oxygen, gradually titrated to oxygen saturation (SpO_2) targets > 94% with an oxygen fraction (FiO_2) <60%. Volume modes are easily understood, have universal acceptance, and ensure the guaranteed delivery of the desired TV and MV. These modes (Volume versus Pressure) are often chosen based on disease etiology, safety limits, the predisposition for ventilator-induced lung injury (VILI), and the user's experience. CMV is a completely controlled mode and does not allow patient participation.

Assisted Ventilation Modes

Modern ventilators have assist-control CMV, which also allows patients participation (assisted breaths). It allows patients to breathe spontaneously (in between the mandatory ventilator breaths) assisted by the ventilator. This ensures the patients' safety by guarding the minute ventilation. A potential disadvantage of A-CMV is its predisposition for iatrogenic hyperventilation and hence requires careful monitoring, especially when the patient's participation (spontaneous breaths) is desired.

Lung Protective Ventilation

The use of low tidal volume (6–8 mL/kg) is recommended, which is lung protective for most medical and surgical patients. The lung protective ventilation strategy ensures the safe delivery of minute ventilation and provides evidence-based protection against the potential mechanical injury which can be transduced by a mechanical ventilator.

Clinical Monitoring Patient on a Ventilator

As a basic standard, patients on mechanical ventilation require a continuous electrocardiogram (ECG), heart rate (HR), blood pressure (BP), SpO_2, and end-tidal carbon dioxide, along with arterial blood gas (ABG) analysis. ABG serves as a useful parameter to understand the disease, its progression, and the response of the given treatment and interventions. It should be performed (if indicated) to objectively document hypoxia, hypercapnia, or acidosis.

Complications

Patients tracheal intubated and in need of mechanical ventilation should be regularly monitored for possible inadvertent tracheal extubation, endobronchial intubation, ventilator-associated pneumonia (VAP), and ventilator-induced lung injury (VILI). VILI has various subsets, including volutrauma, barotrauma, atelectrauma, and biotrauma. Recently VILI has been well understood, and various protocols have been stated, including low tidal volume and regular protocoled monitoring of plateau (<30 cm H_2O) and driving pressure (<15 cm H_2O). VILI complications could be life-threatening, including pneumothorax, pneumomediastinum, acute respiratory distress syndrome (ARDS), and cardiovascular instability.

Initiating Weaning off Mechanical Ventilation

The transition to other ventilation modes depends on disease progression, oxygen requirements, and hemodynamic stability. Once the patient has a partial resolution to the underlying illness and there is NO underlying instability of oxygenation, ventilation, and circulation, the ventilation mode is transitioned to modes that allow patients participation. This process is referred to as weaning. It has two aspects: progressive liberation from mechanical ventilation (and hence more patient participation) and tracheal extubation. Patient-ventilator synchronization is an important consideration to allow safe ventilation, and it hastens early weaning from the ventilator.

Weaning Modes in Ventilators

There are several modes to wean patients off mechanical ventilation. They include pressure support ventilation (PSV) and synchronized intermittent mandatory ventilation (SIMV). As a standard practice, once the patient has acceptable physiology, including a stable acid-base gas milieu, a trial of spontaneous breathing trial (SBT) through pressure support ventilation (PSV) is offered. Many intensivists use a T-piece trial before extubating the trachea and liberating the patient from mechanical ventilation. Placing the patient on continuous positive airway pressure (CPAP) before tracheal extubation ensures avoidance of atelectasis and improves respiratory outcomes.

Before Changing to a Weaning Mode

Patient's spontaneous breaths are a mandatory prerequisite before initiation to PSV or T-piece trial. Appropriate strategies, including sedation vacation, are standard care to facilitate spontaneous breaths. The pressure support is supplemented to the degree of the patient's efforts and neuromuscular strength and in close monitoring of the tidal volume and minute ventilation. Since patients' spontaneous breaths are a prerequisite, these modes may serve as a disadvantage in poor patients' spontaneous efforts. They can lead to dangerous hypoventilation, apnea, and clinically significant desaturation (hypoxemia) if patients are not carefully selected and monitored. To overcome the above disadvantages, some clinicians recommend transitioning to synchronized mandatory minute ventilation (SIMV) before giving a PSV trial. The attractive advantages include it giving mandatory intermittent breaths in between, which ensures minimum mandatory minute ventilation and circumvents the problem of hypoventilation.

Neuromuscular Blockade

Patients needing respiratory support should preferably not be placed on infusions of neuromuscular blockers. Prolonged use of neuromuscular blockers is associated with muscle weakness and wasting. Mechanical ventilation in the ICU is best facilitated by adequate sedation and the preferred use of assisted ventilation modes.

Monitoring Ventilator Function

These challenges are far from real and have not been intensively supported by evidence. Every patient on a ventilator requires intensive monitoring, including scalar waveforms and loops, demonstrating the relationship between volume, pressure, and flow with time. PV and FV loops help the physician to understand the integral relationship between pulmonary functions. Some of the regular variables which need monitoring apart from the patient's vitals include peak airway pressure, plateau pressure, compliance, resistance, auto-peep, and driving pressure.

Weaning off Ventilator

As and when the underlying condition has resolved, chest radiograph, bedside lung ultrasound, and arterial blood gas examination are within an acceptable limit. Stable hemodynamics and normal acid-base and electrolytes balance are mandatory before weaning the patient off the ventilator. Standardized protocols have been recommended to facilitate early weaning and extubation, including daily spontaneous awakening trial (SAT) and daily spontaneous breathing trial (SBT). Not to mention, these protocols are required a meticulous understanding of the disease physiology and have to be practiced bedside, under the supervision of trained intensivists.

HEMODYNAMIC MANAGEMENT AND VASOACTIVE DRUG THERAPY

Shock

Shock is one of the commonest causes of ICU admission. It has been consistently associated with high morbidity and mortality among all admissions in ICU patients. Various etiologies of shock must be understood and clinically mastered as one of the essential skills in intensive care practice. Broadly shock can be categorized as hypovolemic, cardiogenic, septic, and obstructive. The purpose of the monitoring is to identify abnormal physiology and intervene before complications, including organ failure and death, occur.

Monitoring in Shock

The monitoring of shock patients can be bifurcated into basic and advanced assessments.

Basic Monitoring

Basic hemodynamic monitoring includes assessing cardiovascular functions, which can be performed bedside without any advanced interventions. It includes continuous ECG, HR, BP, SpO_2, capillary refill time (normal or delayed), urine output, surface body temperature, and temperature gradient between core and extremities (e.g., patients in septic shock have warm extremities while those in cardiogenic shock have cold extremities), the appearance of mottling, and livedo reticularis.

Advanced Monitoring

It is not uncommon to have complex shock and undifferentiated shock, which have mixed etiologies and hence warrant an advanced assessment of hemodynamic functions, including right side heart functions (CVP; often referred to as preload) and left side heart functions independently (pulmonary artery occlusion pressure, cardiac output), cardiac contractility (systolic versus diastolic dysfunction), systemic vascular resistance (SVR) and pulmonary vascular resistance (PVR). This data assessment requires the placement of an invasive Swan Ganz catheter (pulmonary artery catheter). However, using a pulmonary catheter and its data assessment have not been associated with consistent patient benefits.

Point of Care Ultrasound

Invasive monitoring has been easily replicated by bedside point of care ultrasound (POCUS), where the trained intensivist derives the above indices noninvasively. The use of bedside POCUS is a desirable standard of practice to assess the patient's cardiac and pulmonary functions at the bedside. Another advantage of POCUS is that it is easily reproducible. The use of POCUS has been consistently increasing in the emergency rooms (ER) and ICUs. Standard protocols, including FALLS (fluid administration limited by lung sonography) and BLUE (bedside lung ultrasonography in emergency), have been devised, which allow early identification of the cause of acute circulatory failure and acute respiratory failure, respectively. The advantages include early, rapid, bedside diagnosis with high sensitivity and specificity, which is often a crucial factor in time-bound emergencies.

Invasive Arterial Monitoring

Shock is a condition in which systemic BP is inadequate to provide adequate tissue perfusion. It usually denotes a mean arterial pressure (MAP) < 60 mm Hg with evidence of organ hypoperfusion. The treatment modalities differ for a different types of shock. To facilitate diagnosis and treatment, continuous invasive monitoring of BP is highly desirable. The invasive arterial catheters, which can be easily placed in the radial or femoral artery, help in the continuous, beat-to-beat assessment of blood pressure. Blood pressure is often taken as a surrogate assessment for the perfusion, and hence to facilitate the treatment of shock, it is pivotal to have a regular, uninterrupted assessment. The arterial catheter, in-situ, allows repeated assessment of blood gas and metabolic milieu, including lactate estimation, to rationalize the therapy, including fluids and vasoactive therapy. Noninvasive blood pressure (NIBP) can be fallacious in shock.

Vasoactive Drug Therapy

Vasoactive drugs are the mainstay of therapy along with fluids in managing shock. The vasoactive therapy has to be seen in conjunction with the fluid assessment. Vasoactive therapy is the choice of treatment in vasoplegic (also known as distributive) and cardiogenic shock. Catecholamines, including norepinephrine, epinephrine, dopamine, and dobutamine, are vasoactive drugs. Other vasopressors, vasopressin, levosimendan, and phenylepinephrine, are used in specific subsets of patients. These drugs are used as a continuous infusion, preferably infused through a central line under continuous hemodynamic monitoring. The doses of commonly used vasoactive drugs are mentioned below:

Norepinephrine (0.05–0.15 mcg/kg/min)
It is administered as the initial vasopressor of choice in septic, cardiogenic, hypovolemic shock in conjunction with fluids, obstructive shock like pulmonary embolism to allow improvement in hemodynamics.

Vasopressin (0.01–0.04 mcg/min)
It is used as 2nd add-on drug to norepinephrine in septic shock. It has a catecholamine sparing effect and, in proper settings, has been associated with a significant decrease in the requirement of other catecholamines. Its use has been associated with improved creatinine clearance among all vasoactive drugs. It is associated with risk reduction in the incidence of tachyarryhithmia because of its vagotonic properties.

Epinephrine (0.01–0.2 mcg/kg/min)
It is the 3rd add-on to norepinephrine in septic shock first add-on to norepinephrine in cases of associated myocardial dysfunction or if there are associated bradyarrhythmia. It is the vasoactive therapy of choice in anaphylactic shock.

Dopamine (2–20 mcg/kg/min)
Its use is declining. However, it can be used as an add-on therapy to norepinephrine in case of associated bradyarrhythmias. Its use has been associated with increased mortality plausibly due to its potential for tachyarrhythmias. Its use is not recommended for renal protection, to promote diuresis or spare other catecholamines.

Dobutamine (2–5 mcg/kg/min)
It is the initial agent of choice in cardiogenic shock and is used as an add-on to norepinephrine in septic shock with myocardial dysfunction.

MONITORING

AS7.5: Observe and describe the principles of monitoring in an ICU.

Basic
Continuous monitoring of patients' vital signs or physiological functions aids in ensuring patient safety through awareness of critical changes in the patient's health status and guides daily therapeutic interventions. Early recognition of patient deterioration and timely intervention are critical in saving patients' lives. Subtle changes in vital signs such as respiratory rate, BP, HR, temperature, and SpO_2 are early signs of clinical deterioration that may eventually lead to adverse events. The staff:patient ratio 1:1 and multifunction monitors available in ICU facilitates monitoring of vitals and ensures patient safety. The NICE guidelines recommend that HR, respiratory rate, BP, SpO_2, level of consciousness, and temperature be measured. Additional monitoring of pain, urine output, and biochemical analysis should be added. The vital cardiorespiratory parameters monitored in almost all patients in ICU are:
- HR with continuous ECG
- NIBP showing systolic, diastolic, and MAP
- SpO_2 with plethysmographic waveform
- Breath rate.

Advanced
In critical patients, invasive monitoring includes invasive BP, central venous pressure (CVP), pulmonary artery occlusion pressure, heart contractility (systolic versus diastolic dysfunction), SVR, and PVR assessment are often required to understand and rationalize the fluid and vasoactive therapy. Various modern monitoring tools have made it possible to obtain parameters like continuous cardiac output assessment, including the global

end-diastolic volume (GEDV), global end-systolic volume (GESV), and the extravascular lung water index (EVLW) through the simple arterial catheter placed in a proximal artery. The monitors help to prevent progressive deterioration in the physiologic state of the patient while the underlying disease is being managed. These monitoring tools must be used to complement the clinical assessment and not as a substitute for the astute clinician.

PREVENTION AND TREATMENT OF INFECTIONS

ICU patients are admitted with infection and sepsis, OR develop hospital-acquired infections while in the hospital. Patients admitted to ICU for infections receive their standard therapy per the disease, the severity of illness, and existing comorbidities.

Nosocomial Infections

Prolonged ICU stay is an independent risk factor for developing nosocomial or hospital-acquired infections. The commonest infections which typically an ICU patient is likely to develop are catheter-associated urinary tract infections (CAUTI), central line-associated bloodstream infections (CLABSI), nosocomial pneumonia, and ventilator-associated pneumonia (VAP). These infections are related to indwelling catheters and central lines, which often become the site for colonization and then infection, which, if worsened, lead to sepsis and septic shock. Risk factors for nosocomial sepsis include poor hand hygiene, lack of asepsis, dysfunctional immune status, ineffective antibiotic stewardship, and delayed weaning protocols for tracheal extubation. The intensivist and ICU staff needs to take all the measures to prevent infections in ICU patients.

Infection Control Bundles

Various bundles of care have been proposed to address the above issues. These bundles are protocols recommended to prevent infection. The common bundles recommended are the VAP, CAUTI, and CLABSI bundles. The elements of the bundle, when implemented together, have been effectively able to reduce hospital-acquired infections by a significant proportion.

Catheter-associated Urinary Tract Infection (CAUTI)

Urine output is one of the most important markers for perfusion marker, which helps determine kidney perfusion. Urine output is often addressed as the "Poor's man CVP or cardiac output." However, the presence of catheters has its demerits. Any 'indwelling' catheter is a foreign body and, by its inherent nature, is likely to get colonized by commensal microbes over time. These commensals, when heavily colonized, alter the local tissue milieu, breach into the tissue or the bloodstream and become the source of infection and bacteremia, respectively. The use of urinary catheters must be rationalized on case to case basis and be used only if the merits outweigh the risks associated. The presence of shock, in patients with acute circulatory failure warrants hourly urine output monitoring. One must assess the need for the catheter daily and remove it as soon as possible.

Ventilator-associated Pneumonia (VAP)

In patients with invasive ventilation, an endotracheal tube (ETT) impedes the upper airway reflexes promoting silent aspiration of oropharyngeal secretions. Apart from the endogenous contamination, there is a risk of exogenous transmission if proper tracheal suction hygiene and asepsis have not been implemented. Improper protocols may cause VAP with hospital-acquired multi-drug resistant (MDR) bacteria like *pseudomonas*, *klebsiella*, and *acinetobacter*. ETT suction is a sterile procedure and must be done strictly on a need basis. To minimize the risk of cross-contamination, closed suction units are available. The patients requiring frequent suctioning are at risk for VAP, and using close suction units can minimize the risk for VAP. All patients must be propped up by 30–45° to minimize the risk of passive regurgitation and silent aspiration. The use of subglottic suction can reduce the burden of subglottic secretions. However, its role in the prevention of VAP has not been established. The incidence of VAP depends on the duration the ETT remains in situ and the duration of invasive ventilation. VAP significantly predisposes the patient to prolonged ventilation, increased duration of ICU stay, and increased cost of treatment. Treatment of VAP is becoming challenging with the evolution of MDR pathogens. Treatment of VAP usually requires covering up for MDR pathogens, including extended-spectrum beta-lactamase inhibitors (ESBL), carbapenems, or polymyxins. VAP bundles care elements must be executed daily to facilitate early tracheal extubation and minimize VAP.

Central Line-associated Bloodstream Infection (CLABSI)

Most severely sick patients require a central venous catheter for vasoactive therapy. Low-dose vasoactive therapy can be administered through peripheral venous catheters. Hemodynamically unstable patients requiring an escalating dose of vasopressors and multiple infusions indicate a central line. The presence of a central venous catheter also facilitates CVP monitoring. The role of CVP has declined as it is a static parameter. The presence of the central venous is a risk factor for microbial colonization and warrants strict aseptic handling. Despite all precautions, there is a definitive risk for bloodstream infections. The need for the central line must be reassessed daily as a part of the CLABSI bundle. The lesser indication and the non-functioning catheter must be removed as a priority to minimize this complication.

NUTRITION

ICU patients are often hyper-catabolic, especially those with high-stress factors including burns, trauma, and sepsis. Nutritional support must be initiated early to preserve muscle mass.

Enteral Nutrition

Oral or enteral nutrition is the preferred mode. Enteral nutrition, besides meeting the calorie and protein requirements, prevents intestinal mucosal atrophy. This concept has been popularized as 'trophic' feeding, where the early, low volume initiation of enteral feeding promotes intestinal IgA production in Peyer's patches and intestinal micro-vili and helps prevents gut bacterial translocation and gut dysbiosis. The bacterial translocation across the intestinal barrier is an independent risk factor for infections, including sepsis. The average daily requirement of calories is about 25–30 kcal/kg and that of proteins around 1–2 gm/kg. To improve gut tolerance, the feeding is started in a stepwise manner. By the end of the first week, the patient should be able to receive the target calories and proteins.

Parenteral Nutrition

Failure to meet the target calories, or persistent gut intolerance, despite optimization of electrolytes and prokinetic therapy, should alert the Intensivist to consider partial or total parenteral nutrition (PN). The indications of the parenteral nutrition are restricted, and the gut should be promoted to tolerate and improve enteral (via nasogastric or nasojejunal tube) nutrition. Initiation of feeding in critically ill patients, who are chronically cachexic, must be slow, graded, and under careful supervision. Patients initiated on feeding (especially parenteral) must be regularly assessed for blood sugar, serum electrolytes including potassium, magnesium, phosphate, and chloride levels, abdominal distension, and ileus. Each patient must be assessed daily for bowel movements and input/output balance.

Supportive Nutrition-related Care

The risk of refeeding syndrome leading to life-threatening arrhythmias due to the transcellular shift of potassium, magnesium, and phosphate is a major morbidity in ICU. Patients with two subsequent blood glucose readings >180 mg% qualify for insulin therapy. Non-tight glycemic control (blood sugar 140–180 mg%) is the standard of care.

GENERAL SUPPORTIVE AND NURSING CARE

Nursing Care

Good nursing care is the backbone of an ICU. It is recommended that the ratio of Nursing staff be 1:1 for mechanically ventilated patients and 1:2 for other patients. Medication administration and implementation of infection care bundles primarily rest on the nurses. The vigilance of nurses ensures early detection of deterioration of patients' condition. Nurses ensure a regular change in patient position and help prevent pressure sores by keeping the bed dry and maintaining skin hygiene.

Oral Care

Patients must receive good oral care with chlorhexidine mouthwash or simple brushing teeth to minimize VAP. This practice of oral care, including decontamination, has recently been challenged. However, at present, it looks pragmatic to provide basic hygiene as a part of ICU nursing care. Oral thrush or candidiasis is common and must be prevented.

Sedation

All critically ill patients must receive appropriate analgesia-based sedation to improve patient comfort in ICU. Daily sedation interruption and spontaneous breathing trials to facilitate early weaning and liberation from the ventilator are standard practices.

Deep Vein Thrombosis

Every patient in ICU is at risk of deep venous thrombosis because of the infection and immobility. Various pharmacological and non-pharmacological methods should be employed unless there is a specific contraindication. Patients must use compression or pneumatic stockings and preferably receive anticoagulants for pharmacological prophylaxis.

Stress-related Prophylaxis

Patients are prone to stress-related acid-peptic mucosal disease. All patients receive a proton-pump inhibitor to prevent it. Patients are also prone to depression and ICU delirium. Patients are also exposed to adverse events of other patients. Measures must be taken to ensure mental health and isolate patients from the patients receiving invasive therapy or resuscitation. Measures must be taken to minimize the adverse effects of noise generated by ICU monitors and other ICU activities.

Ambulation

Early bedside ambulation protocols are increasingly being implemented to preserve the muscles' strength and minimize delirium. Patients must receive general and respiratory physiotherapy.

MULTIPLE CHOICE QUESTIONS

1. **To qualify for ICU care, the essential criteria to meet is:**
   a. Patients with end-stage severe disease
   b. Patients with terminal cancer
   c. Patients with a reasonable chance of a meaningful functional recovery
   d. All the above

2. **The following mechanical ventilation mode is an assisted mode:**
   a. Synchronized intermittent mandatory ventilation
   b. Pressure support ventilation
   c. Assist-Control controlled mechanical ventilation
   d. All the above

3. **In lung protective ventilation:**
   a. A tidal volume of 5 mL/kg is set
   b. A tidal volume of 6–8 mL/kg is set
   c. A tidal volume of 10 mL/kg is set with a pressure limitation of 30 cm H_2O
   d. A tidal volume of 10 mL/kg is set with a pressure limitation of 20 cm H_2O

4. **The following ventilation modes are advocated for weaning a patient off the ventilator *except*:**
   a. Synchronized intermittent control ventilation
   b. Pressure support ventilation
   c. Assist control-controlled mechanical ventilation
   d. Continuous positive airway pressure

5. **The recommended modes of ventilation for long-term support include:**
   a. Controlled mechanical ventilation with neuromuscular blockade
   b. Assisted mechanical ventilation facilitated by adequate sedation
   c. Continuous positive airway pressure
   d. None of the above

OSCE

A patient with multiple injuries is shifted to the intensive care unit (ICU) as he develops shortness of breath. On arrival in the ICU, he has a heart rate of 120/min, BP 86/50 mm Hg, SpO_2 86% and respiratory rate of 30/min. He had dyspnea and was seen to be using accessory respiratory muscles for breathing. He was immediately placed on mechanical ventilation support. His biochemical parameters indicated a septic shock. Advanced monitoring was initiated.

6. **Use of which of the following monitoring modes will not benefit this patient?**
   a. Preload assessment
   b. Afterload assessment
   c. Cardiac output assessment
   d. Pulmonary artery pressure assessment

7. **Point of care ultrasound (POCUS) can be used in this case for:**
   a. Lung ultrasonography
   b. Estimating cardiac output
   c. Estimating fluid volume
   d. None of the above

8. **If this patient develops severe vasoplegic shock, which of the following drug combinations can be used?**
   a. Adrenaline with dopamine
   b. Dobutamine with nitroglycerine
   c. Noradrenaline with vasopressin
   d. Noradrenaline with dobutamine

9. **The use of the following infection control bundles is indicated in this case:**
   a. CAUTI
   b. CLABSI
   c. VAP
   d. All the above

10. **Parenteral nutrition is indicated in:**
    a. Failure to meet the target calories
    b. Persistent gut intolerance
    c. Major gut resection
    d. All of the above

Answers
1. c
2. d
3. b
4. c
5. b
6. d
7. a
8. c
9. d
10. d

CHAPTER 14

Special Anesthesia Techniques

Deepak Kumar Sreevastava, Siddharth Chaki

Learning Objectives

- Principles of total intravenous anesthesia (TIVA)
- Conduct of total intravenous anesthesia
- Drug delivery systems for total intravenous anesthesia
- Management of total intravenous anesthesia
- Anesthesia outside the operating room
- Dissociative anesthesia

TOTAL INTRAVENOUS ANESTHESIA

Anesthesia has several components, which include suppression of consciousness, suppression of physiologic response to noxious stimuli, muscle relaxation, and provision of postoperative analgesia. However, there is no ideal drug on the horizon that can meet all the requirements of anesthesia. The concept of balanced anesthesia was popularized by Dundee, where each requirement is met with different agents. Thus, optimal conditions of anesthesia can be achieved by various techniques such as regional anesthesia (RA), RA with minimal general anesthesia (GA), inhalation GA, or total intravenous anesthesia (TIVA). TIVA is now an established technique of anesthesia and is indicated in several situations, which include anesthesia at remote locations.

What is Total Intravenous Anesthesia (TIVA)?

TIVA is a general term for a process by which induction and maintenance of anesthesia are achieved by a combination of drugs-infused intravenous (IV) where the patient either breathes spontaneously or is artificially ventilated in the absence of inhalation drugs including nitrous oxide. TIVA is a natural extension of the process of anesthesia where all the components are provided with IV anesthetic agents.

Current Status

TIVA has received impetus because of newer 'designer' anesthetic drugs with a suitable pharmacokinetic profile which allow reliable anesthesia to be produced when given intravenously and rapid recovery to occur even after long infusions. Additionally, hardware and software are now available, which permit delivery of these agents in a manner superior to manual infusions. The 5th National Audit Project (NAP5) has recently noted that TIVA was being practiced inadequately, causing accidental awareness. It was recommended that *'the relevant anesthetic organizations should establish a set of standards and recommendations for best practice in the use of TIVA.'*

Indications of TIVA

Although TIVA can be used as an alternative anesthetic technique in all situations, it is specifically indicated where there is a need to avoid using volatile anesthetic agents (**Box 1**). TIVA is the technique of choice in patients susceptible to malignant hyperthermia. The major potential advantages of TIVA are the reduction of operating room pollution and the consequent adverse effects on the ozone layer. The technique also scores over inhalation anesthesia in scoliosis surgery (where intraoperative wake-up testing is required), awake craniotomy, recurrent laryngeal nerve monitoring in thyroid surgeries, and cases of the atonic uterus. TIVA is also indicated when inhalation technique is not possible during transfer or for some operations on the airway.

Box 1: Indications of TIVA.
- Malignant hyperthermia (susceptibility or known history)
- History of severe postoperative nausea vomiting (PONV)
- Long QT syndrome (QTc ≥500 ms)
- Surgery on the airway
- Anesthesia in locations away from the operation theater
- Day-care surgery
- Patients with anticipated difficult tracheal intubation/extubation
- Neurosurgical anesthesia to manage intracranial pressure
- Surgery requiring neurophysiological monitoring
- Patients with neuromuscular disorder
- Intrahospital or interhospital transfer of anesthetized patients

TIVA: total intravenous anesthesia

Pharmacokinetic Principles

To maintain a steady level of drugs in plasma and thus maintain the clinical effect without undulations, it is important to understand the disposition of any drug in the body. A three-compartment model (**Fig. 1**) explains the distribution, metabolism, and elimination of a drug in the body. The drug is administered into the central compartment (V_1), from where it passes to the second (highly perfused V_2) and

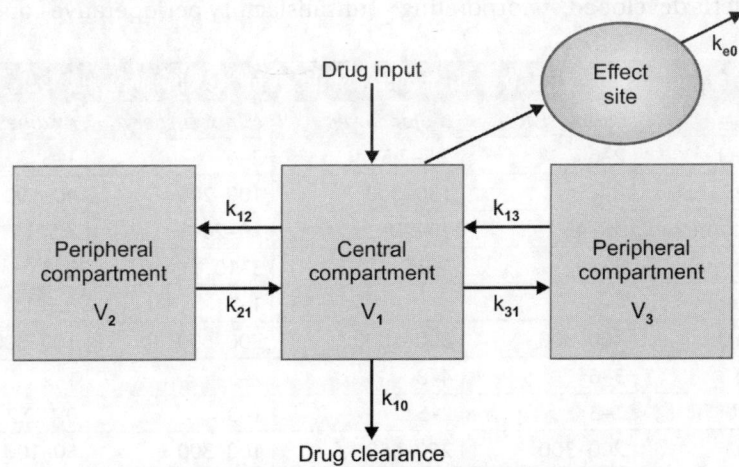

Fig. 1: The three-compartment pharmacokinetic model.

Table 1: Pharmacokinetic models.

Drug	Model
Propofol	• Marsh • Schneider • Schuttler and White-Kenny • Kataria model for children • Paedfusor model for children • Eleveld (Not yet commercially available)
Remifentanil	Minto
Sufentanil	Gepts

third (less well perfused V_3) compartments following rapid and slow redistribution of the drug from the central compartment. Rate constants describe the proportion of drugs moving between compartments. A metabolic rate constant (k_{10}) describes the proportion of the drug in V_1 that is metabolized or eliminated in any unit of time. Finally, a rate constant k_{eo} describes the transfer from the central compartment to the effect site (brain).

These volumes and rate constants are determined from studies. Mathematical modeling software is used to estimate these pharmacokinetic variables in individual subjects and then to estimate the influence of potential covariates such as age, weight, height, and sex on these variables. Finally, a population model is developed, incorporating significant covariates. Commonly used models are given in **Table 1**.

CONDUCT OF TIVA

The basic aim of TIVA is to ensure that the effective plasma concentration of the drug (hypnotic/narcotic or relaxant) is achieved rapidly and is maintained within the range for the entire duration of surgery. In the strict sense of the word, drugs can be administered as periodic boluses or as continuous infusions manually or using infusion pumps.

Manual System

In the manual system, anesthesia is induced and maintained by the anesthetist, who determines the bolus dose(s) and infusion rates. For such a system, it is essential to know standard dosages (**Table 2**). A commonly used manual infusion scheme is the one described by Roberts. It involves a loading bolus of 1 mg/kg followed by a step-down infusion scheme (10 mg/kg/h for the first 10 min, 8 mg/kg/h for the next 10 min, and then 6 mg/kg/h after that). For all the drugs in common use, manual dosing regimens are available. Manual infusions are, however, not error-free, and there is a significant possibility of undulations in the blood levels of anesthetic drugs and unsatisfactory perioperative conditions.

Table 2: Desired target plasma concentration of different drugs for specific clinical effects.

Drug	Skin incision	Major surgery	Minor surgery	Analgesia/Sedation
Propofol (mcg/mL)	2–6	2.5–7.5	2–6	1–3
Midazolam (ng/mL)	—	150–300	100–200	40–100
Thiopentone (mcg/mL)	35–45	10–20	10–20	7.5–15
Methohexital (ng/mL)	5–10	5–15	5–10	2–5
Ketamine (mcg/mL)	—	—	1–2	0.5–1
Etomidate (ng/mL)	400–600	500–1000	300–600	100–300
Fentanyl (ng/mL)	3–6	4–8	2–5	1–2
Sufentanil (ng/mL)	1–3	2–5	1–3	0.1–0.2
Alfentanil (ng/mL)	200–300	250–450	100–300	50–100
Remifentanil (ng/mL)	4–8	4–8	2–4	1–2

Target Controlled Infusion (TCI) System

A TIVA technique has to ensure adequate drug concentration at the effect site (the site where any drug acts). A drug bolus is given initially, followed by an infusion at a rate that alters according to the drug's elimination from the body and two-way transfers from central to multiple peripheral compartments. This involves complex pharmacokinetic equations which are impractical and need frequent pump adjustments to meet the need of a rapidly changing and complex infusion regime till a steady state is achieved.

Computer Assistance

The TCI system is an infusion pump interfaced with a computer and hence also known as a computer-assisted continuous infusion (CACI) device. It is programmed to perform these complex calculations using a model (See **Table 1**) and to adjust the infusion rate accordingly to achieve accurate plasma concentration. These computerized microprocessor-controlled infusion pumps are equipped with drug-specific pharmacokinetic models that also allow for documentation of delivered drugs, fluid balance, and central control of multiple infusion pumps. The TCI system for propofol is now standard equipment in the operating room and considered a standard of anesthetic care in many parts of the world.

Working Principle

The user selects the drug and pharmacokinetic model to be used by that TCI pump and inputs the patient characteristics (covariates) and the desired ('target') initial blood concentration plasma (Cp) or 'brain' (effect-site) concentration of an agent known to be associated with a specific clinical effect. The infusion rates are altered automatically according to the pharmacokinetic model. The computer periodically calculates or predicts Cp based on the pharmacokinetic model and matches it with desired target concentration for specific clinical effects. In case the infusion rate is changed, the computer again predicts the Cp as per the desired target plasma concentration for specific clinical effects, and thus, the cycle goes on. The target plasma concentrations of various drugs are given in **Table 2**.

Current Status

TCI systems have been shown to produce better perioperative conditions than volatile agents. A TCI system improves the convenience of administration and ease of control of anesthesia compared with conventional infusion techniques. It is now recommended that when GA is to be maintained by propofol infusion, target-controlled infusion (TCI) systems should be used.

EQUIPMENT USED IN TIVA/TCI SYSTEM

Several types of equipment are needed for TIVA. An infusion pump is a central requirement (**Fig. 2**). These can be conventional or pharmacokinetic model-driven ones. Usually, syringe infusion pumps are used. One also needs non-compliant tubings with Luer lock, infusion set, an anti-siphon valve on the drug delivery line(s), and an anti-reflux valve on any fluid administration line. Drug and fluid lines should join as close to the patient as possible to minimize dead space. The pump must have instrument occlusion alarms, low battery infusion alarm, bolus delivery alarm, and absent syringe alarm As stated above, the TCI system consists of the user interface, microprocessor(s) with pharmacokinetic software, and infusion pump which delivers up to 1200 mL/h along with visual and audible safety systems.

TYPES OF AUTOMATED DRUG DELIVERY SYSTEMS

Two types of automated drug delivery systems are available: open-loop control and closed-

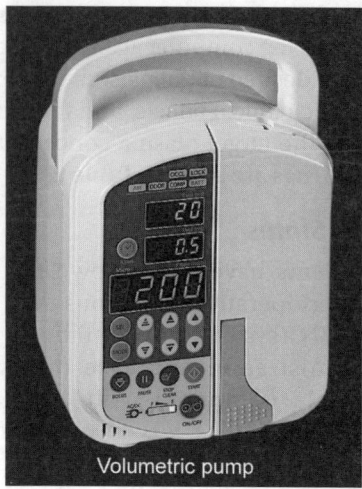 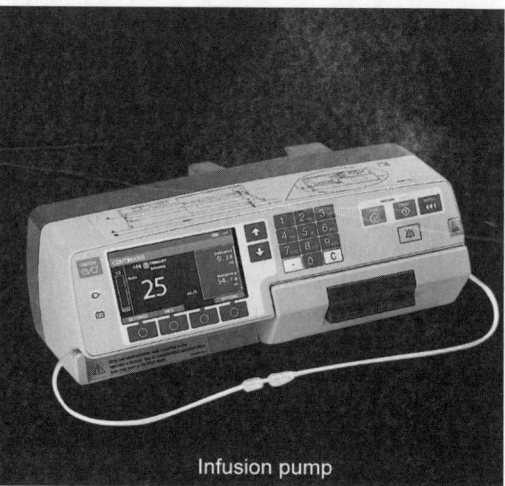

Fig. 2: Types of pumps used in TIVA/TCI.

loop control. The main difference between the open and the closed system is the lack of feedback signal in the former. In the open-loop system, the final response, i.e., the depth of anesthesia, has to be assessed by the anesthesiologist, and necessary changes must be made. However, the closed-loop systems can measure the response after intervention and then automatically generate a new control signal to prescribe a new intervention till the desired target is achieved and maintained.

The performance of the TCI system is judged by the difference between predicted plasma concentration and the measured concentration of the drug. All models incorporate assumptions and elements of inaccuracy in the prediction of plasma and effect-site targets. However, inter-individual variability in pharmacodynamic response represents a more challenging aspect of using TIVA. Practical tips while using TIVA are described in **Box 2**.

Box 2: Practical tips during the conduct of TIVA.
- Before starting, ensure that drug catheters are connected and tubings have been purged, syringes are loaded and the pump settings are correct.
- Infuse through a three-way and check all connections.
- Check repeatedly for adequate flow of the carrier liquid (as patient may wake up in minutes after cessation of infusion).
- Begin with high rates of infusion and then reduce over certain period (based on the knowledge of drugs).
- Be ready to recognize the signs of light as well as deep anesthesia and take steps as necessary.
- Movement is good sign of light anesthesia so avoid complete paralysis. It can be achieved by an infusion of neuromuscular relaxing drugs to maintain adequate surgical relaxation.
- Know the principles of pharmacokinetics and pharmacodynamics well and apply them gainfully.
- A reasonable time sequence for terminating a properly titrated infusion is opioid: 15 to 20 min; muscle relaxants: 5 to 15 min; and propofol: 5 to 10 min prior to the end of surgery. Small boluses of propofol may be required in the end.
- Appropriate reduction in infusion rates can be done for elderly or those who are heavily premedicated.
- The technique should be practiced with dedicated infusion pumps in order to ensure accurate infusion rates and to avoid cumbersome calculations in the operating theaters.
- **It should be remembered however that there are no cook-book approaches.**

DRUGS USED

The hypnotic element of TIVA is achieved by drugs such as propofol. Other common drugs used in TIVA are midazolam, thiopentone, ketamine, etomidate, and dexmedetomidine. Analgesia is achieved with opioids. The most popular opioid for TIVA is remifentanil. Fentanyl, alfentanil, and sufentanil are also suitable for TIVA. Atracurium is the most popular muscle relaxant, followed by rocuronium. The dosage scheme of various drugs has been given in **Table 3**.

Table 3: Dosage regime of various IV anesthetic agents.

Drug	Loading dose (mcg/kg)	Maintenance rate (mcg/kg/min)
Anesthesia		
Propofol	1000–2500	50–150
Midazolam	50–150	0.25–1.5
Thiopentone	2000–4000	150–300
Methohexital	1500–2500	50–150
Ketamine	1000–2000	10–50
Fentanyl	5–15	0.03–0.1
Sufentanil	1–5	0.01–0.05
Alfentanil	50–150	0.5–3
Remifentanil	1–2	0.25–3
Sedation/Analgesia		
Propofol	250–1000	10–50
Midazolam	25–100	0.25–1
Ketamine	200–750	5–20
Fentanyl	1–3	0.01–0.03
Sufentanil	0.1–0.5	0.005–0.01
Alfentanil	10–25	0.25–1
Remifentanil	0.5–1	0.025–0.1
Muscle relaxants		
Succinylcholine	500–1000	50–150
Atracurium	200–400	4–8
Vecuronium	40–80	0.5–1.7
Mivacurium	150–250	5–8

An ideal drug for TIVA should have the following properties:
- Rapid onset and offset
- Non-cumulative
- Non-active metabolites
- Short context-sensitive half-time
- Short context-sensitive decrement time.

MONITORING IN TIVA

The monitoring standards during anesthesia include electrocardiography, pulse oximetry, blood pressure, capnography, and temperature monitoring. Monitoring of depth of anesthesia remains a matter of concern since there is yet no satisfactory method of ascertaining the effective plasma concentration of drugs. Inhalation agent concentrations are readily quantified by mean alveolar concentration values, which are impossible with TIVA. It is thus strongly recommended that the depth of anesthesia be monitored to avoid awareness.

Depth of Anesthesia Monitoring

Several monitors to assess the depth of anesthesia are available, but none is universally acceptable. Depth of anesthesia is usually monitored by measuring physiological parameters such as pulse, electrocardiogram (ECG), blood pressure, respiration rate, and tears. Methods based on the measurement of brain electrical activity are preferred. Clinically the anesthetic depth is assessed by monitoring processed electroencephalogram (EEG) and electromyography activity. A processed EEG monitor is recommended, especially when a neuromuscular blocking drug is used with TIVA.

Depth of Anesthesia Monitors

Commercially, bispectral index (BIS), patient safety index, entropy, and narkotrend provide a numerological value between 0 and 100 to indicate the depth of anesthesia. All these methods measure the spontaneous electrical activity of the brain. BIS was one of the first monitoring modalities for depth of anesthesia and has been studied extensively. It has been used to titrate the level of anesthesia however, the benefits of BIS-titrated TCI or any other anesthetic technique are not established.

Auditory evoked potential monitors assess the depth of anesthesia based on evoked brain electrical activity. Two new EEG-based indices have been described (qCON and qNOX), which also measure nociception. Methods such as lower esophagus contractility also have been described. Closed-loop delivery of anesthetics using these depths of anesthesia monitors has been described, but these systems are still not approved.

ADVANTAGES OF TIVA

- Significant reduction in postoperative nausea and vomiting (PONV), leading to early recovery and discharge.
- Attenuates stress response to surgery and anesthesia better than other techniques.
- Preferable in cases with ventilation-perfusion (V/Q) mismatch, as in pulmonary surgery or in patients afflicted with cystic fibrosis, as it does not affect hypoxic vasoconstriction.
- Preferable in patients with heart disease and low left ventricular ejection fraction (LVEF) as it causes minimal myocardial depression and hemodynamic instability.
- In neurosurgery, it offers a favorable pharmacodynamic effect on intracranial pressure.
- There is also no danger of organ toxicity, e.g., liver damage because of fluoride ions.
- The technique of choice for high-frequency jet ventilation (HFJV) and bronchoscopy.
- Preferred in patients suffering from myopathies and having malignant hyperthermia susceptibility.
- Does not cause atmospheric pollution and so there is no need for scavenging devices.

DISADVANTAGES OF TIVA

- It is expensive because of the requirements of drugs, disposables, and specialized equipment.
- Conduct requires dedicated IV access and considerable organizational effort.
- The setup process is time-consuming and generates quite a lot of waste.
- Despite some control over drug compatibility and interactions, there is a possibility of awareness.
- There is no end point yet which can be easily monitored, and the depths of anesthesia monitors are still not approved.
- If muscle relaxants are used, it may further predispose to awareness.
- Does not have the flexibility of inhalation anesthesia.
- There is significant inter-patient dose variability, and hence plasma concentrations are difficult to predict or are difficult to measure quickly.
- Depth of anesthesia cannot be controlled as easily as with volatile agents.
- There is a danger of anaphylactoid reactions to IV agents (overall incidence of anaphylactoid reactions from IV agents is 1 in 5000–20000).
- Administration by computer-assisted continuous infusion (CACI) has significant problems, including complexity, because of several pumps and programs.

ANESTHESIA AT REMOTE LOCATIONS

Nonoperating Room Anesthesia (NORA)

Several procedures requiring anesthesia are being performed in locations outside the operating room (OR), such as endoscopy suites, cardiac catheterization laboratories, and invasive radiology units. More and more debilitated patients are being managed in these non-OR locations. Administering anesthesia in such locations is referred to as nonoperating room anesthesia (NORA). NORA is challenging and requires an adequate understanding of the principles of anesthetic management to ensure a successful outcome. The American Society of Anesthesiologists (ASA) published its clinical guidelines in 2018 to standardize NORA in routine practice. The NORA procedure location facilities should be augmented on the lines of a conventional OR to ensure patient safety.

Difficulties Associated with NORA

- Lack of familiarization with a new place makes the anesthesiologist uncomfortable.
- Nonavailability of critical equipment and supplies and trained assistants.
- The operator is usually a physician and not a surgeon.
- Risk of radiation exposure.
- Many of them are darkroom procedures.
- Patients are sicker and less optimized and cannot be subjected to major procedures in OR. It has been estimated that NORA sites tend to have a greater proportion of the patients in ASA Physical Status Class III-V.
- Designs of NORA sites are different from that of a regular OR, which further restricts the approach to safe anesthetic care.
- These places are essentially non-standardized OR where the environment is suited to the proceduralist and not the anesthesiologists.
- The NORA suite also does not have scavenging devices.

Preanesthetic Evaluation

The patient population is usually at high-risk for surgery and planned for interventional procedures in NORA suites. Preanesthetic evaluation of patients is a critical step in managing these patients, including past medical, surgical, anesthesia, family, medication, and allergic reactions along with procedure-related problems. A thorough preanesthetic evaluation may not have been performed. A thorough medical evaluation is mandatory, along with consultation with other specialists given their comorbidities.

Preprocedural Diagnostics

Pre-procedural diagnostic testing should be individualized besides baseline laboratory tests, including blood count, hepatic and renal function parameters, and coagulation profile. The need for a chest X-ray and electrocardiogram can be ascertained as dictated by the patient's condition.

Preprocedural Examination

Special attention must be paid to airway assessment since hypoxia and desaturation are the most common respiratory events during the periprocedural period. Smoking, lung disease, older age, malnutrition, chronic obstructive pulmonary disease, higher ASA scores, impaired sensorium, and obstructive sleep apnea are the other medical risk factors. Pulmonary function tests and/or consultation from the department of pulmonary diseases may be useful in patients with bronchial asthma or chronic obstructive pulmonary disease. Bronchodilators should be continued. Cardiac evaluation is equally significant since ischemic heart disease, cardiac failure, diabetes, stroke, peripheral vascular disease, renal insufficiency (creatinine above 2 mg/dL), high-risk surgery, and older age have been determined as risk factors.

Preprocedural Medications

The current medications, especially anticoagulants, antiplatelets, and antihypertensives, should be reviewed. While it is advisable to continue most of the drugs, it will be prudent to avoid immediate initiation of beta-blocker drugs. However, these drugs should be continued if patients are already receiving these. Angiotensin-converting enzyme inhibitors and angiotensin receptor blockers may be withheld 12–24 hours before the procedure due to the concerns of causing hypotension. Diuretics may also be withheld on the day of the procedure. Other antihypertensive drugs should be continued during the periprocedural period.

Preprocedural Fasting

The fasting status for NORA patients should be similar to the practice in general anesthesia. It is important to confirm the fasting status of patients for NORA. In patients for NORA, clear fluids, such as water, and non-particulate juices, such as apple juice, can be taken until two hours before the procedure. Preoperative substrate administration helps improve diabetic control and helps alleviate the discomfort of fasting, especially in the elderly.

Anesthetic Concerns

All anesthetic techniques, including sedation, GA with endotracheal intubation or laryngeal mask, and RA can be used in NORA. Sedation techniques can be divided into mild sedation, moderate sedation, and deep sedation. Since the surgical or interventional procedures are often of short duration and with a lesser degree of tissue handling, drugs with rapid onset and offset must be used. If needed, only short-acting neuromuscular blocking agents should be used. Patient-controlled sedation has also been described. Propofol, midazolam, fentanyl, and remifentanil are popular drug choices. New drugs have been described, which include fospropofol and remimezolam. Remimezolam deserves special mention since it has a faster onset of action and shorter duration than midazolam. Both these drugs are yet to be approved. Paracetamol is safe for postoperative pain relief. Regional nerve blocks can be used, but spinal anesthesia and supraclavicular brachial plexus blocks should be avoided.

Standard monitoring of patients undergoing NORA includes ECG, blood pressure measurement, oxygen saturation, exhaled carbon dioxide, and temperature. Regular end-tidal carbon dioxide ($EtCO_2$) measurement is strongly recommended.

Postprocedural Patient Care

All patients undergoing a non-OR procedure should be closely monitored for any airway-related event, hemodynamic stability, and adequacy of pain control. Possible adverse events such as PONV should be also followed up carefully. Respiratory events are the leading causes of morbidity and mortality. Difficult or esophageal intubation and aspiration of gastric contents were the other common complications.

DISSOCIATIVE ANESTHESIA

The term dissociative anesthesia is given to a state where there is a feeling of detachment or dissociation from the environment and/or self due to dissociation between the thalamo-neocortical system with the limbic system. It is characterized by catalepsy, catatonia, amnesia, and analgesia. Dissociative anesthesia is most commonly used for short surgical procedures that do not require muscle relaxants but where analgesia and amnesia are desired. Dissociative drugs distort perceptions of sight and sound and create feelings of detachment or dissociation from a person's environment and self. Although these effects are mind-altering, they are not technically hallucinations. Dissociative drugs are thought to work by disrupting the action of glutamate throughout the brain, thereby affecting the perception of pain, responses to environmental stimuli, and memory.

Dissociative Drugs

Ketamine is the anesthetic agent clinically used for dissociative anesthesia. Ketamine is a racemic mixture of R(-) Ketamine and S(+) Ketamine. S(+)Ketamine is a three to four times more potent analgesic that has faster clearance and causes lesser psychomimetic reactions.

Ketamine

Ketamine is the only anesthetic available with analgesic, hypnotic and amnesic properties. It is available in 10 mg/mL and 50 mg/mL concentrations and can be administered IV and intramuscularly. The details of the pharmacology of ketamine are described in Chapter 5. While recovering from the effects of ketamine, patients experience hallucinations which can be reduced by premedication with benzodiazepines (usually oral diazepam 0.15 mg/kg an hour preoperative or 0.1 mg/kg IV) and by recovering the patient in a quiet area. Ketamine increases the intracranial pressure and, for this reason, should be avoided wherever possible in those patients with recent head injuries.

Ketamine has been used for induction and maintenance of anesthesia, as an antidepressant, in TIVA, as an analgesic, for management of chronic pain, for neuroprotection, and for treatment of postoperative shivering. Ketamine, when used as an anesthetic agent, is associated with the emergence delirium, which is characterized by undesirable psychotic reactions, vivid dreaming, a sensation of floating, illusions, and a sense of euphoria. Emergence delirium is more common in females and is treated by administration of benzodiazepines.

MULTIPLE CHOICE QUESTIONS

1. **Total intra-venous anesthesia (TIVA) is indicated explicitly in all *except*:**
   a. Long QT syndrome (QTc ≥500 ms)
   b. Patients with pseudocholinesterase deficiency
   c. Patients with malignant hyperthermia
   d. Patients with a history of severe postoperative nausea and vomiting

2. **In the target controlled infusion (TCI) system is a type of total intravenous anesthesia (TIVA) in which:**
   a. Adequate drug concentration is ensured at the effect site
   b. A drug bolus is given initially, followed by an infusion at a rate that alters according to the drug's elimination from the body
   c. Two-way transfers are done from central to multiple peripheral compartments
   d. All of the above

3. **In the closed loop automated drug delivery system:**
   a. An anesthesiologist has to assess the depth of anesthesia and make necessary changes
   b. There is intervention response capability and automatic generation of a new control signal
   c. There is no feedback signal
   d. All of the above

4. **An ideal drug for total intravenous anesthesia (TIVA) should have:**
   a. Prolonged context-sensitive half-time
   b. Active metabolites
   c. Rapid onset and offset
   d. Prolonged context-sensitive decrement time

5. **In total intravenous anesthesia (TIVA) depth of anesthesia can be monitored by:**
   a. Processed electroencephalogram (EEG) monitoring
   b. Minimum alveolar concentration monitoring
   c. Measuring blood levels of the drugs
   d. Physiological parameter monitoring

6. **The advantages of total intravenous anesthesia (TIVA) include all *except*:**
   a. It is not expensive because of the lesser requirements of drugs, disposables, and specialized equipment
   b. Significant reduction in postoperative nausea and vomiting
   c. Better attenuation of stress response to surgery and anesthesia

CHAPTER 14 ♦ Special Anesthesia Techniques

d. Preferable in cases with ventilation-perfusion (V/Q) mismatch
7. **The difficulties associated with non-operating room anesthesia (NORA) include all** *except*:
   a. Lack of familiarization with a new place makes the anesthesiologist uncomfortable
   b. Non-availability of critical equipment and supplies and trained assistants
   c. The operator is usually a physician and not a surgeon
   d. Patients tend to get hypothermic

8. **All are correct for dissociative anesthesia** *except*:
   a. There is a dissociation between the thalamoneocortical system with the limbic system
   b. Remifentanil is popularly used for dissociative anesthesia
   c. It is characterized by catalepsy, catatonia, amnesia, and analgesia
   d. Dissociative drugs distort perceptions of sight and sound

Answers
1. b
2. d
3. b
4. c
5. a
6. a
7. d
8. b

CHAPTER 15

Daycare Anesthesia

Pratibha Panjiar

Learning Objectives

- Set up for daycare surgery
- Principles of daycare anesthesia
- Patient selection and assessment for daycare anesthesia
- Anesthetic technique for daycare anesthesia
- Postoperative management
- Discharge to home
- Procedural sedation outside the operating room

INTRODUCTION

AS4.6: Observe and describe the principles and the steps/techniques involved in daycare anesthesia.

Daycare surgery (DCS) (also known as ambulatory surgery and outpatient surgery) refers to admitting patients on the day of operation and discharging them within 12–24 hours of operation, meaning that the patient does not require overnight stay in a hospital bed. Anesthesia administered to the patient posted for daycare surgery is known as daycare anesthesia (DCA) or ambulatory (outpatient) anesthesia.

James H Nicoll, a pediatric surgeon from Glasgow, is fondly referred to as the 'Father of Day Surgery.' He performed DCS at the Glasgow Hospital for Sick Children between 1894 to 1914. Ambulatory anesthesia was a recognized post-subspecialty after the Society for Ambulatory anesthesia (SAMBA) was established in 1984. Ambulatory surgery now accounts for nearly 80% of elective surgeries in the United States.

SET UP FOR DAYCARE SURGERY

There are four types of setup that provide the facility of DCS.

Hospital Integrated

In this, DCS and inpatient surgeries share the surgical facilities like operation room or surgical equipment. However, a separate area is assigned for preoperative preparation and recovery of ambulatory patients. This setup offers the advantage of being cost-effective and permits sharing of surgical equipment. The potential disadvantage of this setup is the risk of ambulatory surgeries getting delayed or canceled in favor of urgent or emergent inpatient procedures.

Hospital Self-contained

In this, DCS is performed structurally and functionally separate from the inpatient facilities of that hospital. The setup has a separate admission area, operating rooms, recovery areas, and administrative facilities. This setup is ideal as it promotes a patient-focused flow of care. However, there is duplication of surgical equipment, and personnel performing DCS may not have the best skills.

Freestanding

These are independent setups that are completely separated from inpatient and emergency facilities. Some of these setups have the facility of overnight stays in case of potential perioperative complications. These centers have a detailed plan to care for patients needing urgent or emergent transfer to a nearby hospital.

Office-based

Ambulatory surgeries or diagnostic procedures are performed in a physician's office. This arrangement is convenient for the patient and doctor and offers a lower total procedure cost. They do not have the capability of managing perioperative complications.

PRINCIPLES OF DAYCARE ANESTHESIA

- The patient selected for daycare anesthesia should meet the medical, surgical, and social criteria enumerated in **Table 1**.
- All patients should be evaluated in a preanesthetic clinic, and all comorbid conditions should be optimized before surgery.
- The patient must understand the planned procedure and postoperative care required at home and give written informed consent.
- Anesthetic techniques and drugs should be chosen in a manner to allow early postoperative recovery and with minimal perioperative complications risk.
- Patients should be monitored following ASA standards as done in inpatient surgeries.
- Effective postoperative analgesia must be ensured.
- Detailed verbal and written instructions about postoperative care must be provided before discharge.

Table 1: Patient selection criteria.

Surgical criteria	Medical criteria	Social criteria
Surgeries that involve less tissue trauma. Except minimally invasive surgery/laparoscopic surgery, avoid major abdominal and thoracic surgeries	Patient selection is not based on ASA physical status but general health status	A responsible adult should be available to escort and also to stay with patient for reasonable time after operation
Surgeries where large perioperative fluid shifts, significant intraoperative or postoperative blood loss, or the need for specialized postoperative care are not to be done as day-care	No upper age limit for ambulatory surgery. Premature babies with post-conceptual age >60 weeks are relatively contraindicated as they are at increased risk of postoperative apnea	A good means of transport and communication should be available to the patient at home
Availability of physician/surgeon for 24 hours in case of any emergency readmission	Obesity is not a contraindication provided appropriate resources and skilled anesthetists are available	

Table 2: Procedures that can be done on a daycare basis.

Specialty	Surgical procedures
General surgery	Laparoscopic cholecystectomy, pilonidal sinus, perianal fistula, hemorrhoidectomy, breast biopsy, simple mastectomy, open or laparoscopic hernia repair, gastric banding, fundoplication
Orthopedics	Carpel tunnel release, arthroscopic surgeries, fracture reductions, minimally invasive hip surgery, implant removal
Gynecology	Laparoscopic tubal ligation, diagnostic laparoscopy and hysteroscopy, hysterectomy, endometrial ablation
Ophthalmology	Cataract surgery, occuloplasty, squint repair
Otolaryngorhinology	Adenotonsillectomy, tympanoplasty, thyroidectomy, parathyroidectomy, Grommet insertion
Pediatric surgery	Circumcision, inguinal hernia repair, orchiopexy, hydrocele resection
Neurosurgery	Cranioplasty, lumbar microdiscectomy, vertebroplasty
Dental surgery	Tooth extraction
Urology	Pyeloplasty, vasectomies, prostatectomy
Vascular surgery	Varicose vein surgery, dialysis fistula creation

The procedures that can be done in daycare are listed in **Table 2**.

GOALS OF DAYCARE ANESTHESIA

- To make surgery convenient, comfortable, and safe for the patient
- To reduce waiting time for elective surgery
- To reduce the cost of surgery
- To reduce hospital-acquired infections
- To encourage early recovery and mobilization in a familiar environment

MODE OF DAYCARE ANESTHESIA

The basic steps of performing day-care anesthesia (preanesthetic checkup, intraoperative anesthesia and monitoring, postoperative care, and discharge) remain the same as required for inpatient surgery. The various modes of performing day-care anesthesia are:
- General anesthesia
- Regional anesthesia (spinal anesthesia, peripheral nerve blocks)
- Monitored anesthesia care
- Monitored anesthesia care with procedural sedation.

PREANESTHETIC CHECKUP (PAC)

All patients planned for ambulatory anesthesia should undergo preoperative assessment well in advance so that all required investigations can be performed to avoid any last-minute cancellations. Moreover, adequate optimization of the patient comorbid conditions can be done so that risk of associated postoperative complications can be reduced.

History and Physical Examination

A detailed history of all comorbid conditions like diabetes, hypertension, asthma, and obstructive sleep apnea (OSA) should be obtained. Medication history like antiplatelets, anticoagulants, and oral hypoglycemic agents should be reviewed. ASA physical status I and II patients are ideal for DCS. However, the lower physical status of a patient is not a contraindication for DCS. ASA III or IV patients can be taken for surgery after adequate optimization. Careful systemic examination, including meticulous airway assessment, is the key element of preoperative assessment.

Investigations

There are no special investigations recommended for DCS, and the institutional protocol for in-patient surgery must be followed.

Preoperative Information

Verbal and written preoperative fasting instructions should be conveyed well before the time of admission for the procedure. The recommended guideline fasting period is listed in **Table 3**. Instructions about medications to continue till the day of surgery and the medications that need to be stopped should be provided.

Premedication

The primary objective of administering premedication is to allay the anxiety of the surgical patient. The use of anxiolytic drugs to allay anxiety is discouraged in ambulatory anesthesia as it can cause postoperative sedation. Short-acting benzodiazepines like midazolam are preferred for anxious adult patients and pediatric patients.

Anesthetic Techniques

As the patients are discharged on the day of surgery, the anesthetic technique and drugs should allow complete postoperative recovery and have minimal side effects like postoperative respiratory depression and postoperative nausea and vomiting. An ideal anesthetic technique for DCS should have the following characteristics:

- *Faster onset (induction) and offset (recovery) of action*: General anesthesia is the most popular technique after the advent of newer and safer anesthetic drugs like propofol, fentanyl, remifentanil, desflurane, etc. (faster induction and recovery with minimum side effects). Spinal anesthesia can also be used with short-acting local anesthetics.
- *Minimal risk of post-anesthesia sedation and respiratory depression*: Anxiolytic drugs like midazolam are usually avoided except in pediatric or adult anxious patients. Short-acting opioids are preferred to avoid postoperative sedation and respiratory depression.
- *Good postoperative pain relief*: Effective postoperative pain control is imperative for the early discharge of the patients. Administration of adequate analgesia before skin incision (preemptive analgesia) provides good intra- and postoperative analgesia. Multimodal analgesia using multiple classes of analgesics like opioids, dexamethasone, local infiltration, non-steroidal anti-inflammatory drugs (NSAIDs), and paracetamol provide excellent analgesia and decreases the side effects of drugs.
- *Minimal risk of postoperative nausea and vomiting (PONV)*: Regional anesthesia is preferred in patients at high-risk of PONV. Avoid emetogenic drugs like nitrous oxide and opioids. The Apfel scoring system is used to predict the risk of PONV (**Table 4**). The drugs used for PONV prophylaxis are listed in **Table 5**. They can be given pre- or intraoperatively, either alone or in combination, depending on the risk of PONV.

Table 3: Fasting period guidelines.

Types of food	Minimum fasting period in hours
Clear fluids	2
Breast milk	4
Formula feed	6
Light meal	6
Fatty meal	8

Table 4: Apfel scoring system.

Risk factors	Score
Female gender	1 point
Non-smoker	1 point
History of the previous PONV	1 point
Postoperative use of opioids	1 point
Risk of PONV	**Number of points**
10%	0
20%	1
40%	2
60%	3
80%	4

PONV: postoperative nausea and vomiting

Table 5: Commonly used drugs for PONV prophylaxis.

Drug	Intravenous dose
Ondansetron	4 mg
Granisetron	0.35–1 mg
Dexamethasone	4-8 mg
Metoclopramide	10 mg
Droperidol	0.625–1.25 mg

PONV: postoperative nausea and vomiting

GENERAL ANESTHESIA

General anesthesia is the preferred technique for DCS.

Induction of Anesthesia

Propofol is the induction agent of choice as the use of long-acting induction agents like thiopental is not desirable. Ketamine is avoided in patients posted for ambulatory surgery as it can cause postoperative hallucinations. Etomidate is also not preferred for these patients as it can cause myoclonus and adrenal suppression and is associated with an increased risk of PONV.

Analgesic Drugs

Opioids should be used with caution in ambulatory surgery to avoid postoperative respiratory depression and PONV. Fentanyl and remifentanil are the commonly used opioids for DCS. Tramadol, paracetamol, NSAIDs, and dexmedetomidine are also used to provide intra- and postoperative pain relief. Local infiltration of the incision site by the local anesthetic is recommended to decrease the need for analgesic drugs.

Muscle Relaxants

Intermediate-acting muscle relaxants like atracurium and rocuronium are used to achieve intraoperative muscle paralysis. Ideally, neuromuscular monitoring should be used to titrate the use of muscle relaxants. Residual postoperative muscle paralysis can delay recovery. Short-acting depolarizing muscle relaxant that is succinylcholine can also be used where indicated.

Inhalation Agents

Newer inhalation agents like desflurane and sevoflurane have faster onset and recovery profiles and are best suited for DCS. Desflurane is the ideal inhalation agent for ambulatory anesthesia as it has the fastest recovery time. Sevoflurane being sweet-smelling, is often used for inhalation induction, especially for pediatric ambulatory surgery. Nitrous oxide is routinely used as an adjuvant inhalation agent for DCS as it deepens the plane of anesthesia and decreases the risk of awareness.

Airway Adjuncts

Supraglottic airway devices are commonly used in DCS as they have the following advantages:
- Muscle relaxants can be avoided
- Less incidence of sore throat, hoarseness, laryngospasm
- Cost-effective.

TOTAL INTRAVENOUS ANESTHESIA (TIVA)

Total intravenous anesthesia is an anesthesia technique wherein infusions

of other intravenous agents like propofol, dexmedetomidine, and remifentanil are commonly used to maintain anesthesia. TIVA is usually used for office-based ambulatory surgeries. It offers the following advantages:
- Reduced incidence of PONV
- Rapid and smooth recovery
- Minimizes operating room pollution.

REGIONAL ANESTHESIA

Spinal Anesthesia

Spinal anesthesia can be safely used in patients posted for daycare lower abdomen or limb surgeries. Short-acting local anesthetic agents (like 2-chloroprocaine and 2% hyperbaric prilocaine) are preferred. Long-acting local anesthetic agents (bupivacaine) can also be used for spinal anesthesia in low doses with adjuvants like fentanyl, dexmedetomidine, and dexamethasone. Administration of low doses of local anesthetic ensures early postoperative motor recovery, whereas adjuvants help prolong the duration of postoperative analgesia. Spinal anesthesia offers better postoperative analgesia, awake and conscious patients, and less incidence of PONV.

Epidural Anesthesia

Epidural anesthesia is rarely used for adult ambulatory anesthesia. It is very cumbersome and needs a lot of care and vigilance. Caudal epidural analgesia in children is commonly used for postoperative pain relief.

Peripheral Nerve Blocks

Various peripheral nerve blocks are commonly used for DCS. Ultrasound guidance has made these blocks safer than before. They provide excellent postoperative analgesia and help avoid complications associated with general anesthesia.

MONITORED ANESTHESIA CARE

Monitored anesthesia care (MAC) is an anesthesia service that includes all aspects of perianesthesia care. It is a specific anesthesia service for diagnostic or therapeutic procedures performed under local anesthesia where anesthesia service is required for monitoring the patient vitals (e.g., during cataract surgery) or to provide sedation and analgesia titrated to a level that preserves spontaneous breathing and airway reflexes.

Intraoperative Monitoring

The ASA standard minimum mandatory monitoring (noninvasive blood pressure, temperature, oxygen saturation, end-tidal carbon dioxide, electrocardiogram) is recommended for all-day care surgeries.

POSTOPERATIVE MANAGEMENT

Postoperative Recovery

The recovery after ambulatory surgery decides how fast a patient can be discharged back home. The recovery can be divided into three stages:

Phase I (Early Recovery)

Includes recovery of protective reflexes and awakening from anesthesia in the postoperative care unit (PACU).

Phase 2 (Intermediate Recovery)

The patients are monitored in the ward and discharged home once they meet the discharge criteria.

Phase 3 (Late Recovery)

Recovery at home.

Fast Track Recovery

When stable patients do not require monitoring in PACU and bypass phase 1 recovery and go directly to the phase 2 unit, it is known as fast-track recovery.

Postoperative Pain Management

Postoperative pain is assessed with the help of various comprehensible pain scores like the visual analog scale and numeric rating scale. Pain is usually managed with non-opioid analgesics like paracetamol, NSAIDs, and tramadol.

PONV

In case of persistent postoperative vomiting despite PONV prophylaxis, alternative treatment should be considered, like correction of hydration status or hypovolemia and bladder catheterization in case of urine retention. The second line drugs like promethazine (6.25 mg) and propofol (20 mg) may be given for symptomatic relief.

OTHER CONSIDERATIONS AND DISCHARGE

All patients are monitored in PACU so that any side effects of anesthetic drugs or postoperative surgical complications can be addressed in time. The patient's readiness for discharge from PACU is commonly assessed by the Modified Aldrete Recovery Score (described in Chapter 18). The abilities to take oral fluids and to void are no longer considered criteria for discharge.

A discharge summary with details of the anesthetic technique used and the specific postoperative instructions should be provided to the patient and the person accompanying the patient. They should be instructed about when and how to contact the doctors. Advice should be given not to drink alcohol, operate machinery or drive for at least 24 h after a procedure performed under general anesthesia.

PROCEDURAL SEDATION INSIDE AND OUTSIDE OPERATION ROOM

> **AS4.7:** Observe and describe the principles and the steps/techniques involved in anesthesia outside the operating room.

Procedural sedation is a 'technique of administering sedative or dissociative agents, with or without analgesics, to a patient so that unpleasant diagnostic/therapeutic procedures are tolerated without adversely affecting cardiorespiratory function.' Procedural sedation is given to allay anxiety or to prevent patient movement and thus provide suitable operating conditions for some procedures, to tolerate some uncomfortable positions, or in some situations, to provide analgesia. Some common procedures where PS is required are:

Inside Operating Room
- Ambulatory procedural centers
- For minimally invasive procedures
- Minor surgeries
- Ophthalmologic procedures

Outside Operating Room
- *Radiological procedure*: Pediatric or uncooperative patient posted for imaging
- Endoscopic procedures
- Bronchoscopic procedures
- Dental procedures

Technique

All prerequisites required for general anesthesia should be followed for procedural sedation, such as preanesthetic checkups, fasting protocols, availability of anesthesia machines, and other equipment required for resuscitation. ASA minimum mandatory monitoring should be followed in all patients posted for procedural sedation. Furthermore, the patient's response to verbal commands should also be monitored during moderate sedation. Administration of supplemental oxygen is recommended for moderate to deep sedation.

Levels of Sedation

Three levels of sedation have been defined:
1. *Minimal sedation:* Anxiolysis is achieved, but the patient is responsive and maintains the airway.

Table 6: Pharmacological properties of drugs used for procedural sedation.

Drug	Intravenous dose	Time of onset	Duration of action	Metabolism
Midazolam	1.0–2.5 mg	30–60 sec	15–80 min	Liver
Fentanyl	1–2 mcg/kg	1–2 min	1–2 h	Liver
Propofol	1–2 mg/kg	15–30 sec	3–5 min	Liver
Ketamine	1–2 mg/kg	30–60 sec	10–20 min	Liver
Dexmedetomidine	1 mcg/kg slow infusion over 15 min	3–5 min	15 min	Liver

2. *Moderate sedation:* Conscious sedation wherein the patient is sleepier but responds purposefully to verbal or tactile stimuli.
3. *Deep sedation:* The patient can respond purposefully to repeated or painful stimuli and may require a degree of airway or ventilatory support.

Drugs used for Procedural Sedation

Short-acting sedative and analgesic drugs are used for procedural sedation. Some relevant pharmacological facts about the commonly used drugs for procedural sedation are listed in **Table 6**.

Midazolam

Most common drug used for procedural sedation. It is a short-acting water-soluble benzodiazepine. As compared to diazepam, midazolam is two to three times more potent, has a faster onset time, with greater amnesia and less postoperative sedation. The amnestic effects of midazolam are more potent than its sedative effects. Its main side effect is depression of ventilation caused by a decrease in the hypoxic drive. Its antidote is Flumazenil.

Fentanyl

Fentanyl is a synthetic opioid with an analgesic potency of 75 to 125 times that of morphine. Used to provide analgesia along with sedation. Has a more rapid onset and shorter duration of action than morphine. Its main side effects are respiratory depression, nausea, and vomiting. Its antidote is Naloxone.

Propofol

Non-barbiturate intravenous anesthetic agent with an excellent sedative-hypnotic effect. The quick recovery without residual sedation and low incidence of nausea and vomiting make propofol an ideal inducing agent for procedural sedation. Its main side effects are pain on injection, hypotension, bradycardia, and pruritus.

Ketamine

Non-barbiturate intravenous anesthetic agent that produces amnesia as well as analgesia. It does not produce significant respiratory depression and maintains the upper airway reflexes. The main side effects are tachycardia, hypertension, and the emergence delirium.

Dexmedetomidine

It is an α 2-adrenergic receptor agonist that provides sedation and analgesia and, at the same time, preserves respiratory function. The common side effects are hypotension and bradycardia.

MULTIPLE CHOICE QUESTIONS

1. The types of daycare surgery facilities include all *except:*
   a. Hospital integrated
   b. Hospital self-contained
   c. Office-based
   d. Independent
2. The patient selection criteria for daycare surgery include all *except:*
   a. No upper age limit
   b. Patient selection is not based on ASA physical status but on general health status
   c. Availability of physician/surgeon for 24 hours for any emergency readmission
   d. Obesity is a contraindication
3. After consumption of clear fluids, the minimum fasting period recommended before anesthesia delivery is:
   a. 1 hour
   b. 2 hours
   c. 4 hours
   d. 6 hours
4. A commonly used scoring system to predict the risk of postoperative nausea and vomiting is:
   a. Bruce scoring system
   b. PONV scoring system
   c. Apfel scoring system
   d. VONA scoring system
5. The drugs used for procedural sedation include all *except:*
   a. Dexmedetomidine
   b. Propofol
   c. Midazolam
   d. Diazepam

Answers
1. d   2. d   3. b   4. c   5. d

16
Anesthesia for the Elderly

Meenu Chadha

Learning Objectives

- Age changes in the cardiovascular system
- Age changes in the respiratory system
- Age changes in liver and kidneys
- Age changes in the cardiovascular system
- Age changes in the nervous system
- Age changes in the endocrine system
- Age changes in the musculoskeletal system
- Age changes in drug pharmacology
- Preoperative evaluation and optimization
- Anesthetic management in elderly
- Postoperative care and rehabilitation

INTRODUCTION

Aging is associated with a reduction in physiological reserve, disease, cognitive decline, frailty, and exposure to polypharmacy. The aged population is increasing, and so is their need for elective and emergency surgery. A reduced margin of safety makes the elderly (arbitrarily defined as over 65 years of age) more vulnerable to anesthetic complications and thereby prone to morbidity and mortality. Complications can, however, be reduced by a careful preoperative assessment, meticulous anesthetic technique, and good post-operative care. Physiological aging is normal and occurs in all organs and systems. After 40 years of age, organ function is thought to reduce by one percent per year. Functional decline of the cardiovascular, respiratory, renal, central nervous system, hematological, immunological, and musculoskeletal influences the outcome after surgery.

CHANGES IN THE CARDIOVASCULAR SYSTEM

Reduction in Cardiac Output

There is a thickening of the arterial walls due to atherosclerosis making arteries rigid and less elastic. There is a reduced cardiac output due to increased myocardial stiffness, interstitial fibrosis, progressive atherosclerosis, and increased amyloid deposit in the myocardium. Autoregulation of blood flow to kidneys and brain is impaired, making them prone to perioperative ischemia.

Impaired Sympathetic Activity

Heart rate is reduced due to decreased sympathetic activity, fibrotic infiltration, and degenerative changes in the conducting system. The heart's response to stress, adrenergic stimulation, diastolic filling, chronotropic stimulation, and inotropic stimulation is impaired. Venous compliance is impaired, making them susceptible to hypotension in case of blood loss or peripheral pooling of blood.

Cardiac Function

Cardiac muscle hypertrophy secondary to increased systolic afterload leads to myocardial thickening and diastolic dysfunction. The pharmacokinetic and pharmacodynamic response of the anesthetic agent is altered with age, so induction agents may cause hypotension. There may also be diminished response to hypovolemia and atropine due to sinus node dysfunction.

CHANGES IN THE RESPIRATORY SYSTEM

Thoracic Compliance

The compliance of the bony thorax reduces with age with a loss of muscle mass and reduction in the strength of respiratory muscles. The collapse of small airways and alveolar hypoventilation, with increased alveolar compliance, results in air trapping and ventilation-perfusion mismatch.

Lung Changes

Residual volume increases while vital capacity decreases by about 25 mL every year after the age of 20 years. FEV1 also decreases by 200 mL per decade after 20 years of age. Ventilatory responses to hypoxemia and hypercapnia are restricted. Atelectasis and pulmonary infections are more common.

Airway Protective Reflexes

Administration of sedative premedication could increase the risk of aspiration, and their cough and laryngeal reflexes are impaired.

There is a decrease in immune response and mucociliary clearance, making them prone to aspirate and develop postoperative pneumonia. Atelectasis, pulmonary embolism, and chest infections are more after thoracic and abdominal surgeries. Early mobilization and good analgesia can prevent this.

CHANGES IN THE HEPATIC AND RENAL SYSTEM

Renal Changes

The glomerular filtration rate decreases by 6-8% per decade. There is a reduced ability to concentrate urine after dehydration and a decreased ability of the kidney to regulate salt balance, especially under stress. The response of the pituitary to dehydration is compromised. Glycosuria may present due to reduced glucose reabsorption. Even a modest rise in creatinine may indicate renal impairment as the creatinine production falls with a decrease in muscle bulk. Changes in renal function influence the pharmacokinetic and pharmacodynamics of anesthetic agents in the elderly.

Hepatic Changes

There is a reduction in liver size with a corresponding decrease in liver and splanchnic blood. The resultant effect on metabolism causes delayed drug clearance. There is a fall in albumin production which leads to decreased plasma protein binding of drugs.

CHANGES IN THE CENTRAL NERVOUS SYSTEM

There is a decrease in neural density and loss of brain mass with a corresponding 10-20% reduction in cerebral blood flow. There is a loss of motor, sensory and autonomic fibers, a decrease in afferent and efferent conduction velocities, and a decline in signal processing rate in the brain stem. They may have impaired temperature regulation and delayed gastric emptying predisposing them to aspiration. Diminution of vision may be seen in more than 30%, and similarly, deafness may occur in about 35% of elderly patients. The elderly are more susceptible to postoperative cognitive dysfunction. Brain neurotransmitters (catecholamines, serotonin, acetylcholine) are depleted. The dose requirement of anesthetic agents reduced sensitivity to centrally acting anticholinergics drugs.

CHANGES IN THE ENDOCRINE SYSTEM

There is decreased secretion of growth hormone, insulin-like growth factor-1, and androgens which may lead to decreased muscle mass and total body water and an increase in adipose tissue. The incidence of diabetes increases by 25% in patients over 80 years, and this may be associated with multisystem involvement.

CHANGES IN THE MUSCULOSKELETAL SYSTEM

The muscle volume and function decrease, limiting exercise tolerance. Exercise tolerance thus cannot be assessed. The elderly are more susceptible to fractures and dislocations, and immobility promotes thromboembolism and pressure necrosis. Care should be taken in patient movement and positioning. Osteoporosis and ligament laxity makes regional technically difficult. Malnutrition is also common, leading to muscle wasting and morbidity, and mortality.

CHANGES IN THE PHARMACOLOGY

The pharmacokinetics of the drugs are altered by decreased renal/hepatic function and protein binding in the elderly. Highly protein-bound drugs, especially central nervous system depressants, have higher free drug levels leading to enhanced drug delivery to the brain. The minimum alveolar concentration of inhalation anesthetic agents decreases by about 4–5% per decade after 40 years of age, making the brain more susceptible to their effects. A higher than expected initial plasma drug concentration is reached due to dispersion of the drug in a contracted blood volume which decreases by 20–30% by the age of 75 years. There is also sequestration of the drugs and delayed excretion as there is an increase in the percentage of adipose tissue.

PREOPERATIVE EVALUATION

Functional physical status, neurocognitive function, evaluation of comorbidities, medication, frailty, and nutrition, must be assessed in addition to routine preoperative evaluation. Attention areas in the preoperative assessment of geriatric patients are summarized in **Table 1**.

Table 1: Attention areas in the elderly.

Category	Assessment
Medical	• Comorbidity/severity • Previous anesthesia • Any addiction
Medication	• Medication review • Anticoagulant drugs • Any allergies
Cognition	• Mental capacity • Decision-making capacity • Communication
Functional capacity	• Gait and balance • Mobility
Dependence on aids	• Visual • Hearing • Mobility • Dentures
Risk score	• Disease specific • Frailty

LABORATORY INVESTIGATIONS

The minimum requirement is an electrocardiogram, complete blood count, kidney function tests, and blood sugar. For low-risk and intermediate-risk surgery, no invasive testing is needed in patients with moderate functional capacity and intermediate clinical predictors. Testing should focus on the nature of comorbidity and the type of surgery.

INTRAOPERATIVE MANAGEMENT

WHO Surgical Safety Checklist

Amendment of the WHO surgical safety checklist has been recommended for patients aged over 75 years (**Table 2**).

ANESTHETIC MANAGEMENT

Anesthesia for the elderly, whether general or regional, should always be performed by an experienced anesthesiologist. The choice of anesthesia depends on the patient's medical condition and the type and duration of surgery.

Inhalation Anesthetics

Most general anesthetic drugs depress cardiovascular and respiratory function. Alterations in pharmacokinetics and pharmacodynamics sometimes lead to adverse effects of the anesthetic drugs. Neurophysiological changes in the brain decrease the MAC linearly and thereby the requirement of the inhalation anesthetic agent.

Intravenous Agents

There is a decrease in the requirement for intravenous anesthetic agents. All drugs must be administered slowly as they may result in significant hemodynamic instability because of the age-related impairment of reflex heart rate response to blood pressure, decreased myocardial contraction, and blood volume contraction. Dose of narcotics should be reduced and short or intermediated acting neuromuscular blocking drugs used.

Regional Anesthesia

Well-performed peripheral blocks are ideal though they are technically difficult because of anatomical changes. Metabolism and clearance of local anesthetic agents may be delayed and so a lower dose should be administered. Regional anesthesia offers advantages like:
- Amelioration of stress response to surgery
- Lessor postoperative thromboembolic complications.
- Decreased blood loss
- Decreased postoperative cognitive dysfunction
- Decreased postoperative pulmonary complications
- Better pain relief.

Table 2: Recommended preoperative amendments to the WHO surgical safety checklist for all patients aged over 75 years.

Sign in: Before induction of anesthesia	Time out: Before surgical incision
Have vital signs been recorded (heart rate, blood pressure, heart rhythm, SpO$_2$, temperature)?	Have possible areas of pressure damage been padded?
Is the patients resucitation status known?	What is patients hemoglobin concentration?
Does the patient have dentures?	What is patient's estimated glomerular filtration rate
Does the patient have any preoperative sores?	
Has the site of any nerve block been confirmed and marked?	

However, regional anesthesia use also has some disadvantages like:
- Complications due to age-related cardiovascular and sympathetic changes and decreased cardiovascular reserve
- Increased risk of nerve palsies and paresthesias.

Monitored Anesthesia Care

Sedation is challenging as these patients are sicker and have comorbid conditions. There is an increased risk of hypoxia, respiratory depression, and apnea with sedative drugs and opioids. Careful and vigilant monitoring by an experienced anesthesiologist is recommended. Oxygen supplementation is needed in most cases.

POINTS TO REMEMBER

- Psychological preparation
- Lessor no premedication
- Difficult intravenous access as veins are fragile
- Preoxygenation as functional residual capacity exceeds the closing capacity.
- Slow intravenous induction
- Difficult airway because of the osteoporotic mandible, loose teeth, edentulous jaw, temporomandibular joint stiffness, cervical spondylosis, atlantoaxial joint arthritis
- Increased sensitivity to inhalation and intravenous agents
- Increased incidence of hypothermia because of impaired ability to sense a cold, less subcutaneous fat, impaired autonomic homeostasis, decreased heat generation, inability to increase metabolic rate, and decreased ability to vasoconstrict and shiver. Forced-air warmers, higher ambient OT temperature, warm intravenous fluid, and covering the patient with blankets are recommended.
- Fluid administration should consider aging, fasting deficit, and the type of surgery. Dehydration may deteriorate the organ function, while fluid overload may cause adverse cardiac events.
- Proper positioning and protection of bony prominences are essential.

Table 3: Recommended supplementary checks to the WHO surgical safety checklist during 'sign-out' for all patients aged over 75 years age.

What is the patients core temperature?
What is the patient's hemoglobin concentration?
Have age adjusted and renal function adjusted doses of postoperative analgesia been prescribed?
Has a postoperative fluid plan been prescribed?
Can the patient be returned safely to ward?

END OF SURGERY CHECKLIST

To "sign-out" the patient before leaving the operation theatre, a supplementary checklist for patients aged more than 75 years should be followed in addition to the completion of the WHO surgical safety checklist (**Table 3**).

POSTOPERATIVE CARE

DVT Prophylaxis

The need depends also on the nature of the surgery. Depending on the need of the patient oral anticoagulants/low molecular weight heparin/mechanical or passive calf compression can be used.

Pain Management

The postoperative analgesia plan must be charted out preoperatively. Nerve blocks, regional anesthesia, and epidural anesthesia should be used to avoid systemic drugs. Multimodal analgesia is recommended. Non-steroid anti-inflammatory drugs (NSAIDs) should be avoided as they may deteriorate the already impaired renal function. Inadequate analgesia may increase postoperative morbidity, such as delirium, cardiorespiratory complications, and risk of thromboembolism because of the inability to mobilize.

Postoperative Cognitive Dysfunction (POCD)

Reduced functional reserve makes the elderly more susceptible to POCD. Etiological factors include hypotension, hypoxia, drug interactions, depression, dementia, alcohol abuse, and metabolic disturbances. Incidence of POCD is lower in day-case surgeries because of fewer medications and early return to familiar surroundings.

REHABILITATION

Geriatric rehabilitation aims to restore function, enhance functional capacity and improve the quality of life, especially in frail patients. Rehabilitation should emphasize maintaining functional mobility and capability, improving balance through exercise, good nutrition, good hygiene, and social and emotional support. The key to rehabilitation in the elderly is to prevent organ disuse.

MULTIPLE CHOICE QUESTIONS

1. **The fall in cardiac output with aging is related to all *except*:**
   a. Atherosclerosis
   b. Myocardial ischemia
   c. Myocardial stiffness
   d. Myocardial amyloid deposits
2. **Heart rate is reduced in the aged due to:**
   a. Decreased sympathetic activity
   b. Fibrotic infiltration
   c. Degenerative changes in the conducting system
   d. All of the above
3. **Vital capacity of the lung decreases after the age of 20 years by about:**
   a. 25 mL every year
   b. 50 mL every year
   c. 75 mL every year
   d. 100 mL every year
4. **Geriatric patients:**
   a. Have impaired temperature regulation
   b. Delayed gastric emptying predisposes them to aspiration
   c. Have a higher incidence of postoperative cognitive dysfunction
   d. All of the above
5. **The brain of the elderly is more susceptible to the effects of inhalation anesthetics as:**
   a. Neurophysiological changes decrease the minimum alveolar concentration
   b. They have cerebral atrophy
   c. Have altered protein binding
   d. The volume of distribution is reduced
6. **The etiological factors implicated in causing postoperative cognitive dysfunction (POCD) include all *except*:**
   a. Depression
   b. Dexmedetomidine
   c. Dementia
   d. Alcohol abuse

Answers
1. b
2. d
3. a
4. d
5. a
6. b

17
Intravenous Access and Fluid Therapy

Rashmi Datta

Learning Objectives

- Peripheral venous access
- Central venous access
- Fluid therapy
- Intravenous fluids
- Perioperative fluids

INTRAVENOUS ACCESS

AS9.1: Establish intravenous access in a simulated environment.

The veins of the body, and thereby the circulation, can be accessed through peripheral or central veins.
- **Peripheral intravenous (IV) access:** These may be divided into:
  - Peripheral venous access
  - Midline access
- **Central venous access:** These may be further divided into:
  - Percutaneous central venous access — non-hemodialysis
  - Peripherally inserted central access
  - Tunneled central venous access
  - Implanted venous access.

PERIPHERAL VENOUS ACCESS

Peripheral vein access is a procedure whereby a cannula with a flexible tube containing a needle is inserted into a small peripheral vein to administer fluids and/or medications or obtain blood samples. It is a basic skill to learn. The catheters placed in the peripheral veins are called peripheral venous access devices (PVAD).

The following steps must be followed to ensure safety and reduce the risk of trauma, infection, discomfort, and complications to the patient.
1. *Identify the correct patient:* Confirm the name, diagnosis, and appropriate hospital identification number of the patient.
2. *Allay anxiety:* Introduce yourself and explain the procedure to the patient.
   - Obtain verbal informed consent before commencing the procedure.
   - Determine the patient's history with IV therapy. On insertion, needle-phobic patients may have a vasovagal attack with bradycardia, and a drop in blood pressure occurs with signs and symptoms of pallor, diaphoresis, and syncope. Needle phobia is a response a result of previous IV insertions.

Box 1: List of items required for setting up an intravenous line.

- Dressing/IV trolley with sharps container and waste bag
- Dressing pack
- Gloves (sterile)
- Alcoholic swabs and chlorhexidine swabs
- 4 × 4 gauze
- Transparent semi-permeable dressing
- Cannula (size depending on need)
- Extension set and prescribed IV fluids
- Syringe 5 or 10 mL with 0.9% normal saline
- Tourniquet

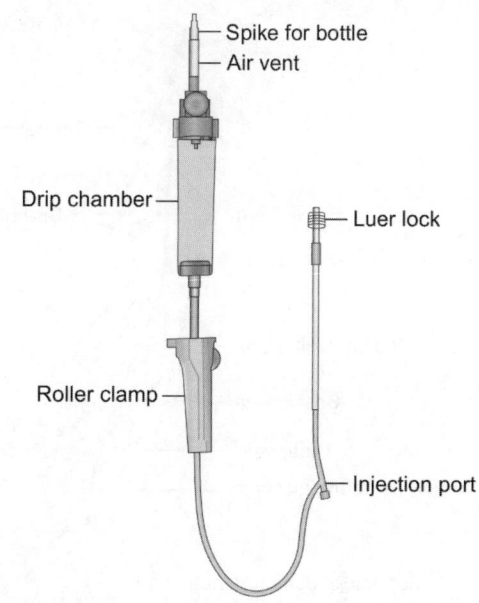

Fig. 1: Components of an intravenous infusion set.

- Ensure the patient is comfortable and sufficiently warm to prevent vasoconstriction.
- Reassure the patient with a soothing tone, educate the patient, keep needles out of sight until the last minute before use, and use topical anesthetics to help manage needle phobia.
- Continually observe the patient.

3. *Ensure:* All equipment and documentation required for the procedure should be at hand (**Box 1**). If an infusion is required, prime the line and de-air it. Connect the IV giving set to the cannula via the appropriate adaptor. The components of an IV set are shown in **Figure 1**.
4. *Position of the patient:* The patient should be lying down.
5. *Choose the right vein:* Preferable choose a vein on the nondominant upper limb, avoiding any joints. The best veins to cannulate are the forearm and the upper arm veins (**Fig. 2**).
    - A well-hydrated person has firm, supple, and easy-to-reach bouncy veins. If you cannot see a suitable vein, palpate for one.
    - You can make the veins more visible by applying a tourniquet. Instruct the patient to clench and unclench his or her fist to compress distal veins and distend them; this helps venous filling. To make veins prominent, tap them gently with the palmar aspect of two fingers. Do not slap the vein or tap them with the dorsal part of the fingers or nails.
    - Bifurcating veins should be accessed below the bifurcation.
    - For difficult IV access (DIVA) in infants, children, obese, and dark-skinned, use equipment like trans-illuminator lights, infrared devices, or ultrasound to facilitate visualization.
6. *Appropriate cannula size:* The cannula size must be smaller than the vein cannulated. The cannula must occupy a maximum of two-thirds of the vein in the cross-section to permit blood drainage around it. The sizes and colors of intravenous cannulae available for clinical use are enumerated in **Table 1**.
7. *Asepsis:* Ensure asepsis throughout the procedure.
    - Before the procedure, wash your hands following your local hand hygiene policy and use an alcohol rub/gel.

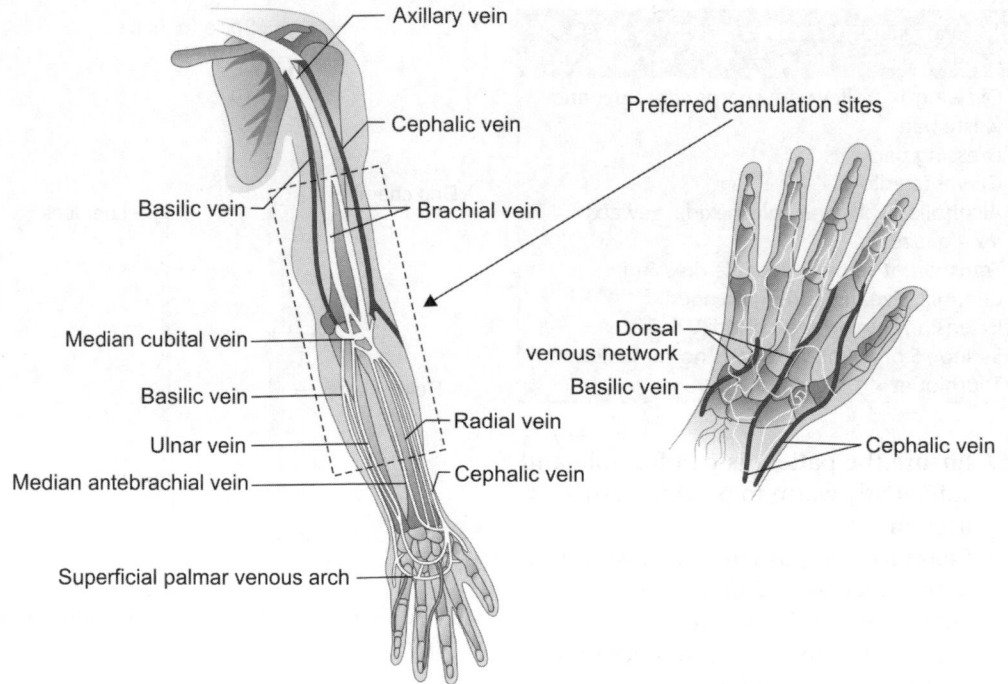

Fig. 2: Common veins of the upper limb.

- Wear disposable gloves.
- Prepare the site by wiping with a chlorhexidine-alcohol swab and allowing it to dry.
- Do not palpate after preparing the skin.

Table 1: Sizes and color of the different intravenous cannulae and their recommended uses.

Size	Colour	Recommended Use
14G	Orange	In massive trauma
16G	Gray	Trauma, surgeries, large volume infusions
18G	Green	Large volume infusions, blood transfusion
20G	Pink	Medications, hydrations, routine therapies
22G	Blue	Chemoinfusions, elderly or pediatric patients
24G	Yellow	Fragile veins, elderly or pediatric patients

8. *Cannulation* (**Fig. 3**)
   - Apply manual skin traction a few centimeters below the proposed cannulation site to immobilize and fix the vein.
   - With the bevel of the cannula facing upwards, insert the needle (and cannula) into the vein at a shallow angle to be in line with the axis of the vein and at an angle <30° to the skin (**Fig. 4**).
   - A flashback of blood is seen in the chamber once you have pierced the vein
   - While maintaining skin traction with the nondominant hand, advance the cannula a few more millimeters, and flatten and push the cannula off the needle.
   - Release the tourniquet and apply pressure to the vein above the cannula

CHAPTER 17 ♦ Intravenous Access and Fluid Therapy

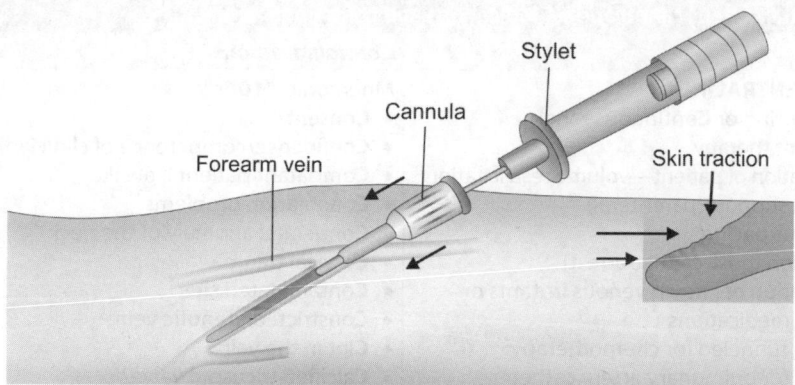

Fig. 3: Cannulation of a peripheral vein.

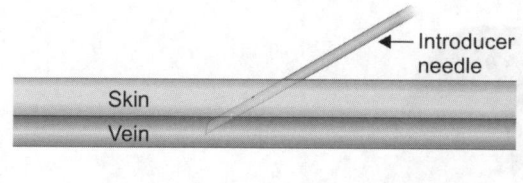

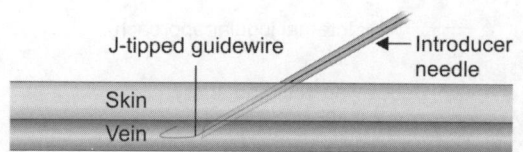

Fig. 4: Seldinger's technique.

tip and withdraw the needle from the cannula and connect the cannula to the IV line assembly.
9. *Securement:* Secure the hub of the cannula with a semi-occlusive or transparent dressing and stress tape to prevent accidental yanking.
10. *Maintain:* The IV cannula must be maintained to prevent blockage and infection by regular site inspection and flushing with normal saline.
11. *Thrombophlebitis prevention:* In case the cannula flow reduces, or redness is seen at the site, it should be removed and a cannula sited at a new location. Heparin-based creams may be applied at these sites of early thrombophlebitis.

CENTRAL VENOUS ACCESS

AS9.2: Establish central venous access in a simulated environment.

To access the central venous system, a central venous catheter (CVC) is peripherally inserted into a large, central vein (commonly the internal jugular, subclavian, or femoral) and advanced until the terminal lumen resides within the inferior vena cava or the superior vena cava. If the central venous pressure has to be measured, then the channel of the CVC used for measurement should open in the intrathoracic part of the great veins. The indications and contraindications of CVC placement are given in **Table 2**.

Techniques of CVC Placement

CVC are placed by the Seldinger technique (**Fig. 4**). The free availability of ultrasound guidance and its safety have made ultrasound-guided CVC placement the standard of care.

Common Sites for CVC Placement (Figs. 5 and 6)

- Internal jugular vein
- Femoral veins
- Subclavian vein

The right internal jugular and left subclavian vein are the most direct paths to the right

Table 2: Central venous cannulation—indications and contraindications.

Indications	Contraindications
Mnemonic **CENTRALINE** • **C**VP monitoring or **C**ontinuous renal replacement therapy • **E**xsanguination of patient—volume resuscitation • **N**utritional support (parenteral) • **T**ransvenous pacing • **R**esuscitation (post-cardiac arrest) • **A**dministration of known venous irritants or vasoactive medications • **L**ong-term tunneled for chemotherapy • **I**ntroducer for pulmonary artery catheter • **N**one/absent peripheral veins • **E**xtraction of air embolus	Mnemonic **"10Cs"** • **C**onsent? • **C**onfidence/competence of clinician? • **C**ombatant patient if awake • **C**oagulation problems • **C**ongenital anomaly of the neck • **C**ervical trauma • **C**ontaminated site • **C**onstricted/stenotic vein • **C**lot in the vein • **C**alcified tricuspid valve?

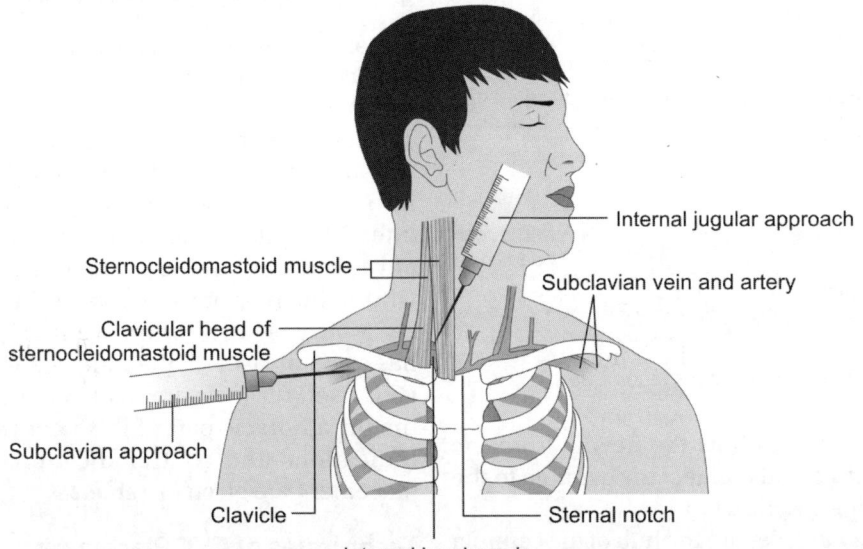

Fig. 5: Cannulation of internal jugular vein and subclavian vein.

atrium via the superior vena cava. Each site has advantages and disadvantages.

Procedure

- Place the patient in the appropriate position for the site selected:
  - For the internal jugular and subclavian approach, place the patient in reverse Trendelenburg with the head turned to the opposite side of the site.
  - For the femoral vein, place the patient in the supine position with the inguinal area exposed with the target leg bent at the knee and the lateral aspect resting on the stretcher or bed.
- CVC should be performed with scrupulous attention to antisepsis and sterile technique to prevent catheter-related infection.
- Prepare the site sterilely using a solution of chlorhexidine and alcohol, sterile gauze, and sterile drapes.

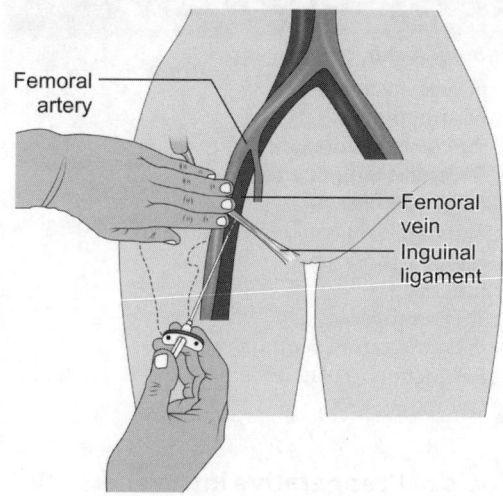

Fig. 6: Cannulation of femoral vein.

- Appropriate draping should be done for asepsis with the surface anatomic landmarks relevant to the venous cannulation exposed.
- It is recommended to place the patient on cardiopulmonary monitoring for the duration of the procedure.
- Equipment/Disposables needed:
  - *Central venous catheter*: In adults, 7 French or larger (the minimum length cannulation of the internal jugular catheter is 15 cm for the right side, 20 cm for the left side)
  - Guidewire, J-tipped
  - Scalpel blade (#11 blade)
  - Dilator
  - Sterile gauze (e.g., 4 × 4 inches [10 × 10 cm] squares)
  - Sterile saline for flushing catheter ports or ports.
  - *Needles*:
    - Small needle for local anesthetic, 25–27 gauge, about 1 inch [3 cm] long.
    - Large finder needle, 22 gauge, about 1.5 inches [4 cm] long. It is used for locating the vein before inserting the introducer needle (recommended for nonultrasound-guided internal jugular vein cannulation).
    - Introducer needle, 18–16 gauge, with an internally beveled hub, about 2.5 inches [6 cm] long.
  - 2- and 5-mL syringes (use slip-tip syringes for the finder and introducer needles)
  - Nonabsorbable nylon or silk suture (e.g., 3-0 or 4-0)
  - Chlorhexidine patch, transparent occlusive dressing
- Infiltrate the skin with 2% lidocaine for local anesthesia around the site of the needle insertion.
- Identify the target vein for cannulation by
  - Landmarks
  - Ultrasound guidance
- Landmarks include:
  - *Internal jugular vein*: The introducer needle should be inserted at a 30° angle at the apex of the triangle formed by the clavicle and the two heads of the sternocleidomastoid. The needle is directed towards the ipsilateral nipple as the vein lies below the medial border of the clavicular head of the sternocleidomastoid. When ultrasound guidance is used, the vein is identified as a compressible structure adjacent to the carotid. The introducer needle is inserted under the vision in-plane.
  - *Subclavian vein*: The introducer needle should be inserted approximately 2 cm inferior to the junction of the middle and lateral third of the clavicle. The needle should be aligned parallel to the clavicular axis and toward the sternal notch. The vein lies posterior to the clavicle.
  - *Femoral vein*: The introducer needle insertion site should be located approximately 1 cm to 3 cm below the inguinal ligament and 0.5 cm to 1 cm medial where the femoral artery is pulsated. The needle is inserted at a 30° angle about 3 cm below the inguinal

ligament and directed superiorly medial to the pulsation of the femoral artery.
- Insert the introducer needle with negative pressure until venous blood is aspirated.
  - The introducer needle should be advanced under ultrasound guidance to ensure the tip does not enter the incorrect vessel or puncture through the distal edge of the vein.
- Once venous blood is aspirated, stop advancing the needle.
- Carefully remove the syringe and thread a J-tipped guidewire through the introducer needle hub. The use of J-tipped guidewire prevents injury to the vessel walls.
- While still holding the guidewire in place, remove the introducer needle.
- Make a small stab in the skin adjacent to the guidewire, just large enough to accommodate the dilator, with a scalpel. Insert the dilator over the guidewire and dilate the track with a twisting motion.
- Advance the CVC over the guidewire.
- Once the CVC is in place, remove the guidewire, check blood aspiration in all ports and flush all ports with sterile saline.
- Secure the CVC in place with the suture and place a sterile dressing over the site.

Complications

Include pain at the cannulation site, local hematoma, infection (both at the site as well as bacteremia), misplacement (possibly causing arterial puncture or cannulation), vessel laceration or dissection, air embolism, thrombosis, and pneumothorax (**Box 2**).

FLUID THERAPY

AS9.3: Describe the principles of fluid therapy in the preoperative period.

Hypovolemia or dehydration is associated with significant postoperative morbidity. The preoperative fluid management strategies aim at maintaining euvolemia in the patient.

Box 2: Complications of CVC insertion.
Mnemonic "**VAS-CATHETER**"
- **V**: Vascular injury
- **A**: Arrhythmias
- **S**: Sepsis and infections
- **C**: Cardiac tamponade
- **A**: Air embolism
- **T**: Thoracic duct injury (chylothorax)
- **H**: Hemothorax, pneumothorax
- **E**: Erosion
- **T**: Thrombosis
- **E**: Embolization of guide-wire
- **R**: Reaction to plastic material and/or antibiotic coating

Goals of Preoperative Intravenous (IV) Fluid Therapy

The goals are:
- To maintain body fluid homeostasis
- To correct preoperative fluid balance (dehydration, hypovolemia).
- To correct plasma constitution (electrolytes)
- To ensure adequate circulatory volume (in combination with vasoactive and/or cardio-active substances)
- To ensure adequate oxygen delivery to organs (in combination with oxygen therapy).

COMMON CAUSES OF PREOPERATIVE HYPOVOLEMIA

Patients coming for surgery may be on maintenance IV fluids before surgery. Certain preoperative conditions and procedures predispose the patient to a hypovolemic state. They are:
- Disorders causing intravascular volume loss due to inflammation and interstitial edema, such as bowel obstruction, gastroenteritis, and pancreatitis.
- Fluid deprivation, such as in the elderly.
- Ongoing hemorrhage.
- Fluid loss from the gastrointestinal tract due to mechanical bowel preparation.

FASTING BEFORE ANESTHESIA AND SURGERY

The risk of aspiration under anesthesia demands preoperative fasting for at least 6 hours before surgery. Water homeostasis is altered by this fasting and other factors like:
- Insensible perspiration contributes to a loss of about 0.3 mL/kg/h of fluids.
- About 500–1,250 mL of fluid is lost in saliva and endogenous gastric secretions during an eight-hour 'fast.'

PREOPERATIVE FLUID INTAKE REDUCES THE RISK OF PULMONARY ASPIRATION

There is a lower risk of aspiration if the gastric volume is less than 25 mL and pH exceeds 2.5. Allowing unrestricted access to clear fluids up to 2 h before surgery:
- Improves patient comfort with reduction of thirst and hunger
- Reduces the acidity of gastric contents
- Does not increase gastric volumes.

Preoperative fasting guidelines have changed the wording from "allow" to "encourage" clear fluids up to 2 h before surgery. Many international guidelines, including those from the American Society of Anesthesiologists, allow the unrestricted intake of clear fluids up to 2 h before elective surgery. Some pediatric centers and adult day-case units have removed all restrictions on clear fluids before surgery. Clear liquids permitted include, but are not limited to:
- Water
- Fruit juices without pulp
- Carbonated beverages
- Carbohydrate-rich nutritional drinks
- Clear tea and black coffee (without milk).

ENHANCED RECOVERY AFTER SURGERY (ERAS)

ERAS pathways recommend oral intake of 200 mL of a maltodextrin carbohydrate drink two hours before surgery. Apart from providing water to the patient, this carbohydrate-rich drink offers the metabolic benefit of:
- Reducing insulin resistance
- Reduction in postoperative nausea and vomiting
- Reduction of postoperative hyperglycemia (a risk factor for nosocomial infections)
- Patients who cannot take or be given fluids orally should be compensated by 1–1.5 mL/kg/h of IV fluids.

INTRAVENOUS FLUIDS

IV fluids are categorized as given below.

Crystalloids

Crystalloids are solutions of low molecular weight substances such as electrolytes or dextrose. Their small molecules can flow easily across semipermeable membranes, which allows for transfer and equilibrium from the bloodstream into the cells and tissues. The equilibrium state of each electrolyte follows the composition of each body compartment. Sodium-containing crystalloids redistribute in the interstitial and intravascular spaces, while glucose-containing crystalloids redistribute in the intracellular, interstitial, and intravascular spaces. The increase in intravascular volume after crystalloid administration is transient, as just about 10–25% of sodium-containing crystalloids remains in the intravascular space after one hour.

Classification of Crystalloids

Isotonic Solutions

- Osmolality 250–310 mOsm/L
- The infusion of isotonic crystalloids creates constant pressure inside and outside the cells, and so the cells remain the same i.e., the cells do not shrink or swell
  - These do not cause any fluid shifts within compartments
  - Isotonic solutions are useful to increase intravascular volume and are utilized

to treat vomiting, diarrhea, shock, and metabolic acidosis, and for resuscitation purposes and the administration of blood and blood products
- Important to monitor patients for fluid volume overload during their administration
- Common isotonic solutions in clinical use include
  - Normal saline (0.9% sodium chloride)
  - Lactated Ringer's solution
  - Hartman's solution
  - Ringer's acetate solution.

Hypotonic solutions
- Osmolality < 250 mOsm/L.
- Have a lower concentration of solutes than plasma. Their infusion lowers the osmolality within the vascular space and causes fluids to shift to the intracellular and interstitial compartments causing cell swelling.
- Rapid infusion requires monitoring for hypovolemia and hypotension due to fluid shifting out of the vascular space.
- Due to potential cellular edema, hypotonic fluids should not be administered to patients with increased intracranial pressure (ICP), by exacerbating cerebral edema.
- Should be used cautiously in patients with burns, liver failure, and trauma.
- Common hypotonic solutions in clinical use include:
  - 5% dextrose
  - 0.45% sodium chloride
  - 0.33% sodium chloride

Hypertonic solutions
- Osmolality > 312 mOsm/L
- The osmotic pressure gradient draws water out of the intracellular space into the extracellular space.
- May cause intravascular fluid volume overload and pulmonary edema, so should not be used for an extended period of time.
- Should not be used in patients with heart or renal disease who are dehydrated.

- Common hypertonic solutions in clinical use include:
  - Dextrose normal saline
  - 5% dextrose and 0.45% sodium chloride
  - 10% dextrose
  - 3% sodium chloride.

Colloids

Colloids are solutions that contain large molecules (nominally MW > 30,000) that cannot pass through semi-permeable membranes. They are used to expand intravascular volume by drawing fluid from extravascular space with their high osmotic pressure. Synthetic colloids are foreign molecules and carry a risk of anaphylaxis.

Classification of Colloids
- *Naturally occurring colloids*
  - Albumin (available as a 5% and 20% solution)
- *Synthetic colloids*
  - Dextrans
  - Hydroxy-ethyl starch (HES)
  - Gelatins: Further sub-classified into:
    - Succinylated fluid gelatins (e.g., Gelofusine)
    - Modified fluid gelatins (e.g., Plasmagel)
    - Urea-cross-linked gelatins (e.g., Haemaccel)
    - Oxy-poly-gelatins (e.g., Gelifundol)

The composition of common IV fluids in clinical use is shown in **Table 3**.

PREOPERATIVE FLUID THERAPY

Fluid therapy can be described based on the different indications for its administration.

Resuscitation
- To restore circulatory volume before surgery, isotonic crystalloids are generally administered as boluses of 20 mL/kg or 500 mL over less than 15 minutes.
- Both 0.9% saline and Ringer's lactate are equally effective. Ringer's lactate may be

Table 3: Composition of common intravenous fluids (all units in mMol/L unless otherwise stated).

	Na⁺	Cl⁻	K⁺	HCO$_3^-$	Energy source	Ca^{+2}	mOsm/L
Normal plasma	135–145	100–110	3.5–5.0	22–26	Glucose 4–7	2.2–2.6	280–295
0.9% NaCl	154	154	—	—	—	—	308
5% Dextrose	—	—	—	—	Glucose 50 g/L	—	154
Hartmann's solution	131	111	5	—	Lactate 29	2	279
Ringer's lactate	130	109	4	—	Lactate 28	1.5	273
Plasmalyte	140	98	4		Acetate 27 Gluconate 23	1.5 (Mg^{2+})	295

preferred in hemorrhagic shock because it minimizes acidosis and does not cause hyperchloremia.
- 0.9% saline is preferred for patients with acute brain injury.
- Hypertonic saline is not recommended for resuscitation.
- Hypotonic fluids are not used for resuscitation since less than 10% of the fluid remains in the vasculature after 1 hour.
- Colloids are to be considered after an infusion of 2 L of isotonic crystalloids, but they offer no major advantage over crystalloids. Complications associated with their use include:
  - Increased risk of renal injury (Hydroxyethyl starch).
  - Poorer outcomes in patients with traumatic brain injury (Albumin).
  - Coagulopathy can occur when > 1.5 L is given (dextrans and hydroxyethyl starch).
- Cross-matched red blood cells are given, but in an urgent situation, 1-2 units of group O Rh-negative blood are an acceptable alternative. Patients receiving > 4 units of blood may require fresh frozen plasma, cryoprecipitate, and platelets to supplement clotting elements.

Routine Maintenance

- The maintenance fluid rate is commonly based on the Holliday-Segar formula. Although it was devised for children admitted to hospitals, based on estimated energy expenditure, it is commonly also used for adults. The formula is based on the assumption that hospitalized patients need more energy. The fluid requirements are determined only by weight.
  - 4 mL/kg/h for the first 10 kg of body mass
  - 2 mL/kg/h for the second 10 kg of body mass (11–20 kg)
  - 1 mL/kg/h for any kg body mass > 20 kg
- If patients need IV fluids for routine maintenance, restrict fluids to:
  - 25-30 mL/kg/day of water
  - Add about 1 mMol/kg/day of potassium, sodium, and chloride
  - Administer 50-100 g/day of glucose for energy.
  - Carbohydrate-containing, hypotonic fluids alone do not address patients' nutritional needs.
- The concept of fluid loss to the third space during surgery has been proved wrong. Replacement of anticipated "third space loss" leads to a worse postoperative outcome due to fluid overload.
- Colloids are not recommended as maintenance fluids.
- Patients receiving prolonged IV fluid therapy need frequent regular monitoring, which includes:
  - Daily clinical fluid status and fluid balance charts

- Daily estimates of urea, creatinine, and electrolytes
- Weight measurement twice weekly
■ Monitoring urinary sodium may be helpful in patients with high-volume gastrointestinal losses
  - Reduced urinary sodium excretion <30 mMol/L indicates body sodium depletion even if plasma sodium levels are normal.
  - Urinary sodium may also indicate the cause of hyponatremia and guide the achievement of a negative sodium balance in patients with edema.
  - Urinary sodium values are, however, misleading in the presence of renal impairment and diuretic therapy.

Reassessment

■ Although the endpoint of resuscitation with fluid therapy is to optimize tissue perfusion, the endpoint is not measured directly.
■ Surrogate clinical endpoints estimated include:
  - Heart rate, mental status, and capillary refill may be affected by the underlying disease process and are less reliable markers.
  - Mean arterial pressure (MAP) is only a rough guideline as compensatory vasoconstriction elevates it in hypovolemia.
  - Clinical indicators of end-organ perfusion
    ♦ Measurements of preload (central venous pressure)
    ♦ Adequate end-organ perfusion is best indicated by urine output of > 0.5 to 1 mL/kg/h.
    ♦ Elevated arterial blood lactate levels may reflect hypoperfusion. However, lactate levels do not decline for several hours after successful resuscitation.
    ♦ Base deficit trend can help indicate whether resuscitation is adequate.
■ Other investigational methods such as measurement of sublingual tissue carbon dioxide or near-infrared spectroscopy to measure tissue oxygenation through the skin may also be considered.

MULTIPLE CHOICE QUESTIONS

1. The recommended method for accessing the internal jugular vein is to insert the introducer needle:
   a. At a 30° angle at the apex of the triangle formed by the clavicle and the two heads of the sternocleidomastoid with the needle directed towards the ipsilateral nipple
   b. With a 30° angle parallel to the lateral edge of the sternal head of the sternocleidomastoid with the needle directed towards the ipsilateral nipple
   c. With a 30° angle at a point just lateral to the carotid pulsation
   d. None of the above

2. There is a lower risk of aspiration if the gastric volume is:
   a. Less than 15 mL and pH exceeds 1.0
   b. Less than 15 mL and pH exceeds 1.5
   c. Less than 25 mL and pH exceeds 2.0
   d. Less than 25 mL and pH exceeds 2.5

3. Clear liquids permitted up to 2 hours before surgery include all *except*:
   a. Fruit juices without pulp
   b. Carbonated beverages
   c. Carbohydrate-rich nutritional drinks
   d. Tea and coffee with milk

4. Crystalloids remain in intravascular space after intravenous administration
   a. For about 3 hours
   b. For about 2 hours
   c. For about one hour
   d. For about 30 min

5. Colloids expand intravascular volume by these methods *except*:
   a. By drawing fluid from extravascular space with high osmotic pressure.

b. By promoting the release of anti-diuretic hormone (ADH).
c. By remaining in the extracellular space for an extended period as their excretion takes time.
d. Their large molecules cannot pass through semi-permeable membranes.

6. **Common hypertonic solutions in clinical use include:**
   a. Urea-cross-linked gelatins
   b. 3% saline
   c. Ringer's Lactate
   d. Hartmann Solution

Answers
1. a
2. d
3. d
4. c
5. a
6. b

CHAPTER 18

Blood and Blood Product Transfusion

Sangeeta Pathak

Learning Objectives

- Importance of blood transfusion
- Blood grouping and cross-matching
- Blood components, their preparation, preservation, use, and shelf-life
- Quality control of blood products
- Safe transfusion
- Monitoring of blood products
- Transfusion reactions
- Challenges in blood transfusion

INTRODUCTION

Blood transfusion involves transferring blood products into one's circulation intravenously. Transfusions are used for various medical conditions to replace lost blood components. Early transfusions used whole blood, but modern medical practice commonly uses only blood components, such as red blood cells, white blood cells, plasma, clotting factors, and platelets. Blood transfusion is a routine, life-saving medical intervention that is generally safe when done appropriately.

Anemia and allogeneic blood transfusions in surgical patients are associated with poor outcomes. Patient blood management (PBM) has been developed as an evidence-based clinical tool by which clinicians can optimize anemia, manage perioperative bleeding, avoid unnecessary blood transfusion and improve patient outcomes. The decision to transfuse should be preceded by careful evaluation of the clinical condition of each patient and not be based exclusively on laboratory results. Transfusion medicine in a hospital setting is mainly focused to ensure that 'the right blood is given to the right patient at the right time and the right place.'

Components of Blood

Red blood cells (RBC) contain hemoglobin, and they supply the body cells with oxygen. White blood cells are not commonly used during transfusion but are part of the immune system and fight infections. Plasma is the "yellowish" liquid part of blood, which acts as a buffer, and contains proteins and important substances needed for the body's overall health. Platelets are involved in blood clotting, preventing the body from bleeding.

Transfusion Trigger

Historically, red blood cell transfusion was considered when the hemoglobin level fell below ten g/dL or the hematocrit fell below 30%. For better patient outcomes, the transfusion trigger level followed today is 7–8 g/dL, as blood transfusion carries risks. The trigger can be higher for patients with poor oxygen saturation and those with symptoms of cardiovascular disease. The outcomes are worsened if large amounts are given. Parenteral iron therapy is preferred in iron deficiency anemia patients with stable cardiovascular parameters. Other blood products are given where appropriate, e.g., to treat clotting deficiencies.

Blood Product Transfusion

It is a general name for a treatment that gives you a component or product of blood. Blood products include red blood cells, plasma, and platelets. A blood product transfusion treats bleeding conditions caused by a lack of blood products, such as anemia and hemophilia. Blood product transfusion is generally safer, but it does have some risks and potential complications. Blood product transfusion is the only method to treat many diseases, disorders, and conditions.

Types of Blood Products

> **AS9.4:** Enumerate blood products and describe the use of blood products in the preoperative period.

Whole blood is rarely transfused today. Blood components are separated and transfused individually, depending on a patient's diagnosis and other factors. Blood products include:

- **Red blood cells:** RBCs have a slightly indented, flattened disk shape. Hemoglobin in RBCs is a protein that contains iron and carries oxygen to its destination. The life span of an RBC is four months, and the body replaces them regularly. RBCs are administered to treat anemia and blood loss.
- **Plasma:** Plasma accounts for around 55% of human blood fluid and is 92% water, and the remaining 8% includes glucose, hormones, proteins, mineral salts, fats, and vitamins. Each of these plays a vital role the blood function. Plasma contains proteins important for blood clotting and fighting infection. Plasma transfusion is indicated in serious burns, liver failure, or clotting disorders, including disseminated intravascular coagulation (DIC).
- **Platelets:** Platelets interact with clotting proteins to prevent or stop bleeding. Platelet transfusions are indicated in thrombocytopenia (marrow suppression, dengue, post-chemotherapy, and radiation therapy).
- **Cryoprecipitate:** Cryoprecipitate contains certain clotting factors and is used to treat bleeding disorders, including hemophilia and von Willebrand disease.
- **White blood cells (WBC):** White blood cells make up less than 1% of blood content but play a vital role in forming defenses against disease and infection. High or low levels of white blood cells indicate disease. White blood cell transfusions are rare and administered to patients with low levels of WBCs, as in cancer patients.

IMPORTANCE OF BLOOD TRANSFUSION

Blood and the components of blood benefit the body in many ways:
1. **Increasing the hemoglobin levels:** Anemia can cause damage to body tissues due to low oxygen delivery.
2. **Help stop bleeding:** Platelets and/or clotting factors help reduce bleeding.
3. **Maintain cardiac output:** Low blood volume can lead to low cardiac output.
4. **Combat blood infections when other methods fail:** Granulocyte transfusions.
5. **Provide red cells and platelets when the bone marrow is compromised:** Blood

cancers, bone marrow transplants, and chemotherapy.
6. **Provide red cells and platelets for patients with blood disorders:** Sickle cell disease, thalassemia, myelodysplasia, and aplastic anemia.

SOURCING BLOOD PRODUCTS

Blood products are sourced either from oneself (autologous transfusion) or someone else's (allogeneic or homologous transfusion), the latter being more common. Using another's blood must first start with the donation of blood. Blood is most commonly donated as whole blood, obtained intravenously, and mixed with an anticoagulant. In developed countries, donations are usually anonymous to the recipient. Still, products in a blood bank are always individually traceable to enable management and investigation of any suspected transfusion-related disease transmission or transfusion reaction. In developing countries, the donor is sometimes specifically recruited by or for the recipient, typically a family member, and the donation occurs before the transfusion.

BLOOD GROUPING AND CROSS-MATCHING

Before a transfusion, compatibility testing between the donor and recipient blood must be done. The first step before a transfusion is to type and screen the recipient's blood. Typing of the recipient's blood determines the ABO and Rh status. The compatibility of different blood groups for transfusion is shown in **Table 1**.

Crossmatching

The goal of blood typing and crossmatching is to find a compatible blood type for transfusion. Crossmatching is performed before a blood transfusion as part of blood compatibility testing, and it involves adding the recipient's blood plasma to a sample of the donor's RBCs. If the blood is incompatible, the antibodies in the recipient's plasma will bind

Table 1: Compatibility of ABO and Rh system for RBC transfusion.

		Donor							
		O-	O+	B-	B+	A-	A+	AB-	AB+
Recipient	AB+	●	●	●	●	●	●	●	●
	AB-	●		●		●		●	
	A+	●	●			●	●		
	A-	●				●			
	B+	●	●	●	●				
	B-	●		●					
	O+	●	●						
	O-	●							

to antigens on the donor's RBCs. This antigen-antibody reaction causes visible clumping or destruction of the RBCs or by reaction with anti-human globulin.

In emergencies, where crossmatching cannot be completed and the risk of dropping hemoglobin outweighs the risk of transfusing uncross matched blood, O-negative blood is used, followed by crossmatch as soon as possible. The laboratory should obtain a pre-transfusion sample in these cases so that a type and screen can be performed to determine the actual blood group of the patient and to check for alloantibodies.

Crossmatching is also used to determine compatibility between a donor and recipient in organ transplantation.

Screening

The sample is also screened for alloantibodies that may react with donor blood. The blood bank also checks for special requirements of the patient (e.g., need for washed, irradiated, or CMV negative blood) and the patient's history to see if they have previously identified antibodies and any other serological anomalies.

Antibody Screening

Commercially prepared RBCs with all the antigens, which direct the production of antibodies causing hemolytic reactions, are mixed with the recipient's serum to detect the presence of those antibodies. It is also carried out with the donor's serum.

Benefits of Typing and Screening

ABO-Rh typing results in a 99.8% chance of a compatible transfusion. Antibody screening increases this safety margin to 99.94%, and an additional cross-match further increases the compatibility to 99.95%.

The distribution of the A, B, O, and AB blood groups in India is 23.16%, 34.10%, 34.56%, and 8.18%, respectively. Rh(D)-positive and Rh(D)-negative populations are 94.13% and 5.87%, respectively. It is important to understand this distribution to cater to blood products in blood banks as per this percentage.

BLOOD COMPONENT PREPARATION AND PRESERVATION

A refrigerated centrifuge was developed in 1960 to separate blood products from units of whole blood and prepare blood components for therapy. Packed RBC (PRBC) and fresh frozen plasma (FFP) are prepared by single-step heavy spin centrifugation. While platelet concentrates (PLTCs), PRBC concentrates, and FFP is prepared by two-step centrifugation. The two main procedures for preparing PLTC are the platelet-rich plasma (PRP) method and the Buffy coat (BC) method. PRP method is simple, comparatively cheaper, and easily done manually, but the platelet and plasma yield is less. BC method is complicated and needs automation. An automated component separator instrument permits the preparation of low-volume BC with a recovery of 90% of whole blood platelets.

The main components are PRBC, PLTC or random donor platelet (RDP), FFP, cryoprecipitate, cryo-poor plasma (CPP), and plasma fractionation products. The last product is produced only in the pharmaceutical industry. 350 mL or 450 mL of whole blood is collected in bags with CPDA-1, or additive solution, and components are separated within 5–8 hours. The component preparation room should be separate and sanitized.

Preservation

Whole blood is collected in containers manufactured from polyolefin or polyvinyl chloride (PVC) bags. The currently used bags provide nearly twice the oxygen permeability of first-generation-plasticized PVC containers and maintain a pH >6 for better platelet survival and function. Proper component storage helps preserve the biological function of the constituents, decrease their metabolic activities, and reduce bacterial growth.

Citrate-Phosphate-Dextrose-Adenine (CPDA) is commonly used for the preservation of blood. Citrate prevents coagulation by chelating calcium. Alkaline pH and phosphate help maintain levels of enzyme 2,3 diphosphoglyceric acid (2,3 DPG), which is essential for oxygen release to tissues. Adenosine helps restore ATP. Dextrose provides nutrition to the banked blood cells. Many other preservative combinations are available commercially.

Storage

As per standard guidelines, the storage temperature for red cells is +2°C to +6°C, for platelets and leucocytes-between +20°C to +24°C, and for plasma products, below −18°C. All components are to be stored in three compartments:
- Untested components
- Tested safe for an issue
- Tested as unsafe or quarantined components for discarding.

Separate equipment is required for keeping safe crossmatched units if available. All components are routinely stored between +20°C and +24°C and transported at the same temperatures. The temperature changes can be monitored and documented either through indicators fixed on units or by checking each component manually for any deterioration.

The storage equipment used is:
- Refrigerators (+4 ± 2°C) for storing whole blood, PRBC, thawed FFP, and other plasma products.
- Platelet incubator-agitators (+22 ± 2°C) with agitation speed at 60 cycles per minute for all platelet products.
- Deep freezers (−80°C) are used for freezing FFP or frozen blood constituents.

The recommended storage conditions and the shelf-life of the commonly used blood components are listed in **Table 2**.

Transport Boxes

During the transport, the components can be stored for a maximum of 24 h, if maintained at the suggested temperatures. PRBC must be maintained between +2°C to +10°C. Transport boxes transport blood or blood components for a short duration between two storage sites. Even bloodmobiles have built-in cold chain storage devices with backup power. All frozen components should be transported in the frozen state. The cold chain maintenance for all blood components should extend to the point of transfusion.

USES OF BLOOD COMPONENTS

RBC

Transfusion of RBCs serves to re-establish the patient's volume of cells after hemorrhage, thereby allowing for an increase in the oxygen-carrying capacity of the blood. RBC transfusion also serves to treat chronically anemic patients.

Plasma

Plasma is mainly transfused to correct deficiencies in clotting factors and to treat shock due to a loss of plasma following severe burns or massive hemorrhages.

Platelets

Platelets are transfused in patients suffering from serious wounds, severe hemorrhaging, aplastic anemia, leukemia, and cancer.

QUALITY CONTROL OF BLOOD PRODUCTION AND STORAGE

Testing of random components to ensure they achieve reliably certain specific standards. It includes analysis of test results and detection of irregularities to identify deficiencies in the

Table 2: Storage recommendations and shelf-life of blood components.

Component	Storage	Expiration
PRBC-component, after apheresis and leucodepletion	4 ± 2 °C	CPDA 1: 35 days
RBCs irradiated	4 ± 2 °C	• With additive solution: 42 days • Open system: 24h • Original expiration or 28 days from date of irradiation, whichever is earlier • To avoid hyperkalemia in neonates 24 h
FFP (Plasma frozen within 24 h of phlebotomy)	≤ -18 °C	12 months
FFP (after thawing)	20–24°C 4 ± 2 °C	• For use for coagulation 6 h • 24 h
Liquid plasma	20–24°C	Open system or pooled 4 h
Cryoprecipitate	≤ –18 °C	12 months
Cryoprecipitate (after thawing)	20–24°C	• 24 h for Factor VIII content • 74 h for fibrinogen content
Platelets and Platelets irradiated	20–24°C with continuous gentle agitation	24 h to 5 days depending on collection system
Apheresis platelets	20–24°C with continuous gentle agitation	24 h to 5 days depending on collection system

PRBC = packed red blood cells; FFP = fresh frozen plasma

production of blood and blood components. Quality control (QC) of blood components is an integral part of the quality management systems in the blood bank. Quality assurance ensures proper yield, functionality, and efficacy of the components for patient care. QC of components is defined as testing random components to ensure they achieve reliably specific standards. It should include analysis of test results and detection of irregularities to identify deficiencies in the production of blood and blood components.

Quality of blood components is achieved only if all aspects of blood collection, component preparation, testing, storage, and transport are controlled and monitored. A blood bank should conform to accommodation and environment standards as per regulation, and the ambient temperature of blood component processing areas should be maintained within a range that should not harm component viability/shelf-life.

SAFE TRANSFUSION AND MONITORING

Essentials for safe blood transfusion are:
- Avoid unnecessary and inappropriate transfusions
- Preventing 'wrong blood and wrong patient' incidents by human error
- The transfusion prescription must contain the minimum patient identifiers and specify components to be transfused, date of transfusion, number of units to be transfused, and the rate or duration of transfusion.
- Preventing identification errors during pretransfusion blood sampling, sample handling in the laboratory, collecting

the component from the blood bank, or transfusion to the patient.
- A final identity check between the patient and blood component is crucial.
- Excellent communication and good documentation at every stage of transfusion.
- Where possible, patients should give 'valid consent' for transfusion.
- Patients should be monitored during transfusion with a minimum of pre-transfusion pulse, blood pressure, temperature, and respiratory rate. The parameters must be checked every 15 min.
- Repeat the administration identity check with each unit.
- Document end of transfusion.

BLOOD TRANSFUSION REACTIONS

Transfusion reactions are adverse events associated with the transfusion of whole blood or one of its components. These may range in severity from minor to life-threatening. Reactions can occur during the transfusion (acute transfusion reactions) or days to weeks later (delayed transfusion reactions) and may be immunologic or nonimmunologic. Immune-mediated transfusion reactions typically occur due to mismatch or incompatibility of the transfused product and the recipient.

A reaction may be difficult to diagnose as it can present with nonspecific, often overlapping symptoms. The most common signs and symptoms include fever, chills, urticaria (hives), and itching. Some symptoms resolve with little or no treatment. Respiratory distress, high fever, hypotension (low blood pressure), and red urine (hemoglobinuria) indicate a more serious reaction.

Types of transfusion reactions include the following: acute hemolytic, delayed hemolytic, febrile non-hemolytic, anaphylactic, simple allergic, septic (bacterial contamination), transfusion-related acute lung injury (TRALI), and transfusion-associated circulatory overload (TACO). All suspected reactions should result in immediately stopping the transfusion and notifying the blood bank, and treating the clinician.

Acute Transfusion Reactions

- *Mild allergic:* Due to hypersensitivity to a foreign protein.
- *Anaphylactic:* A more severe reaction occurs in a patient with IgA deficiency who makes alloantibodies against IgA and receives blood products containing IgA.
- *Febrile non-hemolytic*: Thought to be caused by cytokines released from donor leukocytes.
- *Septic:* Caused by bacteria or bacterial byproducts in contaminated blood.
- *Acute hemolytic transfusion reactions:* Intravascular or extravascular hemolysis.
- *Transfusion-associated circulatory overload (TACO):* When the transfused volume causes volume overload.
- *Transfusion-related acute lung injury (TRALI):* Acute lung injury is due to antibodies in the donor product reacting with antigens in the recipient. The recipient's immune system responds and causes the release of mediators that lead to pulmonary edema.

Delayed Transfusion Reactions

- *Delayed hemolytic transfusion reaction*: Typically caused by an anamnestic response to a previously exposed foreign antigen.
- *Transfusion-associated graft-versus-host disease:* Results from engraftment of donor lymphocytes (commonly found in cellular blood products) into an immunocompromised recipient's bone marrow.

CHALLENGES IN BLOOD TRANSFUSION

The main challenges are adequacy and safety of the blood supply. Attempts to resolve these challenges led to the evolution of blood transfusion into a multidisciplinary field, beyond issues related to blood procurement and storage. Blood transfusion now involves several aspects, including but not limited to the adequate and safe blood supply, appropriate use of blood and blood products, development of novel cellular therapies, manipulation, and prevention of immune responses. The blood supply is now safer largely due to conversion from paid to voluntary non-remunerated blood donors, improvements in donor screening, improvement of assays that detect transfusion-transmissible infections in donor blood, regular quality control on blood units, leukoreduction techniques, blood management, hospital transfusion committees, and hemovigilance.

MULTIPLE CHOICE QUESTIONS

1. **For better patient outcomes, the transfusion trigger level followed in healthy adults is:**
   a. Hemoglobin 7 to 8 g/dL
   b. Hemoglobin 8 to 9 g/dL
   c. Hemoglobin 10 g/dL
   d. Hemoglobin 11 g/dL

2. **Blood and the blood components benefit the body in these ways *except*:**
   a. Increasing the hemoglobin levels
   b. Increasing protein levels
   c. Help stop bleeding
   d. Maintain cardiac output

3. **Cross-matching before a blood transfusion:**
   a. It is a method to choose the same blood group for transfusion
   b. It is a method to determine if the different components of the donor blood match the recipient
   c. It is a test performed for blood compatibility testing
   d. None of the above

4. **A common preservative used for the storage of blood is:**
   a. Citrate-Phosphate-Dextrose-Adenine (CPDA)
   b. 2,3 diphosphoglyceric acid (2,3 DPG)
   c. Sodium meta-bisulphide
   d. Rhesus factor

5. **As per standard guidelines, the storage temperature for red cells is:**
   a. +2°C to +6°C
   b. +20°C to +24°C
   c. +30°C to +36°C
   d. +37°C to +38°C

6. **In Citrate-Phosphate-Dextrose-Adenine (CPDA), used for blood preservation, citrate:**
   a. Helps maintain levels of enzyme 2,3 diphosphoglyceric acid (2,3 DPG)
   b. Helps restore ATP
   c. Helps prevent coagulation by chelating calcium
   d. Provides nutrition to the banked blood cells

7. **Plasma is mainly transfused to:**
   a. To correct severe hypoalbuminemia
   b. As a supplement to platelet transfusion
   c. Correct deficiencies in clotting factors
   d. To treat hypovolemic shock

8. **Essentials for safe blood transfusion include all *except*:**
   a. Always using leukoreduction techniques
   b. Avoid unnecessary and inappropriate transfusions
   c. 'Wrong-blood and Wrong-patient' prevention
   d. A final identity check between the patient and blood component

Answers
1. a
2. b
3. c
4. a
5. a
6. c
7. c
8. a

CHAPTER 19

Pain Pathways and Chronic Pain

Jyotsna Agarwal

Learning Objectives

- Pain and nociception
- Pain processing
- Pain pathways
- Pain inhibitory mechanisms
- Pain assessment
- Pain management
- Principles of pain management in palliative care in the terminally ill
- Interventions for pain relief
- Bio-psycho-social therapy

INTRODUCTION

Pain is defined by the International Association for the Study of Pain, 2020 as "an unpleasant sensory and emotional experience associated with, or resembling that associated with, actual or potential tissue damage."

This definition is expanded upon by the addition of six keynotes:

1. Pain is always a personal experience that is influenced to varying degrees by biological, psychological, and social factors.
2. Pain and nociception are different phenomena. Pain cannot be inferred solely from activity in sensory neurons.
3. Through their life experiences, individuals learn the concept of pain.
4. A person's report of an experience of pain should be respected.
5. Although pain usually serves an adaptive role, it may adversely affect function and social and psychological well-being.
6. Verbal description is only one of several behaviors to express pain; the inability to communicate does not negate the possibility that a human or a nonhuman animal experiences pain.

NOCICEPTION

The "neural process of encoding noxious stimuli" is called nociception. Nociception is not synonymous with pain. Nociception is the neurophysiological activity in peripheral sensory neurons (nociceptors) and higher nociceptive pathways.

PAIN

AS8.1: Describe the anatomical correlates and physiologic principles of pain.

On the other hand, pain is more subjective and involves perception. Pain can be physiologic or pathologic. Physiologic pain is 'protective.'

It is a mechanism to prevent further injury to the organism. Physiologic pain includes acute pain and nociceptive pain. Physiologic pain is mediated by a sensory system consisting of primary afferent neurons, spinal interneurons and ascending tracts, and supraspinal areas (**Fig. 1**). Pain can be classified in various ways, such as acute or chronic pain, malignant or non-malignant pain.

Chronic Pain

Alterations and maladaptations in the nervous system during acute pain can lead to pathologic, long-standing, or chronic pain. When pain becomes pathologic, it can be considered a disease. Since it is considered a disease, chronic pain was included in the International Classification of Diseases (ICD) for the first time in 2019. Pain is considered to become chronic when it is "extending in duration beyond the expected temporal boundary of tissue injury and normal healing, and adversely affecting the function or well-being of the individual." Normal tissue healing time is usually taken to be three months.

Malignant Pain

'Cancer pain' or 'malignant pain' occurs due to the invasion of tumor cells in pain-sensitive structures such as the pleura, peritoneum, peripheral nerves, and nerve plexus. Symptoms will be dictated by the structure invaded, such as predominantly neuropathic pain will be seen in case of invasion of nerve plexus, pleuritic pain symptoms. Cancer treatment therapies such as radiotherapy and chemotherapy can be associated with severe pain conditions such as mucositis.

Nonmalignant Pain

Types of non-malignant pain are described in **Table 1**.

Allodynia

'Pain due to a stimulus that does not normally provoke pain' is called allodynia. For example, a feather touch can be perceived as painful.

Hyperalgesia

An exaggerated response to a normally painful stimulus is called hyperalgesia. For example,

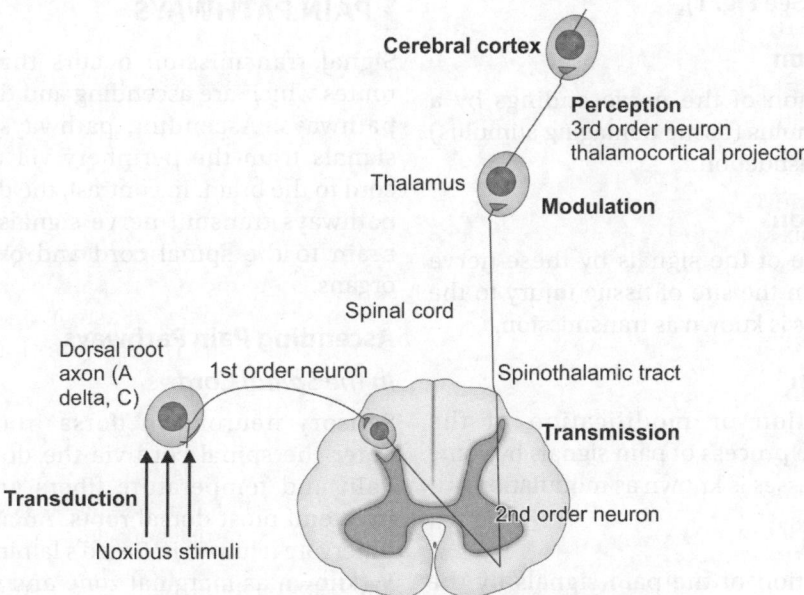

Fig. 1: Ascending pain pathway and pain processes.

Table 1: Types of nonmalignant pain.

Types of non-malignant pain	Features/Examples
Inflammatory	Chronic inflammatory pain, arthritis
Musculoskeletal	• Low back pain, ligaments or muscle injuries • Usually localized to the injured muscle or tendon or myotomes
Neuropathic pain	• Postherpetic neuralgia, complex regional pain syndrome, radiculopathy, trigeminal neuralgia • Pain is typically lancinating, shooting or burning in character. Hyperalgesia and allodynia may also be associated
Post-traumatic pain	Persistent pain developing after injury as trauma, accident, surgery
Orofacial pain or headache	Headaches and orofacial pain can be persistent and become chronic. It can be of various origins such as atypical fascial pain, migraine, cervical pain, trigeminal neuralgia
Visceral pain	Caused by visceral injury or inflammation

light pressure can be perceived as very painful. Secondary hyperalgesia is said to occur if the pain spreads beyond the injury site.

PAIN PROCESSING

The process by which brain perceives the pain-related information involves four main steps: transduction, transmission, modulation, and perception (See **Fig. 1**).

Transduction
The activation of the nerve endings by a noxious stimulus (tissue damaging stimulus) is called transduction.

Transmission
The carriage of the signals by these nerve endings from the site of tissue injury to the brain regions is known as transmission.

Modulation
The reduction or modification of the transmission process of pain signals by some neural processes is known as modulation.

Perception
The perception of the pain signals by the brain is known as perception. Perception is the subjective awareness of pain. The sensory and neural messages are acknowledged by the brain. This is a complex process and involves various functions such as attention, interpretation, and expectation. The initial three processes can be measured objectively, but pain perception is subjective and exhibits inter-individual variability.

PAIN PATHWAYS

Signal transmission occurs through two routes which are ascending and descending pathways. Ascending pathways transmit signals from the periphery via the spinal cord to the brain. In contrast, the descending pathways transmit nerve signals from the brain to the spinal cord and other reflex organs.

Ascending Pain Pathways
In the Spinal Cord
Sensory neurons in dorsal root ganglia enter the spinal cord via the dorsal roots. Pain and temperature fibers are present in lateral most dorsal roots. Aδ and C fiber innervate neurons in Rexed's lamina I, II, and V (known as marginal zone and substantia gelatinosa of grey matter in the spinal cord)

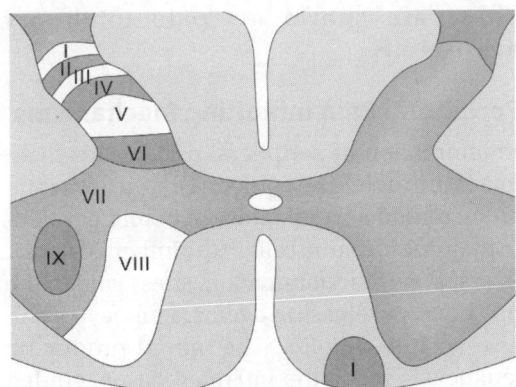

Fig 2: Cross-section of the spinal cord showing Rexed laminae.

(Fig. 2). These fibers carry information about pain and temperature. They cross the midline (decussation) and ascend to the thalamus in the anterolateral spinal cord, forming the spinothalamic tract.

In the Brain

Thalamocortical projections from the thalamus to the somatosensory cortex lead to pain perception in the cortex. Other cortical structures also receive input from pain pathways. These areas include the anterior cingulate gyrus, insula, prefrontal cortex, ventrolateral orbital cortex, and motor cortex. Collateral communication is present between the spinothalamic tract with the hypothalamus and the limbic system.

Integration and Response

These projections mediate affective and autonomic responses associated with pain and lead to the integration of sensory-discriminative and affective components of the noxious stimulation, including pain localization and emotional, autonomic, and motor responses to a noxious stimulus. Symptoms such as anxiety, depression, fear, tachycardia, hypertension, and stress response associated with pain are mediated by these pathways.

Nociceptors

Free nerve endings in peripheral tissues have polymodal nociceptors. These receptors can transduce various categories of noxious stimuli such as electrical, mechanical, chemical, and thermal. Aδ and C fibers arise from dorsal root ganglion (DRG) and innervate the peripheral tissues such as skin, joints, muscle, and viscera. These fibers transmit noxious stimuli from free nerve endings to the spinal cord.

Aδ Fibers

Aδ fibers are thinly myelinated, medium diameter, and rapidly conducting. They mediate the initial sharp, well-localized pain, also known as delta pain, first pain, or epicritic pain. In chronic pain, A β fibers, which normally transmit touch, can also transmit pain.

C Fibers

The C fibers are unmyelinated, have small diameters, and are slow conducting. These carry the slow aching pain, also known as 'second pain' or 'protopathic pain.' This pain is poorly localized, dull, and aching in character. It occurs due to the activation of C fibers by the local chemicals released due to tissue injury.

Blockade by Local Anesthetics

The clinical differences in Aδ and C fibers are seen in certain situations, such as external pressure and local anesthetics injection. Pressure blocks larger axons first. Therefore, a needle prick may be perceived as a dull sensation under external pressure. Local anesthetics block unmyelinated fibers earlier than myelinated fibers. During the phase of blockage of only unmyelinated fibers, needle prick pain is perceived as sharp pain and is not followed by residual, aching pain.

No Pain in a Population Subgroup

A subgroup of the population who have mutations in the tyrosine kinase protein A gene cannot sense pain, as it leads to the non-development of pain conducting fibers (Aβ, Aδ, and C fibers).

Pain Mediators

Chemical mediators that mediate pain are elaborated on in **Figure 3**. Some chemicals triggering pain receptors are:
- Glutamate activates postsynaptic N-methyl-D-aspartate (NMDA) receptors
- Substance P activates neurokinin (NK1)
- Neurotrophic factors activate tyrosine kinase receptors.

Central Sensitization of Pain

Repeated nociceptive stimulus leads to sensitization of peripheral and central neurons. This results in a reduction in activation threshold and amplification in response, as compared to a normally noxious stimulus. The output in spinal neurons can increase progressively and frequency-dependent in response to persistent nociceptor excitation. This is known as the 'Wind Up' phenomenon.

PAIN INHIBITORY MECHANISMS

Certain peripheral and central mechanisms in our body help in reducing the pain sensation. These are known as "pain inhibitory mechanisms."

Peripheral Pain Inhibiting Mechanisms

Inflammation of peripheral tissue leads to an increase in opioid receptors in DRG neurons and an increased accumulation of opioid peptide-containing immune cells in the inflamed tissue. In response to inflammation, stress, and in the presence of releasing agents, leukocytes can also secrete opioids. The opioid-producing leukocytes reach the inflamed tissue, guided by chemokines and adhesion molecules, and secrete opioids. Endogenous opioid production is up-regulated in inflamed tissue.

Central Pain Inhibiting Mechanisms (Flowchart 1)

These pathways mediate pain modulation. The descending inhibitory pathways travel from the brainstem to the dorsal horn (**Fig. 4**). Important "triad" of regions mediating central inhibiting mechanisms include periaqueductal gray (PAG), dorsolateral pontine tegmentum (DLPT), and rostral ventral medulla (RVM). Signals descend from the cerebral cortex to PAG in the midbrain. From here, the signals travel to locus ceruleus,

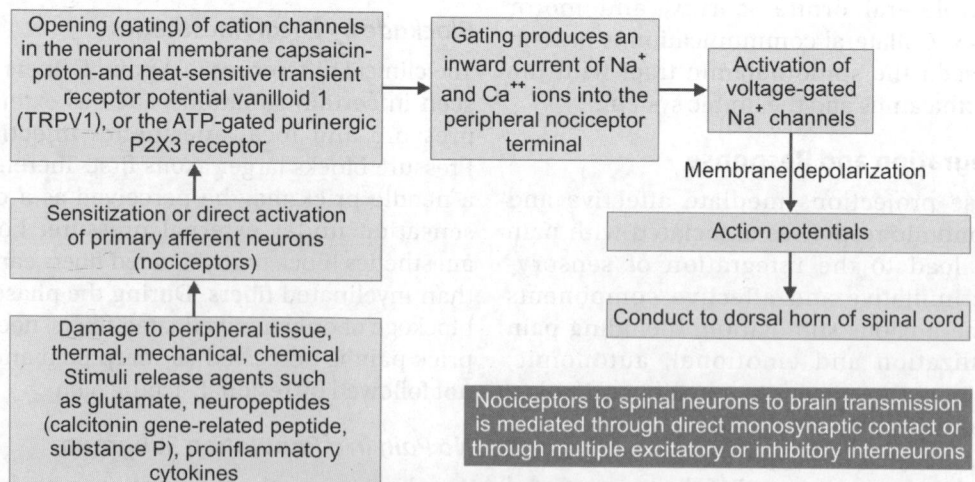

Fig. 3: Pain mediators.

CHAPTER 19 ♦ Pain Pathways and Chronic Pain

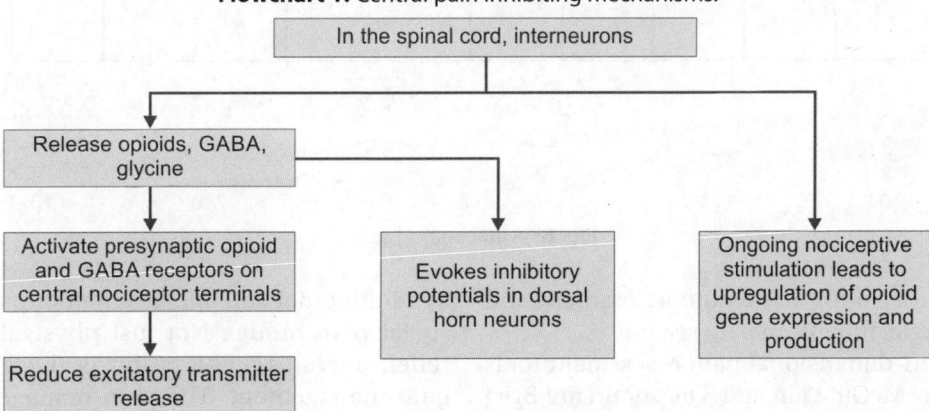

Flowchart 1: Central pain inhibiting mechanisms.

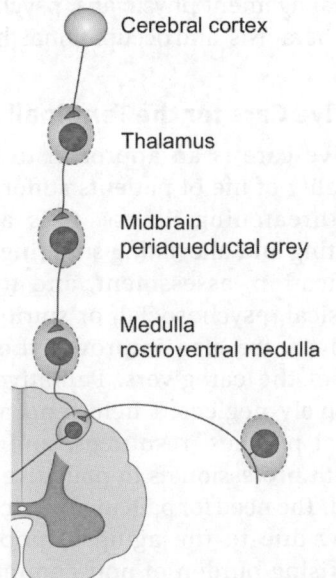

Fig. 4: Descending pain pathways.

located in DLPT, and further to locus raphe magnus in RVM. The action potentials generated here travel down the dorsolateral tracts in the spinal cord and terminate at the interneuron, where primary and secondary afferent fibers synapse. Here it inhibits pain transmission by decreasing the excitatory mediators such as glutamate and substance-P and reducing excitatory signals generation. These inhibitory pathways function through noradrenergic, serotonergic, and opioid systems. This pathway also forms a part of the "gate control theory of pain" described in 1965 by Melzack and Wall.

PAIN ASSESSMENT

AS8.2: Elicit and determine the level, quality and quantity of pain and its tolerance in patient or surrogate.

Various pain assessment scales are available. Common scales used are the Numeric Rating Scale (NRS) (**Fig. 5**) and the visual analog scale (VAS) (**Fig. 6**). The NRS and VAS are usually 11-point scales with 0 signifying 'no pain' and 10 signifying 'worst pain.' NRS and VAS are

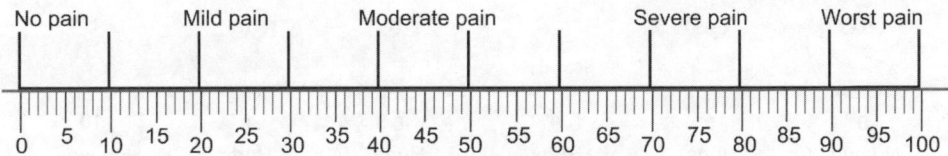

Fig. 5: Numeric analog scale.

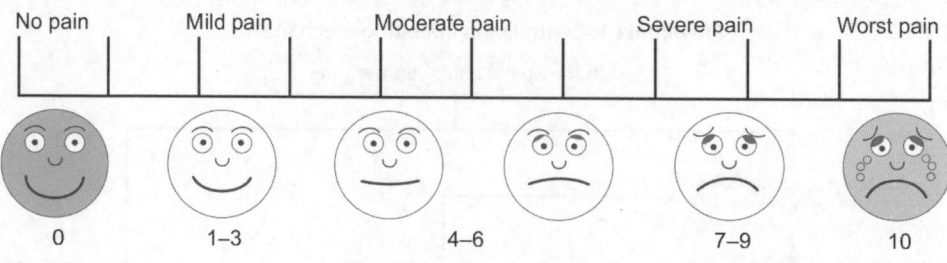

Fig. 6: Visual analog scale.

mostly used for acute pain assessment and are single dimension pain scales.

Multi-dimensional pain assessment tools such as McGill Pain and Questionnaire Brief Pain Inventory (BPI) are used to assess chronic and cancer pain. Wong-Baker Face pain rating scale (**Fig. 7**) and FLACC (face, leg, activity, cry, and consolability) are commonly used in the pediatric population.

PAIN MANAGEMENT

> **AS8.4**: Describe the principles of pain management in palliative care.
> **AS8.5**: Describe the principles of pain management in the terminally ill.

Pain is multifactorial and has complex underlying mechanisms. It is the subjective endpoint of various physical, social, and psychological factors. Physical pain is just a symptom of comprehensive pain syndrome. This particularly relates to cancer pain and palliative care.

Chronic pain is caused by an interaction of biological (tissue damage), psychological (cognition, memory, conditioning), and social factors (attention, reinforcement). Therefore, effective pain management programs must be multimodal and address the bio-psycho-social pain model. Not just physical pain relief, overall rehabilitation is the aim of pain management. The pain management team is ideally multi-specialty, including pain management physicians, psychologists, physiotherapists, and occupational therapists.

Palliative Care for the Terminally Ill

Palliative care is an approach to improve the quality of life of patients suffering from a life-threatening illness. It is aimed at preventing and alleviating suffering by early identification, assessment, and treatment of physical, psychosocial, or spiritual pain. Palliative care also improves the quality of life of the caregivers. Palliative care is a relatively neglected field, and adequate national policies, resources, and training of health professionals in palliative care are needed. The need for palliative care continues to grow due to the aging of populations and a rising burden of non-communicable diseases. Palliative care involves a range of professionals supporting the patients and their families, including physicians, nursing, support workers, paramedics, pharmacists, physiotherapists, and volunteers.

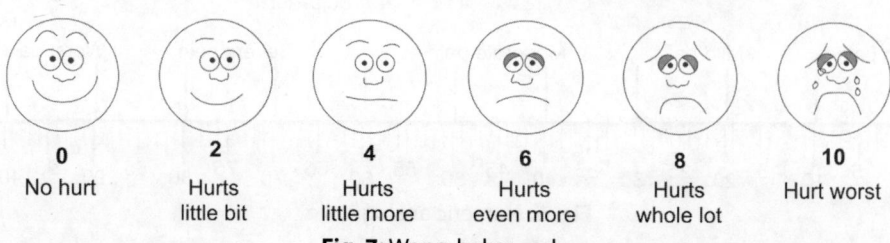

Fig. 7: Wong-baker scale.

Methods of Pain Management

The methods include:
- Analgesic medication
- Intervention
- Cognitive-behavior therapy (addresses the maladaptive cognitive and behavioral patterns and helps patients actively participate in their recovery)
- Functional restoration such as occupational and physical therapy (helps restore movements and body functions and improves confidence)
- Social support (financial, legal, employment, and family support concerns need to be addressed)
- Relaxation therapy.

Analgesic Medications

> **AS8.3:** Describe the pharmacology and use of drugs in the management of pain.

In 1986, the World Health Organization (WHO) proposed the three-step analgesic ladder approach for rational use of analgesics in pain relief for cancer patients (**Fig. 8**). This has undergone several modifications over the years and is now also used for the management of non-cancer pain.

Routes of Administration

Medications can be administered through various routes. These medications inhibit impulse generation and transmission, which cause pain. These can act at peripheral and central sites (**Fig. 9**). There are various routes of different analgesic drug administration, such as oral, intravenous, topical, subcutaneous, transmucosal, transnasal, intrathecal, epidural, and intraarticular. Analgesic medications used and their mechanism of action are listed in **Table 2**.

Opioid Analgesia

Opioids are the most favored analgesics in chronic pain. Some adverse features seen with opioid analgesics use are:
- Tolerance (drug effect decreases with repeated administration of the same dose of the drug, and increasing doses are required to achieve the same effect)
- Physical dependence (withdrawal symptoms on abrupt drug cessation or dose reduction or by administering an antagonist). Physical dependence is seen with all opioids, even after short administration periods.
- Need for opioid rotation (sometimes used in improving pain relief or reducing side effects)
- Opioid-induced hyperalgesia (including Allodynia) (attributed to the neuroexcitatory effects of opioid metabolites)
- Opioid withdrawal-induced hyperalgesia (occurs following the abrupt cessation of opioids).

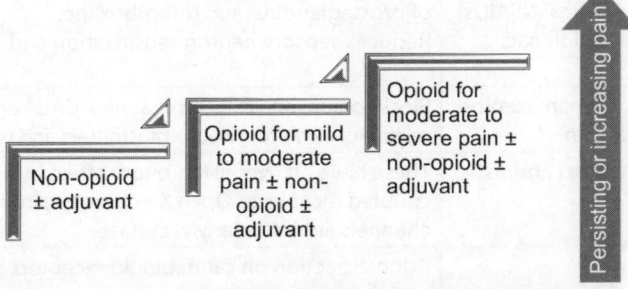

A fourth 'interventional' step has been proposed which includes invasive and minimally invasive techniques. A 'Bidirectional apporoach' has also been proposed which indicates that analgesics should be stepped down when pain relief is achieved

Fig. 8: WHO three-step analgesic ladder.

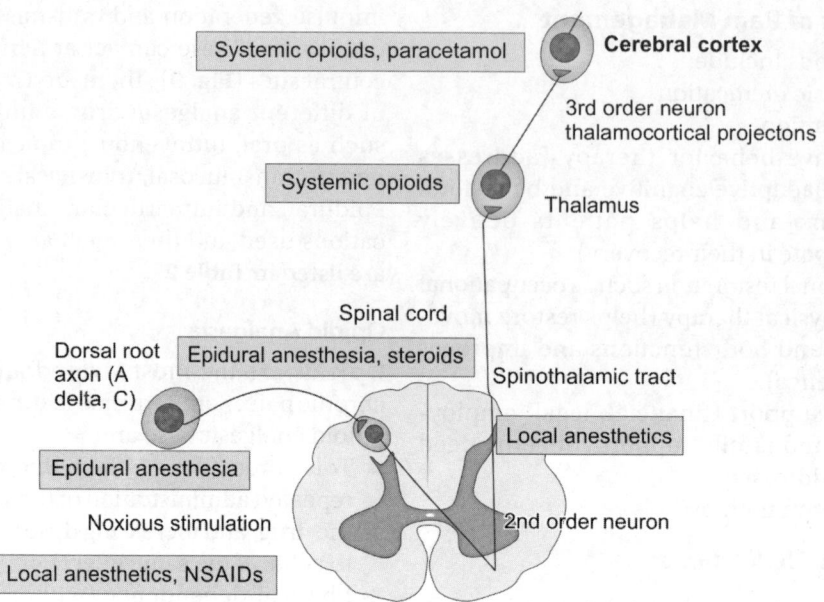

Fig. 9: Site of action of various analgesic drugs.
NSAIDs: nonsteroidal anti-inflammatory drugs

Table 2: Analgesic medications.

Drugs	Action
Opioids e.g. Morphine, Fentanyl	Act on μ-, δ-, κ-receptors, Inhibit release of excitatory neurotransmitters and reduce neuron excitability
Serotonin agonists e.g. Triptans	Act on G-protein coupled 5-HT receptors and inhibit release of excitatory neuropeptides, reduces inflammation. Cause vasoconstriction.
Antidepressants e.g. Venlafaxine, duloxetine, amitrytiline, nortryptiline	Act on Noradrenaline/5-HT transporters and sodium and potassium channels causing reduction in neuron excitability
Acetaminophen and Non-Steroidal Anti-Inflammatory Drugs (NSAIDs) e.g. indomethacin, diclofenac, ibuprofen	Inhibits cyclooxygenases (COX-1, COX-2) and reduces production of prostaglandins and thromboxane. Reduces sensory neuron sensitization and inhibits spinal neurons.
Antiepileptics e.g. Carbamazepine, Gabapentin, Pregabalin	Block sodium and calcium channels. GABA agonistic activity. Inhibit release of excitatory neurotransmitters and reduce neuron excitability.
α2-Adrenergic receptors agonists e.g. clonidine	These have an overall inhibitory effect by action on G-protein coupled receptors, Open K+ channels, inhibit presynaptic Ca++ channels, inhibit adenylyl cyclase.
Cannabinoids	Agnostic action on cannabinoid receptors in brain, spinal cord and periphery
Benzodiazepines	Reduce muscle spasm, useful in musculoskeletal pain and muscle spasticity states

Contd...

Contd...

Drugs	Action
Baclofen	Reduce muscle spasm, useful in musculoskeletal pain and muscle spasticity states. Activates both presynpatic and post synaptic GABA-B receptors, leading to a decrease in excitatory and an increase in inhibitory neurotransmission.
Botulinum toxin	Inhibits acetylcholine release at the neuromuscular junction.
Ziconotide	It is a synthetic peptide which blocks N-type voltage-sensitive Ca^{++} channels and inhibits release of excitatory neurotransmitters.
Topical Analgesics e.g. Diclofenac, Capsaicin, local anesthetics, opioids	These preparations act locally at peripheral nerve endings and mediate analgesia
Anti-depressants (tricyclic antidepressants, doxepin)	Used in post-herpetic neuralgia, post-mastectomy pain, neuropathic pains

Interventions for Pain Relief

Common interventions performed are:
- Nerve blocks
- Stimulation techniques
- Acupuncture
- Spinal cord stimulation (SCS)
- Transcutaneous electrical nerve stimulation (TENS).

Nerve Blocks

Nerve blocks can be diagnostic or therapeutic. They can help diagnose or locate a pain source by blocking specific nerves. They help in pain relief by blocking nerves, act as an adjuvant to medical treatment, help in improving therapeutic effect, and help in physical therapy and rehabilitation of the patient. Nerve blocks can be administered both in cancer pain and in non-malignant neuropathic pain also. Common blocks include celiac plexus block and lumbar sympathetic ganglia block.

Nerve blocks can be done using local anesthetics or permanent neurolysis or ablation. Neurolytic blocks involve the application of alcohol, phenol, or radiofrequency ablation. They are used in trigeminal neuralgia and cancer pain.

Nondestructive nerve blocks cause temporary nerve blocks, which help in healing and physiotherapy. They involve the administration of local anesthetics and steroids. Some examples are epidural steroids injections, trigger point injections, intraarticular injections, and sympathetic nerve blocks.

Bio-psycho-social Therapy

Pain is a complex phenomenon having underlying bio-psycho-social factors. Alterations in the nervous system can cause pain to become persistent and chronic. Pain pathways and processing occur through ascending and descending pathways involving peripheral, spinal, and supraspinal neural structures. Pain modulation helps in reducing the pain sensation. Various scales are available to assess pain objectively. However, due to its multidimensional pathology and clinical manifestation, accurate and reproducible pain assessment remains a challenge. Pain management involves multimodal therapy, including medications, interventions, and behavioral and social therapies.

MULTIPLE CHOICE QUESTIONS

1. **The term nociception is used for:**
   a. Physiological pain
   b. Neural process of encoding noxious stimuli
   c. Pain perception
   d. All of the above

2. **Allodynia is:**
   a. Chronic pain after surgery
   b. Pain after a stimulus that does not normally provoke pain
   c. A term used for ischemic pain in the limbs
   d. Excruciating neuropathic pain

3. **Hyperalgesia is:**
   a. Radiation of pain beyond the injury site
   b. No pain despite a painful stimulus due to sensory loss
   c. Exaggerated response to a typically painful stimulus
   d. Persisting of pain despite analgesics

4. **Pain pathways ascend in the spinal cord to the thalamus via the:**
   a. The anterolateral spinal cord
   b. The posterolateral spinal cord
   c. The dorsal spinal tracks
   d. Anterior spinal tracks

5. **Aδ fibers mediate:**
   a. The protopathic pain
   b. The slow aching pain
   c. The initial sharp, well-localized pain
   d. All of the above

6. **Which of the following is a pain assessment scale:**
   a. Visual analog scale
   b. Numeric analog scale
   c. Wong-baker scale
   d. All of the above

7. **Palliative care involves:**
   a. Improving the quality of life of patients suffering from a life-threatening illness
   b. Treatment of physical, psychosocial, or spiritual pain
   c. Improves the quality of life of the caregivers
   d. All of the above

8. **The World Health Organization (WHO) the three-step analgesic ladder approach was proposed for:**
   a. Reducing the chances of opioid addiction
   b. Following a step-wise approach for acute pain relief
   c. Rational use of analgesics in pain relief for cancer patients
   d. All of the above

9. **Neurolytic blocks with the application of alcohol, phenol, or radiofrequency ablation can be administered for:**
   a. Coeliac plexus block
   b. Trigeminal neuralgia
   c. Cancer pain
   d. All of the above

Answers
1. b
2. b
3. c
4. a
5. c
6. d
7. d
8. c
9. d

CHAPTER 20
Patient Safety in Operation Theatre

Manish Jagia

Learning Objectives

- Patient identification safety
- Role of communication—WHO surgical safety checklist
- Safety in patient positioning
- Preventing medical and medication errors
- Safety in glycemic control
- Safety under anesthesia
- General safety measures

INTRODUCTION

Patient safety is fundamental to any healthcare system. Millions of surgery take place every year, and adverse events due to negligence during surgery can lead to temporary or permanent disability and death. A safe operating theatre is achieved only through careful planning, maintenance, periodic checks, and proper ongoing training for staff. By definition, errors are unintentional. They occur due to wrong decisions or failure to execute an intended, planned action. Errors result from overriding or overlooking protocols by medical staff in an emergency or in haste.

To address the issue of surgical safety, World Health Organization (WHO) undertook several global and regional initiatives. The WHO Second Global Patient Safety Challenge, "Safe Surgery Saves Lives," sets standards to improve the safety of surgical care around the world. The first global patient safety initiative was "Clean care is safer care," which set standards for hand hygiene to prevent healthcare-associated infections.

Patient safety is primely important to medical personnel, especially in the operation theatre (OR). Standard protocols should be followed religiously to ensure well-being of the patients. Communication between team members is integral to preventing and managing complications in OR. Patient safety measures not only prevent complications but also improve the patient's outcome.

PATIENT IDENTIFICATION SAFETY

Safety measures start in the ward before the patient is shifted to the OR. Proper communication and hand-over between the ward and OR staff are important before shifting the patient.

Patient Identification

A hospital identification (ID) band mentioning name, hospital registration number, age and sex must be worn by all inpatients. These

standards are more important when patients are unaccompanied by relatives, in a new environment, or anxious. The staff shifting the patient checks the hospital ID band to verify:
- Taking over the right patient with documented surgery
- Preanesthesia clearance is given with proper consent for anesthesia and surgery, risk stratification, and blood transfusion signed by the patient and one adult witness.
- The operative site and side should be marked with an arrow pointing at it with a marker pen by the surgical team member to avoid the wrong site/side surgery.

Patient Identification Bands

The patient's identity is confirmed by the OR staff. If the patient is unable to speak or mentally unfit, the identity is confirmed from the identification wristband worn by all hospitalized patients once admitted. Color-coded wristbands are often used as part of a multi-component approach to patient safety. Wristbands of different colors are used for ease in identification of patients needing special care, e.g., red (signifies allergy), yellow (elevated risk of fall), purple (do not resuscitate), and green (prior anaphylactic reaction to latex).

ROLE OF COMMUNICATION IN SAFETY

AS10.3: Describe the role of communication in patient safety.

WHO Surgical Safety Checklist

Mishaps have been reported due to errors in patient identification before surgery, wrong site of surgery, and wrong surgery, which caused unfortunate morbidity in patients. The most vital step in OR patient safety was the introduction of the WHO surgical safety checklist (**Fig. 1**). WHO surgical safety list is based on improving communication amongst the surgical team members to ensure patient safety. Strict adherence to the WHO safety checklist ensures correct patient, correct site, and proper coordination among the team members.

SAFETY IN PATIENT POSITIONING

AS 10.1: Enumerate the hazards of incorrect patient positioning.

The responsibility of patient positioning for surgery is shared by the surgeon, anesthetist, technician, and nurses in the OR. The patient's position can affect physiologic changes and result in soft tissue injury (e.g., nerve damage, pressure-induced injury or ulceration, or compartment syndrome). The consequences of position-related injuries can be profound, but the injuries are preventable.

Preventing Iatrogenic Patient Injury

AS10.2: Enumerate the hazards encountered in the perioperative period and steps/techniques taken to prevent them.

Patient falls, and limb injuries in surgeries in odd positions are prevented by strapping the torso and, at times, the head and limbs to the operating table. Prone position can result in transient or rarely permanent visual loss due to eyeball compression. Neurological, vascular, musculoskeletal, and pressure ulcers are the most common position-related injuries in surgical patients. The patient's head should be placed in a neutral position and extreme flexion/extension of the neck avoided. To avoid brachial plexus injury, the arm should not be abducted more than 90°. Neurological complications can be avoided by placing forearms in a neutral position or slightly supinated to minimize pressure. To prevent ischemia and compartment syndrome, straps should not be too tight. Padding under bony prominences helps prevent pressure-related complications. Gel pads or soft cotton rolls are used under the head, forearm, knees, and ankles to prevent pressure injuries.

Surgical safety checklist

World Health Organization — Patient safety: A world alliance for safer health care

Before induction of anesthesia
(with at least nurse and anesthetist)

Has the patient confirmed his/her identity, site, procedure, and consent?
☐ Yes

Is the site marked?
☐ Yes
☐ Not applicable

Is the anesthesia machine and medication check complete?
☐ Yes

Is the pulse oximeter on the patient and functioning?
☐ Yes

Does the patient have a:
Know allergy?
☐ No
☐ Yes

Difficult airway or aspiration risk?
☐ No
☐ Yes, and equipment/assistance available

Risk of >500 mL blood loss (7 mL/kg in children)?
☐ No
☐ Yes, and two IVs/central access and fluids planned

Before skin incision
(with nurse, anesthetist and surgeon)

☐ Confirm all team members have introduced themselves by name and role

☐ Confirm the patient's name, procedure, and where the incision will be made

Has antibiotic prophylaxis been given within the last 60 minutes?
☐ Yes
☐ Not applicable

Anticipated critical events
To surgeon:
☐ What are the critical or non-routine steps?
☐ How long will the case take?
☐ What is the anticipated blood loss?

To Anesthetist:
☐ Are there any patient-specific concerns?

To nursing team:
☐ Has sterility (including indicator results) been confirmed?
☐ Are there equipment issues or any concerns?

Is essential imaging displayed?
☐ Yes
☐ Not applicable

Before patient leaves operating room
(with nurse, anesthetist and surgeon)

Nurse verbally confirms:
☐ The name of the procedure
☐ Completion of instrument, sponge and needle counts
☐ Specimen labeling (read speimen lables aloud, including patient name)
☐ Whether there are any equipment problems to be addressed

To surgeon, anesthetist and nurse:
☐ What are the key concerns for recovery and management of this patient?

Fig. 1: WHO surgical safety checklist.

Preventing Medical and Medication Errors

AS10.4: Define and describe common medical and medication errors in anesthesia.

Medication safety is ensured by applying the five R's: right drug, right route, right time, right dose, and right patient. Modern systems of information technology, such as computerized order entry, barcode medication administration, and personal health records, are essential in the prevention of medication errors. A proper history of drug allergies or reactions must be taken from patients before initiating treatment. The most common prescribing errors are incorrect drugs, incorrect doses, allergies, and drug-drug interactions. Prescribing the generic name of drugs simplifies communication among healthcare workers, reducing errors. A separate closet is maintained for drugs that "look-alike and sound-alike." Similarly, separate cabinets are maintained for high-risk medication and concentrated electrolytes solutions like 3% hydroxyethyl starch, etc.

Safety in Glycemic Control

Stress of surgery and anesthesia causes hyperglycemia which alters fluid balance, tissue homeostasis, and wound healing and makes the patient prone to infection and resulting in poorer surgical outcomes, morbidity, and mortality. Maintenance of normoglycemia is especially important in diabetic patients. Hypoglycemia is associated with higher mortality than hyperglycemia. Intraoperative normoglycemia is ensured by regular blood glucose monitoring with a glucometer and administration of insulin and dextrose solutions.

SAFETY UNDER ANESTHESIA

Anesthesia Machine Safety

Anesthesiologist must check the anesthesia machine for proper delivery of oxygen and anesthesia gases. The machine must undergo a calibration check every day before use. Anesthesia workstations are designed to ensure hypoxia prevention and fire safety. The workstations and monitors have inbuilt monitoring systems and alarms.

Anesthesia Drug Safety

All anesthetic drugs must be prepared by an anesthetist after checking the drug name and expiry date. The drug name, its concentration, and date of preparation must be labeled on the syringes used. A medication error can occur when drug labels look-alike or sound-alike are administered. Color-coding labels of drug ampoules, vials, and syringes enhance safety.

Patient Safety Under Anesthesia

The patient's airway patency and breathing are ensured. Adequate hemodynamics for perfusion of body organs is maintained. Basic monitoring, as recommended by American Society of Anesthesiologists standards (electrocardiography, pulse oximetry, capnography, and blood pressure monitors), is applied to all patients. Arterial or central venous lines are placed for invasive pressure monitoring if indicated by the patient's clinical condition or surgery.

Preventing Deep Vein Thrombosis

In prolonged surgeries (such as hip arthroplasty, knee replacement surgeries, and cancer surgeries), patients are immobilized for a long duration. This immobility promotes deep vein thrombosis (DVT). DVT is the most common preventable cause of death in surgical patients. DVT can be prevented by the administration of anticoagulants like low molecular weight heparin or ultra fractionated heparin preoperatively and/or the use of intermittent pneumatic compression or compression stockings. Pharmacological measures are usually withheld before surgery according to their metabolism, but intermittent pneumatic compression is continued during surgery. Postoperatively, anticoagulants are initiated to prevent DVT.

INFECTION CONTROL

Operation theater environment should have a sterile surgical environment to ensure asepsis and prevent infection during surgery. Measures to control include:
- Proper scrubbing technique with an alcohol-based solution for at least 5 minutes, as shown in **Figure 2**.
- Using personal protective equipment (e.g., gloves, masks, eyewear).
- Using clean, disinfected, and sterilized instruments and linen in the OR. All the instruments are cleaned of blood or secretions in free-flowing water and disinfected. The processes commonly used for sterilization are autoclaving, ethylene oxide gas, chemicals, and plasma.
- Preoperative skin preparation is done with povidone-iodine or chlorhexidine for 5 min for aseptic part preparation for surgery, invasive lines, and catheterization.
- The process of covering a patient and surrounding areas with a sterile barrier to create and maintain a sterile field during a surgical procedure is called draping. Draping restricts the passage of microorganisms from nonsterile to sterile areas.
- Devices like operation tables, anesthesia machines, endoscopes, floors, and doors are cleaned or chemically disinfected regularly.
- Safe injection practices and maintenance of intravenous cannula (i.e., an aseptic technique for parenteral medications).

CHAPTER 20 • Patient Safety in Operation Theatre

- Handwash with soap and water on arrival to or, after having donned theatre clothing (cap/hat/bonnel and mask)
- Use an alcohol-based handrub (ABHR) product for surgical hand preparation, by carefully following the technique illustrated in images 1 to 17, before every surgical procedure
- If any residual talc or biological fluids are present when gloves are removed following the operation, handwash with soap and water.

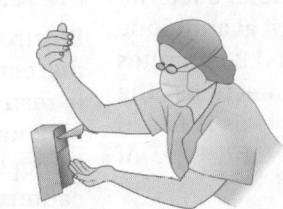

1
Put approximately 5 mL (3 doses) of ABHR in the palm of your left hand, using the elbow of your other arm to operate the dispenser.

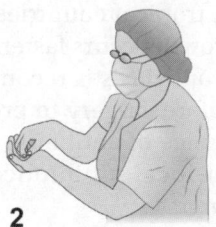

2
Dip the fingertips of your right hand in the handrub to decontaminate under the nails (5 seconds).

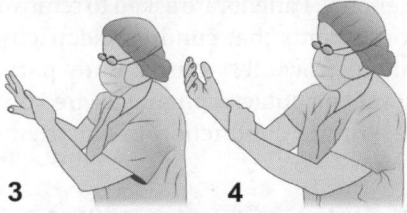

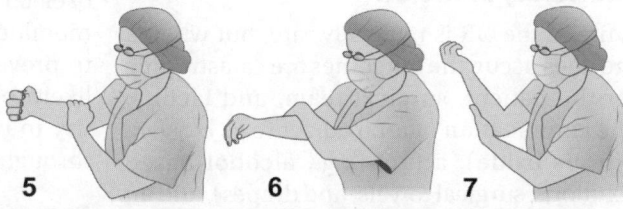

3 4 5 6 7

Images 3–7: Smear the handrub on the right forearm up to the elbow. Ensure that the whole skin area is covered by using circular movements around the forearm until the handrub has fully evaporated (10–15 seconds).

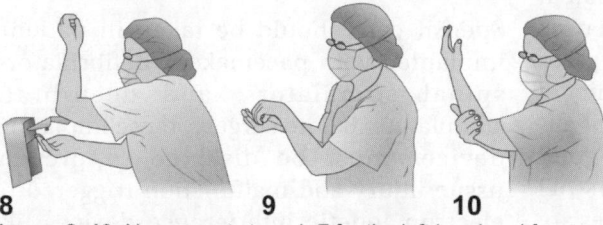

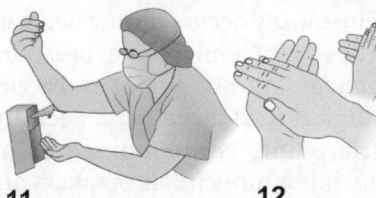

8 9 10 11 12

Image 8–10: Now repeat steps 1–7 for the left hand and forearm.

11 Put approximately 5 mL (3 doses) of ABHR in the palm of your left hand, as illustrated, to rub both hands at the same time up to the wrists, following all steps in images 12–17 (20–30 seconds).

12 Cover the whole surface of the hands up to the wrist with ABHR, rubbing palm against palm with a rotating movement.

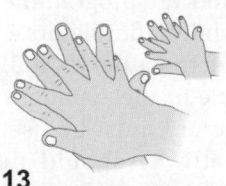

13
Rub the back of the left hand, including the wrist, moving the right palm back and forth and vice versa.

14
Rub palm against palm back and forth with fingers interlinked.

15
Rub the back of the fingers by holding them in the palm of the other hand with a sideways back and forth movement.

16
Rub the thumb of the left hand by rotating it in the clasped palm of the right hand and vice versa.

17
When the hands are dry, sterile surgical clothing and gloves can be donned.

Repeat this sequence (average 60 sec) the number of times that adds up to the total duration recommended by the ABHR manufacturer's instruction. This could be two or even three times

Fig. 2: WHO recommended surgical hand hygiene technique.

- In tropical countries like India, bacterial growth occurs faster. Empirical antibiotic prophylaxis is recommended 30 minutes before surgery to prevent infections. The choice of antibiotic prophylaxis is based on local antibiotic policy and type of surgery.

GENERAL SAFETY MEASURES

Fire Safety in the OR

A fire in the OR is relatively rare, but when a fire does occur, the outcomes are catastrophic for the patient, surgical team, and facility. The combination of an oxidizer (e.g., oxygen, nitrous oxide), a fuel (e.g., alcohol-based solutions, surgical towels, and drapes), and an ignition source (e.g., electrosurgery unit and LASER) in a closed environment can result in fire. Fire mostly occurs during head and neck surgeries by inflammation of breathing gases (oxygen and nitrous oxide) in the vicinity of the surgical field by cautery. Security of all-electric points is maintained using good quality miniature circuit breakers and strict compliance to ensure that no loose wires are used at plug points.

Temperature Safety

In the OR, the temperature and humidity of the OR are maintained low to prevent infection. Patients (especially those undergoing prolonged surgery, debilitated, geriatric and pediatric) are prone to hypothermia by exposure to the cold OR environment. The environmental temperature and humidity are displayed in all modern ORs. Hypothermia can result in delayed recovery from general anesthesia, leads to shivering, increased oxygen demand, and makes the patient uncomfortable. To maintain normothermia, active body warming is done using heating disposable blankets, convective warm air blowers, heated water mattresses, and using warm intravenous fluids.

Preventing Electrocautery Burns

Electrocautery is used intraoperatively for dissection and hemostasis. Current flow is restricted to between the two poles, and making is safer as the current does not pass through the adjoining tissues. In monopolar cautery, on the other hand, current passes between the site of touch of the cautery pencil and the earthing pad. The earthing pad should be properly placed to prevent the dissipation of electric energy. Patients are asked to remove metallic ornaments that conduct electricity to prevent electrocautery burns. Body parts likely to come in contact with metals are kept dry to prevent the conduction of electricity through water.

Preventing Injury Related to Artificial Implants

Special care should be taken in patients implanted with pacemakers, defibrillators, spinal stimulators, and deep-brain stimulators. Before surgery, these implanted devices must be disabled to prevent tissue injury and malfunction triggered by electromagnetic interference devices like electrocautery. Pacemakers are programmed to asynchronous mode while defibrillators are switched off. Bipolar electrocautery should be used as far as possible in these patients. If monopolar electrocautery must be used, the cautery current pathway should not flow towards the medical device or its leads. The electrocautery grounding plate should be placed so the current flows away from the device.

Preventing Needle Stick Injury

Surgeons, anesthesiologists, and paramedical workers can inadvertently sustain needle stick injuries. All personnel must take precautions to prevent needle stick injury and follow recommended OR protocols. All used needles must be disposed of in a "sharp disposable container" present in every

OR. In case of an injury, the site should be immediately washed with soap and water. The incident should be reported and an exposure report sheet documented. The exposure should be assessed like the type of fluid, type of needle, amount of blood on the needle, etc. The source of exposure should be evaluated for the potential of infection transmission [such as human immunodeficiency virus (HIV), hepatitis B virus (HBV), and hepatitis C virus (HCV)]. Appropriate post-exposure prophylaxis should be started within 24 hrs in case the exposure source is infective.

Collection of Biopsy and Surgical Specimens

Wrong labeling, mixing of samples, and misplacement of biopsy and surgical samples compromise patient outcomes and safety. Tissue biopsy or pus, blood, and fluids must be collected in a sterile manner intraoperatively. Samples must be labeled properly with the name of the patient, hospital registration number, site of sample collection, and type of sample like pus, tissue, tumor, etc. The patient's history must be properly documented and dispatched to the pathology or microbiology laboratory.

MULTIPLE CHOICE QUESTIONS

OSCE

A patient has been received in the operation theater (OT) directly from the admission desk for routine listed surgery of a Ganglion wrist right under daycare. His admission papers state that he has diabetes mellitus and hypertension. He has reported after overnight fasting for surgery as instructed by the surgical team. He has not taken any medication on the morning of surgery. On arrival in the OT, his pulse rate is recorded as 86/min and blood pressure as 180/100 mm Hg. He is wheeled into the OT immediately for surgery as per schedule.

1. **What protocol should have been taken for the identification of the patient?**
   a. His identity should have been confirmed with any of his identification cards
   b. He should have been identified by the surgeon before being wheeled into the OT
   c. His identity should have been verified from his hospital identification band
   d. His identity should have been confirmed by him verbally

2. **What is the correct method to confirm the site and side of surgery?**
   a. Verbal confirmation of the patient
   b. Checking the site and side of surgery from the medical documents
   c. Asking the surgeon about the site and side of surgery
   d. The site marked by the surgical team is verified before shifting the patient to the operating room

3. **Apart from the parameters recorded, which other vital parameter should be checked before shifting the patient to the operating room?**
   a. Respiratory rate
   b. Temperature
   c. Oxygen saturation
   d. Electrocardiogram

4. **As per the WHO surgical safety checklist, the following need to be verified before induction of anesthesia, *except*:**
   a. Patient identity
   b. Surgical site marking
   c. Anesthesia machine check
   d. Antibiotic prophylaxis administration

5. **As per the WHO surgical safety checklist, the following need to be verified before the start of surgery:**
   a. Confirming all members have introduced themselves
   b. The estimated case duration
   c. The estimated blood loss
   d. All of the above

6. **The anesthetist asks the technician to administer mezolam (generic name midazolam), but he administers morphine by mistake. How do you avoid such errors?**

a. By keeping 'sound-alike look-alike' drugs in separate closets
   b. By using generic names rather than brand names
   c. By ensuring proper labeling of syringes
   d. All of the above
7. **Empirical antibiotic prophylaxis is recommended for all surgeries. To ensure adequate antibiotic blood levels, the recommended timing of administration of the empirical antibiotic dose is:**
   a. Morning of surgery
   b. 2 hours before surgery
   c. Less than 30 min before surgical incision
   d. At the time of surgical incision
8. **Patients are prone to hypothermia by exposure to the cold operating room environment. Hypothermia can cause:**
   a. Shivering
   b. Increased oxygen demand
   c. Delayed recovery
   d. All of the above
9. **To prevent needle-stick injury:**
   a. All sharps must be disposed of immediately in the sharps container
   b. All hypodermic needles must be recapped after use
   c. All sharp objects must be broken after use and placed in a polybag
   d. None of the above
10. **For surgical scrubbing, the hands and the arms must be scrubbed and cleaned with an antiseptic for a period of at least:**
    a. 2 min
    b. 3 min
    c. 4 min
    d. 5 min

Answers
1. c
2. d
3. c
4. d
5. d
6. d
7. c
8. d
9. a
10. d

CHAPTER 21

Resuscitation

Rakesh Garg, Indu Bala Maurya

Learning Objectives

- Causes of cardiac arrest
- Basic cardiopulmonary life support
- Comprehensive cardiopulmonary life support
- Early comprehensive life support and postresuscitation care
- Pediatric cardiopulmonary resuscitation
- Neonatal cardiopulmonary resuscitation
- Trauma care

INTODUCTION

Cardiopulmonary resuscitation (CPR) is an emergency lifesaving procedure done for a victim of cardiac arrest to sustain vital organ function. Recovery after cardiac arrest depends on early algorithmic step-wise resuscitation. Various CPR guidelines have been developed by professional bodies, including the American Heart Association, European Resuscitation Council, and Australian Resuscitation Council. In 2017, the Indian Resuscitation Council (IRC) framed the resuscitation algorithm for adult victims. Basic cardiopulmonary life support (BCLS) provides an evidence-based algorithmic stepwise approach for managing cardiac arrest victims outside the hospital, while comprehensive cardiopulmonary life support (CCLS) for inside the hospital by a trained health care worker.

Cause of Cardiac Arrest in Adults

CPR is not a definitive treatment for cardiac arrest but rather a means of maintaining ventilation and tissue oxygenation until the underlying cause is identified and corrected. The most common cause of sudden cardiac arrest in an adult is ventricular fibrillation. Others are pulseless ventricular tachycardia, asystole, and pulseless electrical activity. The various reversible condition can predispose to sudden cardiac arrest in adults, which can be remembered as a mnemonic '**HIT THE TARGET**' (**Table 1**).

The major components of CPR are chest compressions for circulation, maintenance of airway/ventilation to ensure oxygenation, electrical therapy or defibrillation, and drugs. This includes basic airway management, rescue breathing, manual chest compressions, and defibrillation.

Table 1: Common reversible causes of cardiac arrest in adult.

HIT	THE	TARGET
• **H**ypoxia • **I**ncreased H ions [Acidosis] • **T**ension pneumothorax	• **T**oxins/Poisons • **H**ypovolaemia • **E**lectrolyte imbalance [Hypo-/Hyperkalaemia]	• **T**amponade cardiac • **A**cute coronary syndrome • **R**aised intracranial pressure (Subarachnoid hemorrhage) • **G**lucose [Hypo/hyperglycemia] • **E**mbolism (Pulmonary thrombosis) • **T**emperature (Hypothermia)

BASIC CARDIOPULMONARY LIFE SUPPORT (BCLS) FOR AN ADULT

AS2.1: Enumerate the indications, describe the steps and demonstrate in a simulated environment, Basic Life Support in adults, children and neonates.

The optimal outcome of CPR outside the hospital would depend on certain focused links that must be followed during CPR. There are four essential 'Core Links' in BCLS as framed by IRC (**Fig. 1**). These core links are followed in a stepwise algorithmic approach to managing a cardiac arrested victim (**Fig. 2**).

Early Recognition and Activation

This is the first link and encompasses various elements.

Scene Safety

The safety of the rescuer along with the victim is very important. The rescuer should immediately proceed for BCLS, only if the site is without any danger such as the risk of fire, electrocution, drowning, etc. The help of concerned authorities (police personnel/fire brigade /lifeguard) must be taken in an unsafe situation (**Fig. 3**).

Check Victim's Response

The rescuer must check the victim's response from the front-facing victim's face. Tap on the shoulder and speak loudly (e.g., "Hello, are you all right?" or "What is your name?") in a language the victim can understand (**Fig. 4**).

Call for Help and Inform the Emergency Medical System

Ask for help from nearby people if available. That person may be instructed to inform the emergency medical service (**Fig. 5**). If alone, the rescuer should inform the emergency medical service and give details of the victim (number of victims, location, etc.), and ask for an automated external defibrillator (AED) and other emergency equipment (**Fig. 6**). Every citizen must know local emergency and hospital contact details (Any local emergency medical service number, e.g., across India 112, and Delhi 102/1099).

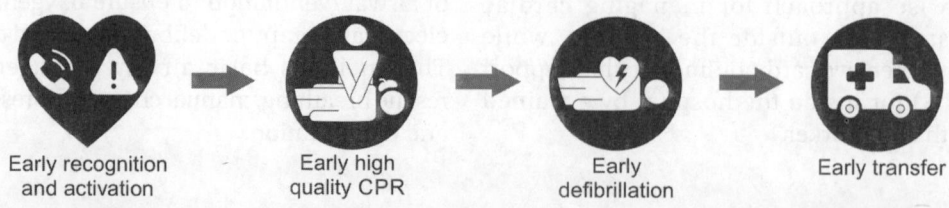

Fig. 1: Core link in adult basic cardiopulmonary life support (BCLS) (Indian resuscitation council).

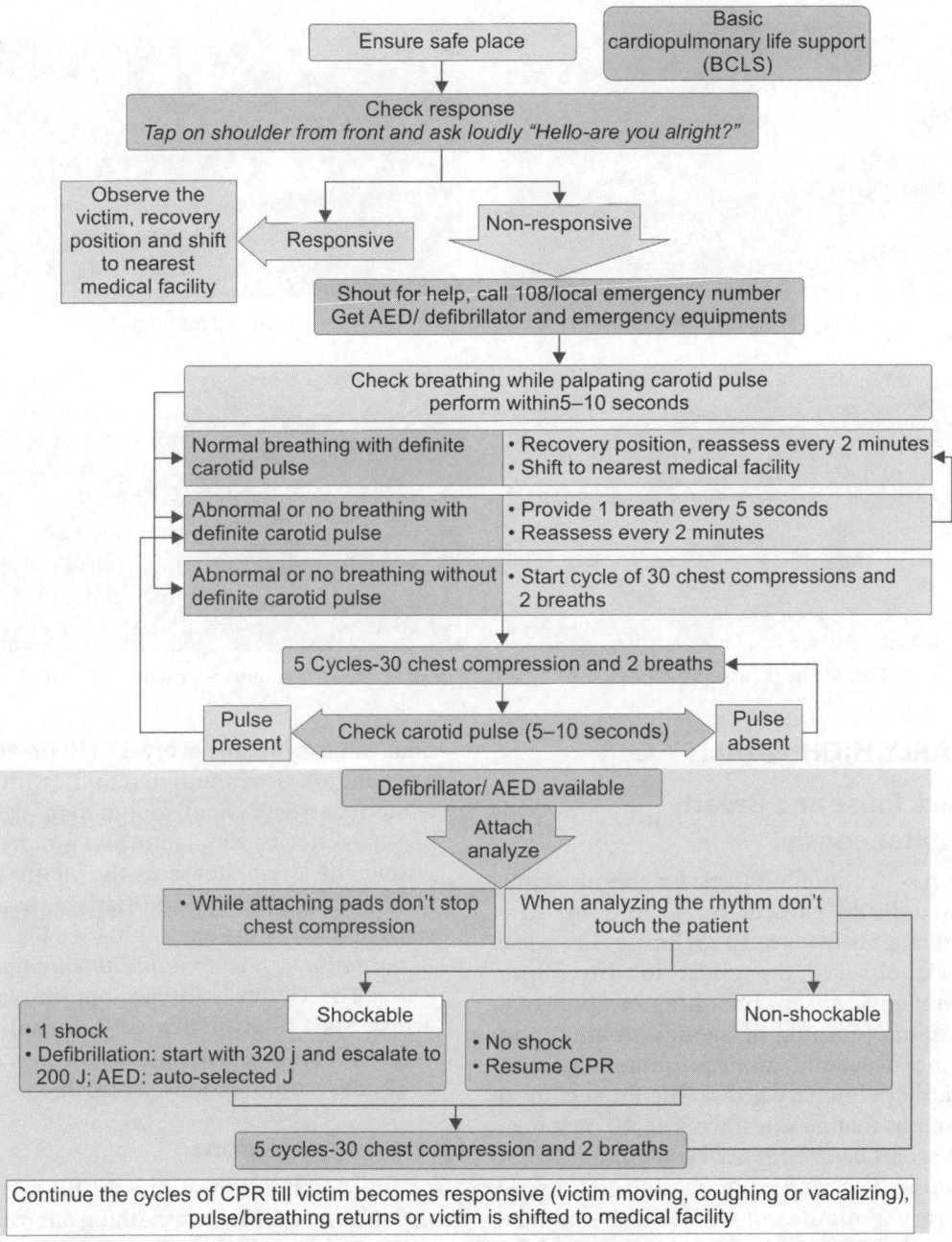

Fig. 2: Adult basic cardiopulmonary life support (BCLS) (Indian resuscitation council).

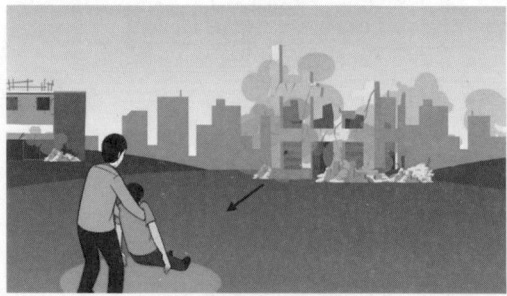

Fig. 3: Scene safety.

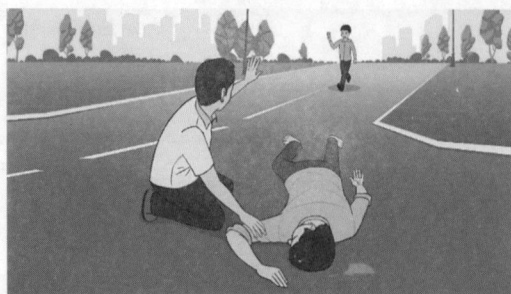

Fig. 5: Call for help.

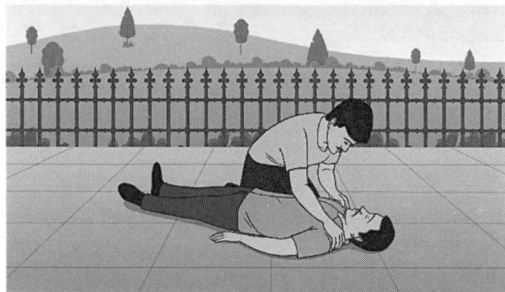

Fig. 4: Check responsiveness.

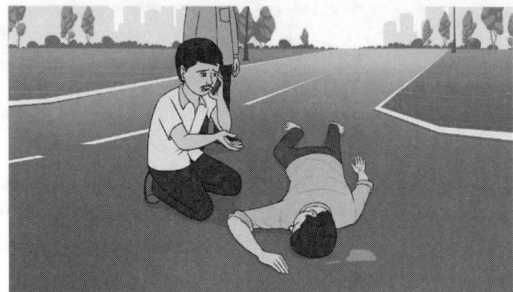

Fig. 6: Activate the emergency medical system (alone).

EARLY HIGH-QUALITY CPR

Check Pulse and Breath Simultaneously

The rescuer should check for the presence of a definite carotid pulse and breathe simultaneously for 5–10 s. During this pulse check, observe the chest for breathing movements. Absent breathing or abnormal breathing (gasping or agonal breaths) and absence of definite carotid pulse are suggestive of cardiopulmonary arrest. The three clinical situations that may be encountered include:
- *Normal breathing with a definite carotid pulse:* The victim needs to be assessed every 2 minutes or earlier if the clinical condition deteriorates and should be managed as per the steps defined in the algorithm (See **Fig. 2**).
- *Abnormal or no breathing with a definite carotid pulse:* The victim is in respiratory arrest. The victim should be provided normal tidal volume breaths every 5 s (12 breaths per minute). Use mouth to mouth (with or without barrier device), mouth to mask, or bag-mask device ventilation and watch the visible chest rise. Reassess the victim for pulse every 2 min should be managed as per steps defined in the algorithm (See **Fig. 2**).
- *Abnormal or no breathing and absent carotid pulse*: The victim is in cardiopulmonary arrest. Start high-quality CPR, including cycles of compression and breaths (cycles of 30 chest compressions: 2 breaths).

Chest Compressions

Place the victim in the supine position on a firm, flat surface and move clothing out of the way. Place the heel of one hand two fingers above the lowest end of the sternum (**Fig. 7**). Place the heel of the other hand directly on top of the first with interlaced fingers and position your shoulders directly over your hands (**Fig. 8**). Immediately give effective 30 chest

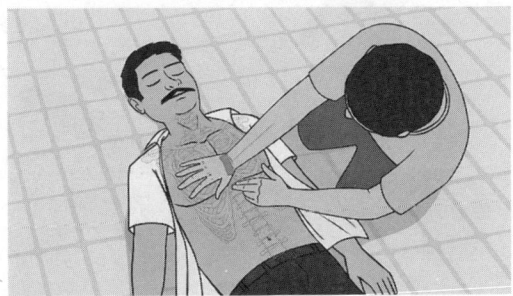

Fig. 7: Chest compression—position of the hand.

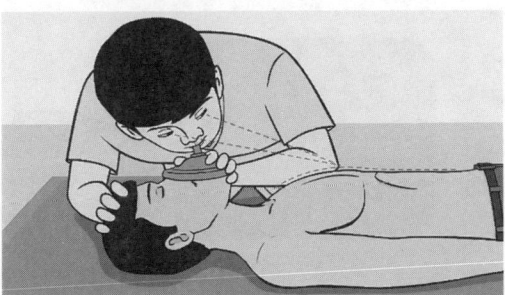

Fig. 9: Mouth to mask ventilation.

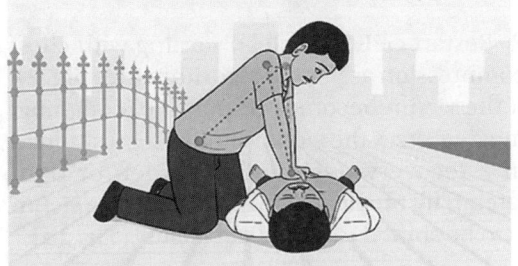

Fig. 8: Chest compression—position of shoulder.

compressions. Compression depth should be 5–6 cm in an adult victim with a rate of 120 compressions per minute. Push hard and fast. Minimize interruptions during compressions.

Breaths

After chest 30 compressions, open the airway by head tilt and chin lift (only jaw thrust/chin lift for suspected cervical spine trauma victim). Place one hand on the forehead and apply backward pressure. Place the fingers of your other hand on the bony part of the jaw and lift the chin. Give two rescue breaths for 1 second each breath using mouth to mouth (with/without barriers device), mouth to mask, or a bag-mask device, and watch for chest rise (**Fig. 9**). Lift your mouth between breaths. After two breaths, immediately resume compressions.

If help is available, then the chest compression and breath can be given by two different rescuers. The rescuer should interchange themselves every five sets of CPR (five cycles of 30 chest compressions and two breaths) to prevent exhaustion. After five sets of CPR, check the carotid pulse and follow the steps shown in the algorithm (**Fig. 2**).

Early Defibrillation

The rescuer or any layperson may retrieve the automated external defibrillator (AED) if nearby. The AED is a device that recognizes heart rhythm, automatically charges, and gives a shock (**Fig. 10**). Once the AED is

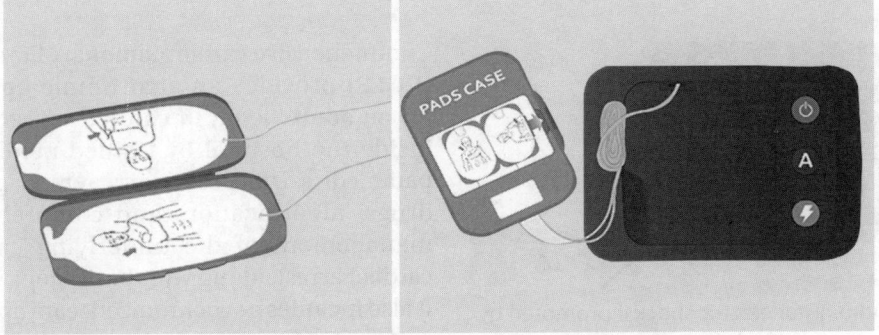

Fig. 10: Automated external defibrillator (AED).

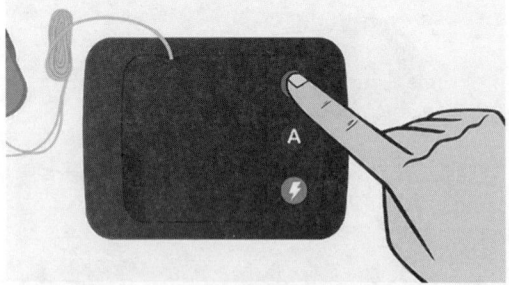

Fig. 11: Switch ON the AED and follow the voice prompts.

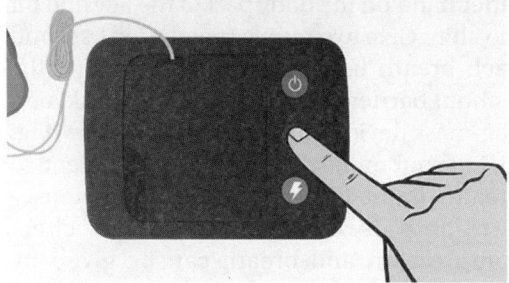

Fig. 12: Analyze the rhythm. (Do not touch the victim during rhythm analysis).

available, rhythm analysis and defibrillation should be done immediately, irrespective of the stage of the CPR cycle.

Attach AED pads (one at the apex of the heart on the left side of the chest and the other below the clavicle on the right side in the mid-clavicular line) without interrupting the chest compressions. The steps of using an automated external defibrillator are shown in **Figures 11 to 13**.

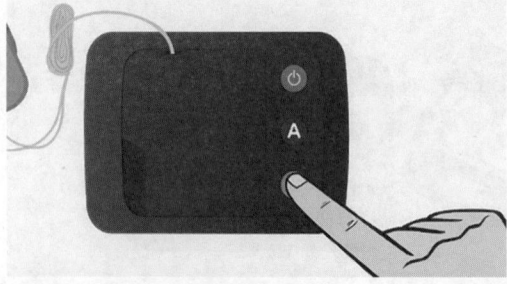

Fig. 13: Administer electric shock if prompted by AED.

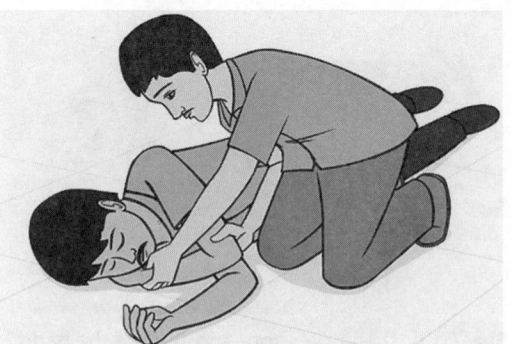

Fig. 14: Recovery position.

Restart CPR (5 cycles), starting with chest compression as per the algorithm (See **Fig. 2**). If the victim becomes responsive (coughing, moving, etc.), the victim should be positioned in a recovery position (either left or right lateral) till medical help arrives and the victim is to be shifted to a medical facility (**Fig. 14**).

Early Transfer

The victim should be transferred to the nearest healthcare facility for medical care and management of the underlying etiology of the cardiopulmonary arrest.

COMPREHENSIVE CARDIOPULMONARY LIFE SUPPORT (CCLS) FOR AN ADULT

AS2.2: Enumerate the indications, describe the steps and demonstrate in a simulated environment, Advanced Life Support in adults and children.

Comprehensive cardiopulmonary life support (CCLS) provides an algorithmic approach for an adult victim in cardiac arrest patient inside the hospital by trained medics and paramedics. It focuses on airway management, drugs, identification, and comprehensive management of the underlying cause of cardiac arrest, along with basic steps of CPR. It also includes a synchronized team approach and post-resuscitation care.

CHAPTER 21 ♦ Resuscitation

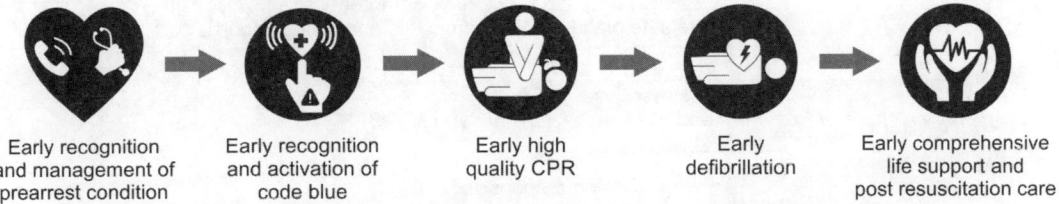

Fig. 15: Core link of CCLS for an adult cardiac arrest victim (Indian resuscitation council).

The CCLS has five essential core links for optimal outcomes in patients with cardiopulmonary arrest (**Fig. 15**). These core links are integrated into a stepwise algorithmic approach for a cardiac arrested victim in the hospital (**Fig. 16**).

EARLY RECOGNITION AND MANAGEMENT OF PRECARDIAC ARREST CONDITION

Early Recognition and Activation of Code Blue

In adults, the various reversible condition can predispose them to sudden cardiac arrest (**Table 1**). Early identification and management of the prearrest condition in hospitalized patients are very important. Thus, sudden cardiac arrest can be avoided.

Ensure a Safe Place for Resuscitation

Though hospital premises are usually safe. However, in certain situations, the victim may have collapsed in a relatively unsafe area such as a bathroom, lift, an area under construction, etc. The victim should be shifted immediately to a safer place for CPR without wasting time. All places inside the hospital are suitable for CCLS, and no specific area is suggested in this guideline.

Check Response

The rescuer should come from the front-facing the victim's face, tap on the shoulder and ask loudly (e.g., Hello! Are You all right?) in a language victim can understand (**Fig. 17**). Do not shake the victim. If the victim is responsive (verbally and/or by purposeful movement), monitoring and evaluation must be done. In the absence of response, activate the Code blue team or any local team (from the Intensive care unit/emergency area) to bring a defibrillator and emergency crash cart (emergency drugs and equipment). Ask someone if available nearby to activate the Code blue or a local team. All hospitals must have a Code blue speed dial number displayed in all areas.

Early High-quality Cardiopulmonary Resuscitation

Check Pulse and Breathe Simultaneously

Check for the presence of carotid pulse for 5-10 s. During this pulse check, watch for any breathing movements (**Fig. 18**).

Following Three Clinical Situations may Arise After Pulse and Breath Check

Normal breathing with a definite carotid pulse: Assessed the patient every 2 min or more frequently for any change in clinical parameters. Shift patients to ward/intensive care (if needed) for continuous monitoring and further evaluation.

Abnormal/no breathing with a definite carotid pulse: This is the situation of respiratory arrest. Opening of the airway by head tilt and chin lift (only jaw thrust or chin lift in suspected cervical spine trauma). Give a normal tidal volume breath every 5 s and watch for visible chest rise using the bag-mask device [**Fig. 19 (a-d)**]. It includes a well-fitting

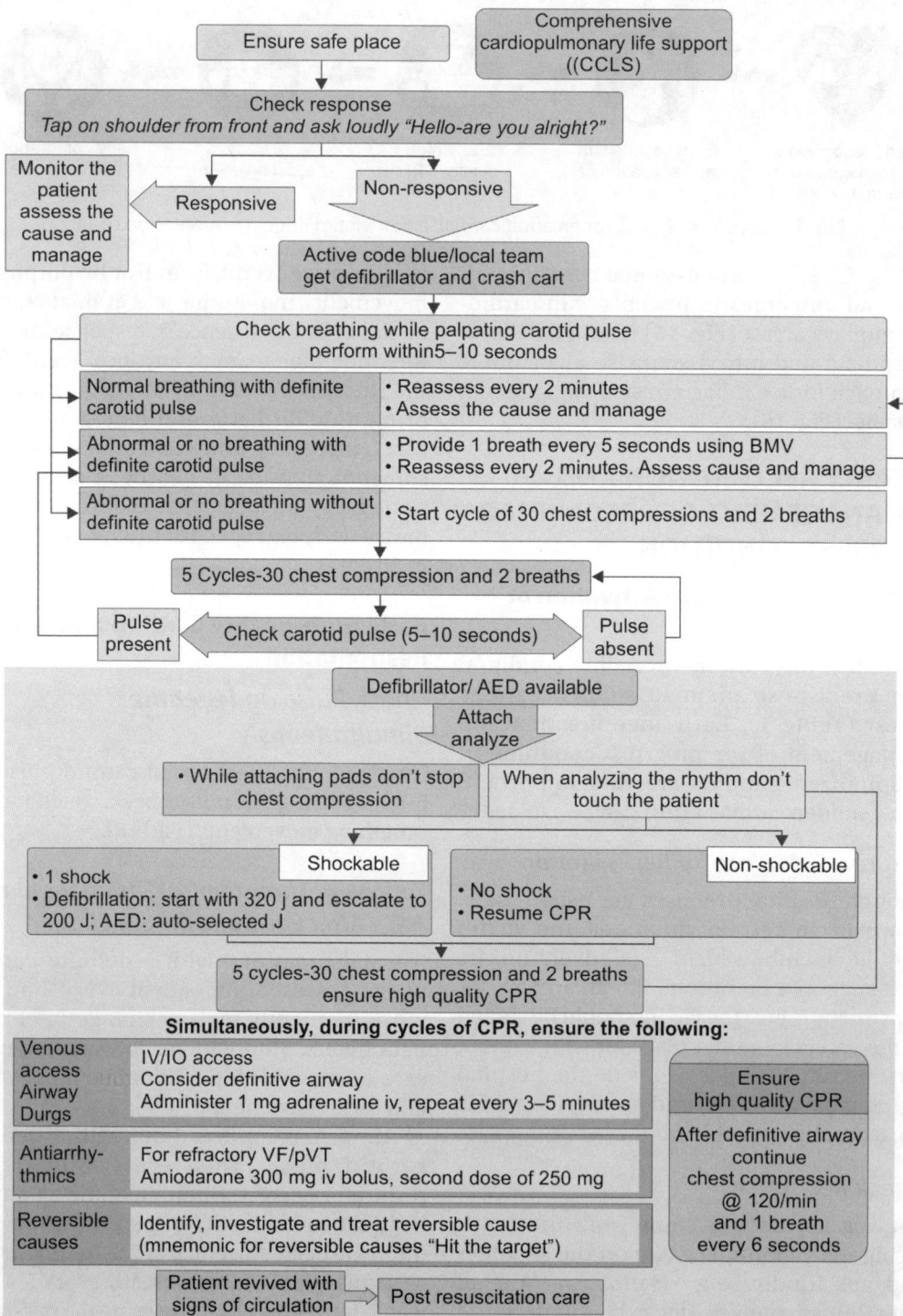

Fig. 16: Comprehensive cardiopulmonary life support (CCLS) for an adult (Indian resuscitation council).

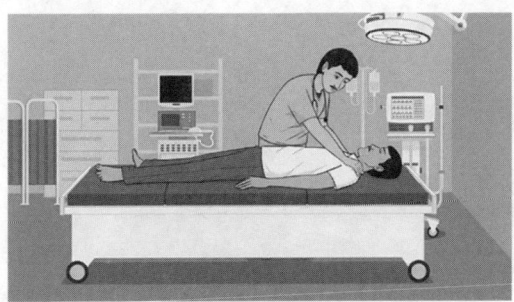

Fig. 17: Check responsiveness.

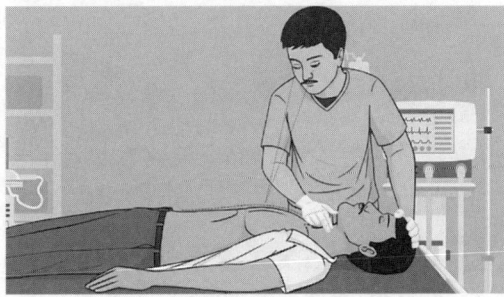

Fig. 18: Check for pulse and breathing.

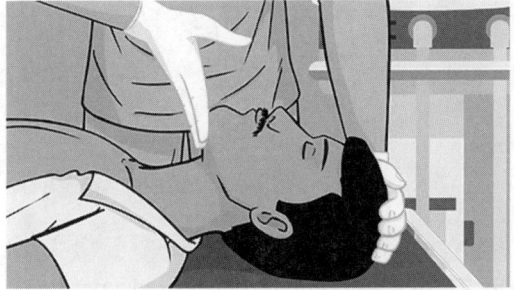

Fig. 19 (a): Head tilt and chin lift.

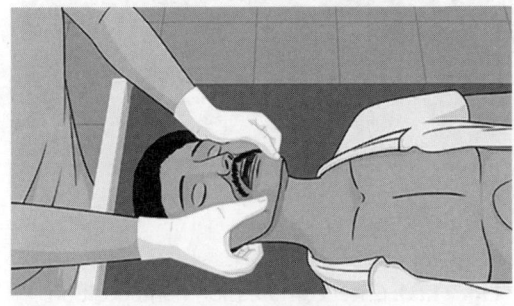

Fig. 19 (b): Jaw thrust.

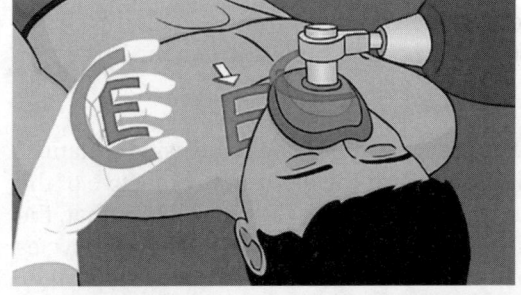

Fig. 19 (c): Mask holding C-E technique - 'C' shape with thumb and index finger over each side of the mask while the 3rd, 4th and 5th fingers hands lift the mandible toward the mask in 'E' shape.

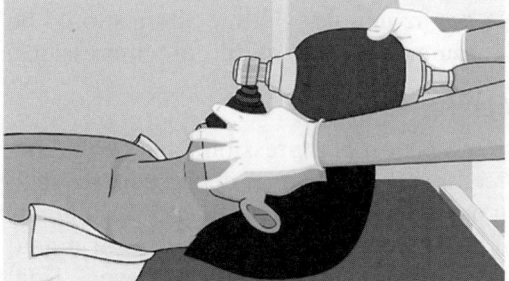

Fig.19 (d): Bag and mask ventilation.

mask covering the mouth and the nose, which is connected to a compressible, self-inflating bag connected to an oxygen source.

The oropharyngeal or nasopharyngeal airway devices may be used during bag and mask if chest rise is not satisfactory (**Figs. 20 a and b**).

Abnormal or no breathing without a definite carotid pulse: The patient is in cardiopulmonary arrest and requires high-quality CPR at the earliest. Start with cycles of 30 chest compressions and two breaths.

Chest Compression

The patients should be placed supine and on a firm bed/surface (a hardboard may be slipped under the patient). Place interlocked hand two fingers above the lowest end of the sternum and position shoulders directly over your hands [**Fig. 21(a–b)**]. Give 30 chest compressions with a rate of 120 compressions

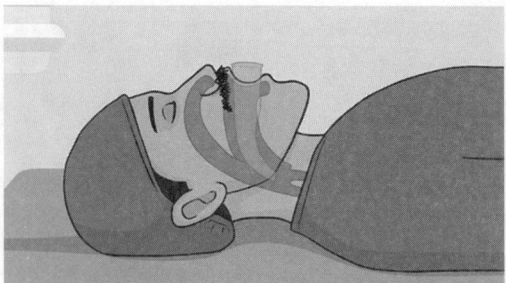

Fig. 20 (a): Oropharyngeal airway.

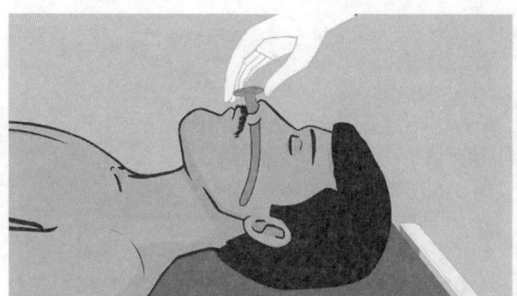

Fig. 20 (b): Nasopharyngeal airway.

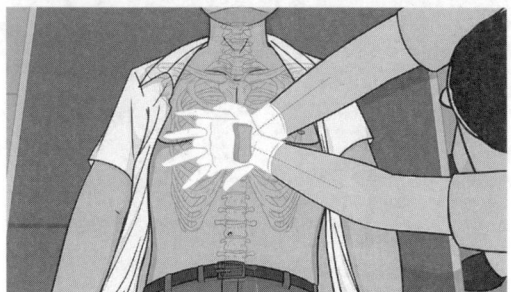

Fig. 21 (a): Chest compression-hand position.

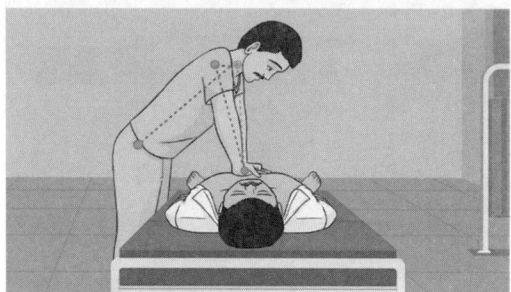

Fig. 21 (b): Chest compression-shoulder position.

per minute. Compression depth should be at 5–6 cm in an adult victim. There should be minimum interruptions during compressions.

Breaths

After 30 chest compression, give two rescue breaths with a bag-mask device connected to an oxygen source. Use basic airway adjuncts such as nasopharyngeal/oropharyngeal airways if chest rise is not achieved. Tidal volume breath should be delivered over 1 s with visible chest rise. After allowing 1 s for exhalation, another breath over 1 s is provided. The chest compression should be immediately resumed to minimize interruption.

The rescuer for chest compressions and the one for breath should interchange themselves after every five cycles of CPR to prevent exhaustion. After five cycles of CPR, check the carotid pulse and follow the steps as shown in the algorithm (See **Fig. 16**). If the patient's airway is already secured with an endotracheal tube, give chest compressions continuously at a rate of 120 compressions/min and ten breaths/min rather than cycles of 30 chest compressions and two breaths.

Early Defibrillation

Defibrillation should be done using a manual defibrillator at the earliest, irrespective of the stage of the ongoing CPR cycle. After that, the defibrillation should be given after five cycles of 30 compressions and two breaths. Follow the steps to prepare for defibrillation:
1. Switch on the defibrillator
2. Attach ECG leads. Keep defibrillator paddles on the chest (one at the apex of the heart on the left side of the chest and the other below the clavicle on the right side in the midclavicular line).
3. Analyze the rhythm. Do not touch the patient during rhythm analysis.
4. Give shock if shockable rhythm (ventricular fibrillation/pulseless ventricular tachycardia) is there. Charge the defibrillator to 120 Joules. Chest compression should

be continued during charging. Deliver the shock while ensuring that no one is touching the patient or bed. Resume CPR with chest compression after delivery of the shock. Non-shockable rhythm (asystole and PEA): Immediately resume CPR cycles, starting with chest compressions.

During ongoing CPR, other aspects such as venous access, airway management, and drug administration should be integrated as early as possible with minimal interruption (See **Fig. 16**).

Table 2: Common drugs used during CPR.

Epinephrine	1 mg (1:10000) intravenous or 2-2.5 mg (1:1000) through an endotracheal tube every 3 to 5 min during CPR
Amiodarone	1st dose: 300 mg bolus, 2nd dose: 150 mg, Max dose: 2.2 grams/day
Lignocaine	1st dose: 1-1.5 mg/kg IV, 2nd dose: 0.5-0.75 mg/kg IV every 5–10 min. Max dose: 3 mg/kg

Venous Access

Peripheral intravenous access is the most preferred. If unable to secure venous access in 3 attempts, an alternative route for administration is intraosseous. Few selected drugs (naloxone, adrenaline, atropine, and lidocaine) may also be administered through the endotracheal route if other routes are not secured. Send investigations based on possible causes of cardiac arrest based on history and medical record.

Advanced Airway Management

Consider definitive/advanced airway, i.e., endotracheal tube if expert help is available and correct placement must be verified using end-tidal capnography.

Drug Administration

Adrenaline (epinephrine) should be administered as boluses and be repeated every 3–5 minutes during ongoing CPR. If, after initial 2-3 sets of 5 cycles of CPR, the arrhythmias persist, then antiarrhythmics drugs are required, such as Amiodarone. Lidocaine may be an alternative drug for persistent arrhythmia (**Table 2**).

EARLY COMPREHENSIVE LIFE SUPPORT AND POST-RESUSCITATION CARE

After the return of spontaneous circulation (palpable carotid artery pulsation, abrupt sustained increase in end-tidal CO_2), the patient should be shifted to a dedicated unit. Post-resuscitation care ensures adequate oxygenation and circulation to avoid further cerebral insult. Ventilatory support may be continued as per patient assessment. The cause of cardiac arrest needs to be investigated and treated. Expert opinion may be needed to assess the need for coronary interventions.

Team Dynamic During CPR

Many healthcare providers (Doctors, Nurses, Technicians, etc.) from different specialties are involved during resuscitations. Teamwork, leadership, and communication are important for an effective outcome. A person who is assigned as a team leader is responsible for the overall management of the resuscitation process and coordinating communication among all team members. All team members should participate actively and speak up if they have concerns.

PEDIATRIC CARDIOPULMONARY RESUSCITATION

The principles of resuscitation discussed in previous sections also apply to a child in cardiac arrest. The CPR for the pediatric age group has been discussed as per the American Heart Association Guidelines 2020.

Causes of Cardiac Arrest in the Pediatric Age Group

Asphyxia is a more common cause of cardiac arrest in children than a primary cardiac

Table 3: Reversible conditions leading to cardiac arrest in children.	
6 H	5 T
• **H**ypovolemia • **H**ypoxia • **H**ydrogen ion (Acidemia) • **H**ypoglycemia • **H**ypo/hyperkalemia • **H**ypothermia	• **T**ension pneumothorax • **T**amponade (cardiac) • **T**oxins • **T**hrombosis (Pulmonary) • **T**hrombosis (Coronary)

cause. Airway and ventilation problems lead to asystole and PEA as the most common presenting rhythms. The common reversible condition which can lead to cardiac arrest in a child can be presented as 6H and 5T (**Table 3**).

In both the out-of-hospital and the in-hospital chain of survival in the pediatric age primary focus is on the prevention of cardiac arrest (**Fig. 22 a and b**). In the out-of-hospital situation, this includes safety measures such as road traffic laws for bikes, helmet laws, and early access to emergency care. In the in-hospital environment, early identification of precardiac arrest conditions and treatment such as acute heart failure, pulmonary hypertension, etc.

The pediatric resuscitation guidelines emphasize high-quality CPR, which includes chest compressions of adequate rate, adequate depth, full chest recoil between compressions, minimum interruptions, and avoiding excessive ventilation. Though the principle is the same as adult CPR, the following modifications are required for pediatric CPR.

Airway and Breathing

Upper airway anatomy is different in children. The head is large with a small face and a short neck. Use an appropriate size face mask and a pediatric manual resuscitator. Avoid undue pressure on soft tissue during mask ventilation which can lead to obstruction.

Circulation

- *Checking pulse*: Check carotid pulse for a child and brachial or femoral pulse for an infant.
- *Hand position during chest compression*: During chest compression, either two hands or one hand (very small child) technique on the lower half of the sternum can be used [**Fig. 23(a)**]. For an infant, the two-finger technique is used for a single rescuer [**Fig. 23(b)**] and the two-thumb technique if two or more rescuer is available [**Fig. 23(c)**].
- *Rate and depth of chest compression:* The chest compression in a child should be at least 1/3 of the anteroposterior diameter of the chest and with a rate of 100–120/min. Give chest compression at a rate of 100-

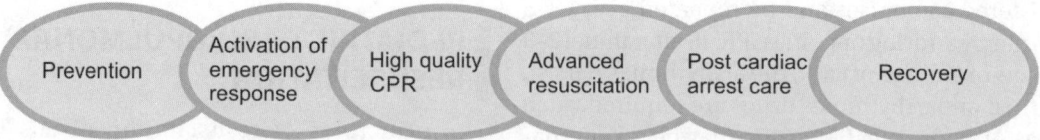

Fig. 22(a): Pediatric chain of survival for out-of-hospital cardiac arrest.

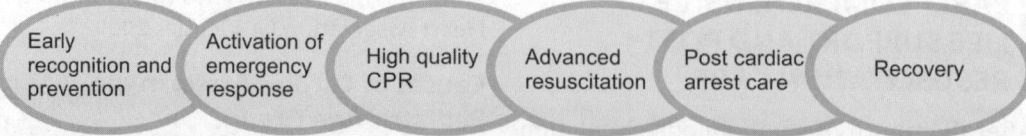

Fig. 22(b): Pediatric chain of survival for in-hospital cardiac arrest.

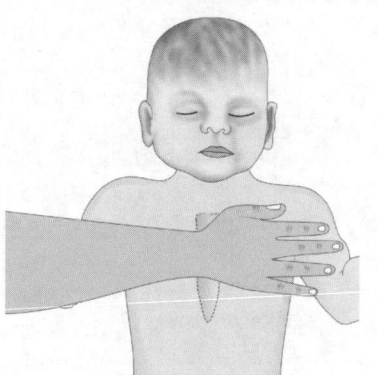 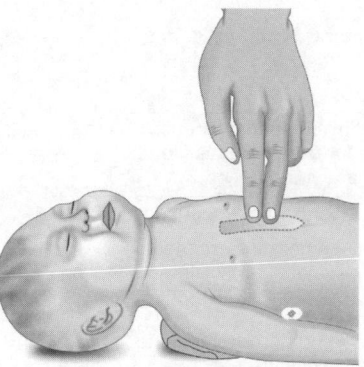 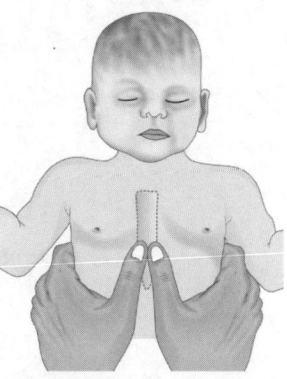

Fig. 23(a): One-hand chest compression.
Fig. 23 (b): Chest compression with two fingers.
Fig. 23 (c): Chest compression. Two thumb Technique.

120/min if the patient is already intubated (advanced airway). Allow complete recoiling of the chest between compression.
- *Chest compression-ventilation ratio:* Single rescuer should follow a 30:2 chest compression – ventilation ratio and a 15:2 chest compression – ventilation ratio in the presence of two or more rescuers.

Electrical Therapy

Consider a pediatric attenuator when using an AED on an infant and child <8 years old. Manual defibrillators are preferred because the shock energy dose can be titrated as per the child's weight.
- First shock: 2 J/kg
- Second Shock: 4 J/kg, Subsequent shocks ≥ 4 J/kg, maximum 10 J/kg or adult dose.

Use the 8 cm adult paddles if they fit on the chest wall with an adequate gap, or use the 4.5 cm pediatric paddles during manual defibrillation.

Drug Therapy

Either intravenous or intraosseous routes may be used for drug administration. The drugs are similar to adult CPR but should be used per the child's weight (**Table 4**).

The resuscitation algorithm for cardiac arrest for a child is shown in **Figures 24 (a) and (b)**.

Table 4: Most common drugs used during pediatric CPR.

Drugs	Dosage
Epinephrine	0.01 mg/kg (0.1 mL/kg of the 0.1 mg/mL concentration), maximum dose 1 mg. Repeat every 3–5 minutes
Amiodarone	5 mg/kg bolus. Repeat up to 3 times for refractory VF/pulseless VT
Lignocaine	Loading dose: 1 mg/kg. Maintenance dose: 20–50 mcg/kg/min

Neonate Cardiopulmonary Resuscitation

The primary goal of neonatal resuscitation at birth is to facilitate the transition from the womb to the outside environment, i.e., the establishment of lung inflation and ventilation after birth, maintenance of cardiovascular, temperature, etc. Approximately 10% of newborn babies need assistance to start breathing immediately after birth, and 1% of newborns may need resuscitative measures to sustain cardiorespiratory function. However, these guidelines apply to newborns during the neonatal period (birth to 28 days). The important points in Neonatal Resuscitation Guidelines are as follows:

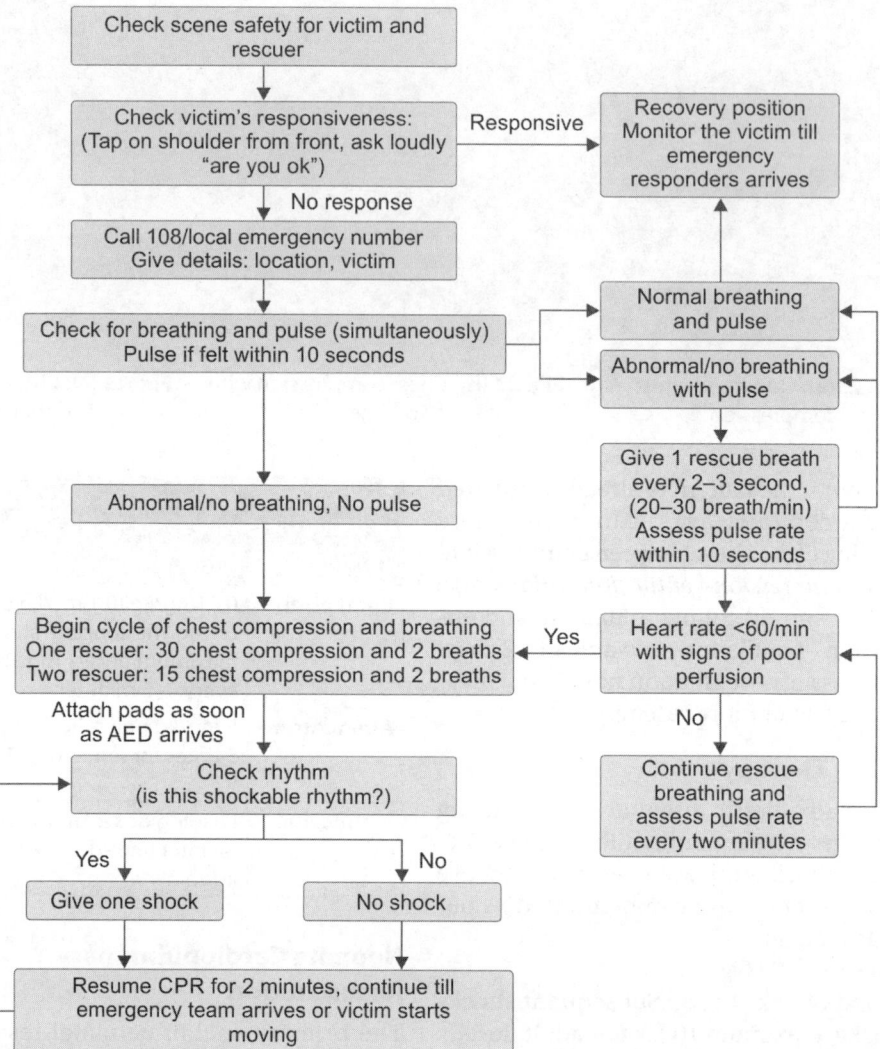

Fig. 24 (a): Pediatric basic life support algorithm.

Anticipation and Preparation

At least one skilled and equipped person should attend to newborn babies. The person should be able to initiate positive pressure ventilation. Standardized necessary equipment in a functional state should be available nearby.

Cord Management

For newborns (Preterm/term) who have not responded to resuscitation, cord clamping can be delayed for longer than 30 sec. For newborns <28 weeks of gestation, cord milking is not recommended.

Positive-pressure Ventilation and Chest Compressions

Positive pressure ventilation is the main intervention to resuscitate newborns who are apneic/bradycardic/poor respiratory effort. Use pulse oximetry to titrate oxygen therapy.

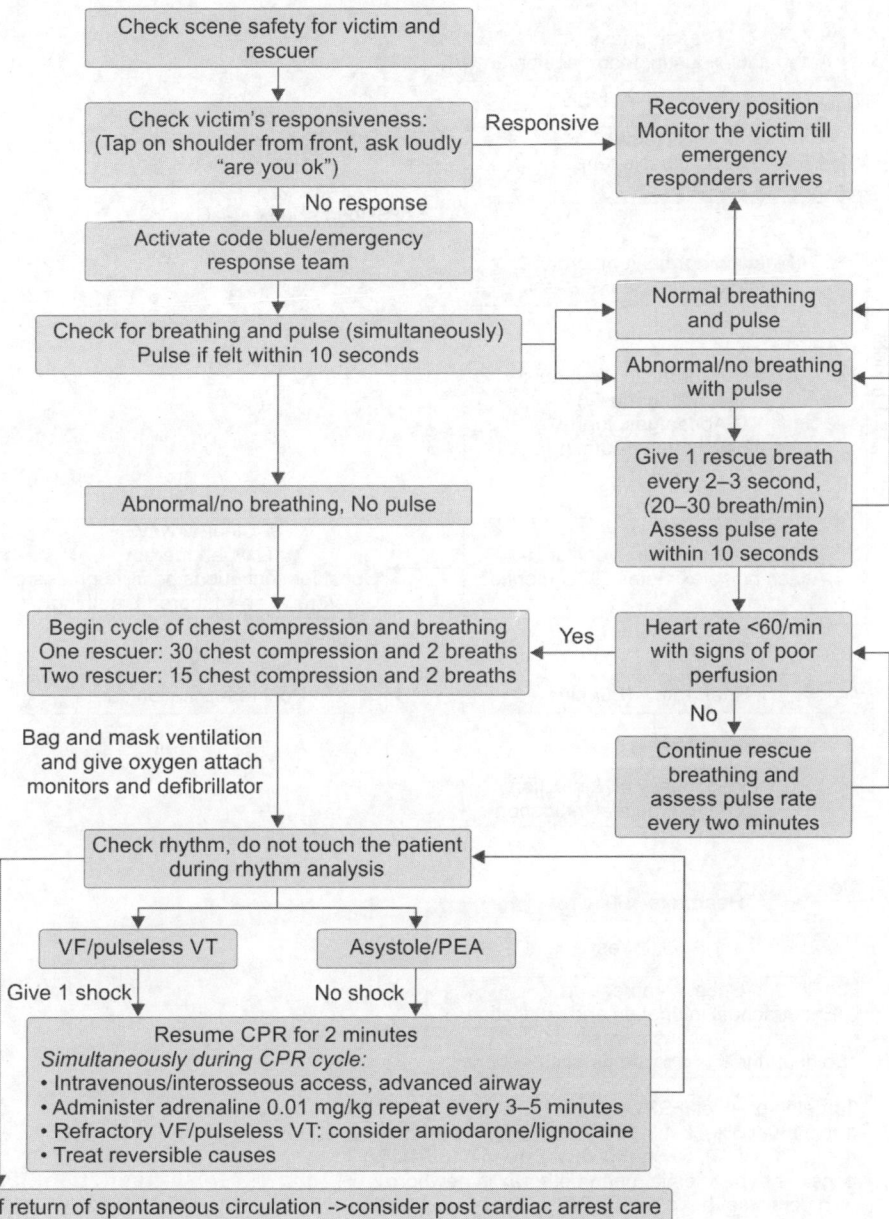

Fig. 24 (b): Pediatric advanced cardiac life support algorithm.

Heart rate is an important indicator of effective ventilation. If the heart rate remains < 60/min despite 30 seconds of ventilation, chest compressions should be performed using two thumbs encircling technique with the ratio of 3 chest compressions: 1 chest compression and rate of 30 ventilation per minute and 90 compressions per minute.

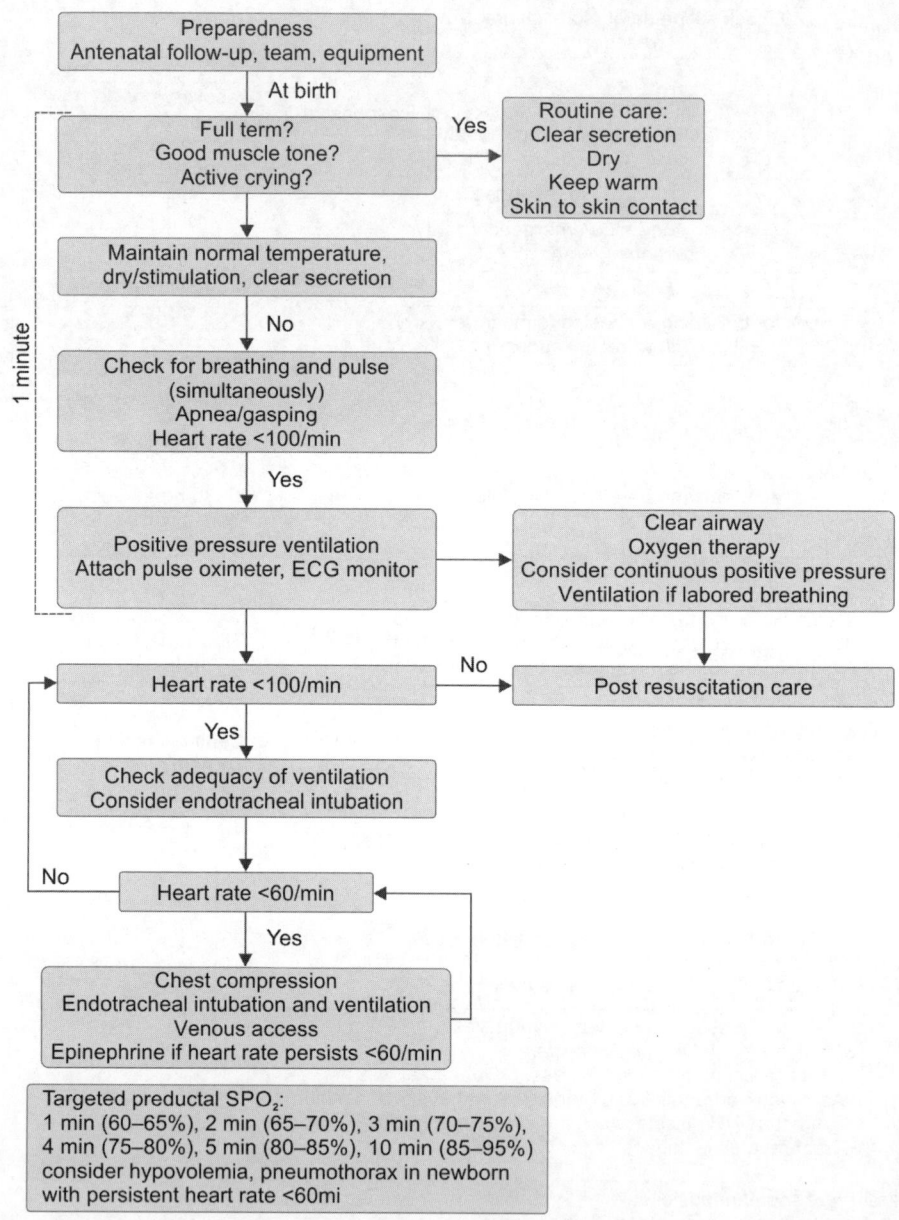

Fig. 25: Neonatal resuscitation algorithm.

Hypothermia Prevention

'Skin-to-skin care after birth effectively promotes breastfeeding and hypothermia prevention.

Vascular Access

The umbilical venous route is preferred in newborns. Alternatively, the intravenous or intraosseous route may be considered.

The Neonatal Resuscitation Algorithm, described in the American Heart Association Guidelines 2020, is shown in **Figure 25**.

TRAUMA CARE

Prehospital Care of Injured Patients

Prehospital care for injured patients is provided by the emergency medical team, which include technician, paramedics, physicians, etc. Airway obstruction and hemorrhage are the most common cause of mortality at the scene. The aims of prehospital trauma care are quick assessment, stabilization, and transport of injured patients to the appropriate nearby trauma facility for further management. Prehospital care depends on the level of training of the emergency medical team and local protocols. The steps of prehospital care are briefly described below.

Airway

Initiate basic airway measures to ensure oxygenation and ventilation. Use suction and airway adjuncts (oropharyngeal/nasopharyngeal airway, supraglottic device) if needed.

Manual in-line Stabilization of the Cervical Spine

All patients with trauma must be considered to have cervical spine injury unless proved otherwise. Neck movements must not be done, and manual in-line stabilization of the spine must be done (**Fig. 26**).

Hemorrhage Control

Immediately identify and control external hemorrhage and achieve intravenous/interosseous access to resuscitate with an intravenous fluid such as Ringer's lactate/0.9% saline.

Drugs and Defibrillation

Administer medication such as analgesics etc. if indicated in the local protocol. Use of AED in case of cardiac arrest.

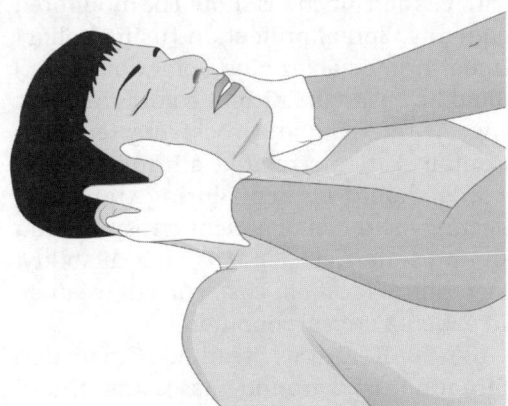

Fig. 26: Manual in-line stabilization.

The prehospital team should notify regarding the number and type of patients injured to the receiving hospital/trauma center before transport. This allows mobilization of all necessary personnel and resources to the emergency department/casualty at the time of the patient's arrival. There must be a smooth hand-over process between prehospital providers and those at the receiving hospital to ensure all important information with the entire team.

Transfer of Injured Patient

Smooth and efficient transfer of the trauma patient should be planned to minimize risk to the patient during the transport process. If the decision for the patient's transfer has been taken, no time should be wasted in tests/procedures. Order only relevant tests to identify life-threatening conditions. Referring team should continue resuscitation measures according to ATLS protocol. Spinal, pelvis, and extremity immobilization should be done if indicated. A cervical collar, pelvic splinting, and long backboard should be used during transport.

During transport, resuscitative equipment and a qualified person should be available. Ensure availability of a sufficient quantity of intravenous fluids, blood products, and drugs.

Vital signs and functions should be monitored frequently. Spinal protection (using collar/manual in-line stabilization, spine board, etc.) should be ensured. Efficient communication between referring and receiving teams is essential. Patients related all documents/records should be kept during transport. Selecting the mode of patient transportation (Ground/water/air) depends on availability, geographical location, cost, current weather, and patient's critical condition.

ABC-SBAR (Airway, Breathing, Circulation - Situation, Background, Assessment, and Recommendation) is a standardized template used for the handover process to improve patient safety (**Table 5**).

Principle of Triage of a Trauma Victim

Triage is the process of prioritizing trauma patients' treatment during mass-casualty or multiple casualties to ensure reasonable treatment for all patients with available resources. Triage is done at a different level and repeated several times. This is first done at the site of the event site, known as field triage. In field triage, all patients are prioritized for treatment and evacuation from the site. Triage is also done in the emergency department or casualty regarding shifting patients for further treatment such as operating room, intensive care unit, ward, etc. Triage is also done for the sequence in which patients are taken for surgical procedures. The triaged is repeated multiple times because the patient's conditions may either improve or worsen with interventions and time. All patients are tagged with color markings as per the triage category. One of the most common and simple methods is tags with the colors of a stoplight: red, yellow, and green (**Table 6**).

Over triage refers to a triage system in which a low-risk trauma patient receives a higher level of patient care that is unnecessary. High-risk trauma patients do not receive the desired

Table 5: Airway, Breathing, Circulation: Situation, Background, Assessment, and Recommendation (ABC-SBAR).

A	Airway	Intervention details
B	Breathing	Intervention details
C	Circulation	Intervention details
S	Situation	Patents' Details: Name, age Referring team details: Names Indication for transfer Site of IV access Type of IV fluid and rate Any interventions
B	Background	AMPLE assessment (Allergies, Medications, Past medical history, Last meal, and Events) Blood products Imaging performed Splinting
A	Assessment	Vital signs Physical exam findings Patient response to intervention
R	Recommendation	Transport mode Level of transport care Medication intervention during transport Further assessments and interventions

Table 6: Triage color coding.

Red	The life-threatening injury that requires immediate intervention, e.g. Tension pneumothorax, Cardiac tamponade
Yellow	Injuries that may become life- or limb-threatening if care is delayed for a few hours. e.g., Femur fracture
Green	Only minor injuries
Black	Deceased patients

Table 7: Recommended equipment and medications in the emergency department.

- Airway cart for intubation, oxygen masks/tubing, suction catheter, NG tubes
- Crystalloid IV fluids, large-bore IV cannula, IV dressing, transfusion set, blood/plasma
- Sterile towels, betadine/chlorhexidine, sutures, thoracostomy tray, central line tray
- Drugs: Sedatives, muscle relaxant, analgesics, naloxone, antiemetic, antiepileptic
- Others: Portable ultrasound, warm blankets

level of care if under-triage is done. Thus, a robust trauma system depends on appropriate triage protocol. Under triage may result in mortality/morbidity due to delay in definitive care, and over triage may result in a burden for trauma centers. Various triage protocol is used at different levels of trauma care. The Centers for Disease Control and Prevention (CDC) published an algorithm which is a four-step assessment process, which includes:

1. Assessment of vital signs and level of consciousness
2. Anatomy of injury
3. Assessment of high-energy mechanisms of trauma
4. Assessment of the special patient (e.g., extremes of age, pregnancy, burns, etc.).

Management of Trauma Victims in an Emergency Department or Casualty

Hypoxia is the most common early cause of mortality in trauma patients and is due to airway obstruction (direct injury to the face/neck, airway hemorrhage, decreased level of consciousness secondary to head injury, etc.) and inadequate ventilation (traumatic brain injury, high cervical spine injury, intoxication, hypothermia, pneumothorax or hemothorax, etc.). Hemorrhage is the second most important cause of death in trauma patients as ongoing blood loss is fatal.

Emergency/casualty trauma teams are generally composed of trauma surgeons, surgical subspecialties, anesthesiologists, emergency medicine physicians, nurses, technicians, and ancillary personnel. The roles and responsibilities of all team members should be defined. Advanced preparation and anticipation of patient conditions are important for the resuscitation of the trauma patient. All necessary equipment and medications should be checked and placed (**Table 7**).

Trauma patients are assessed and managed per advanced trauma life support (ATLS) guidelines. The ATLS consists of a rapid primary survey with simultaneous resuscitation and a more detailed secondary survey, and the initiation of definitive care. The primary survey consists of the ABCDEs (mnemonic—airway, breathing, circulation, disability, and exposure) of trauma care. It can identify life-threatening conditions by following this sequence, as shown in **Table 8** (Primary survey). The secondary survey is a head-to-toe assessment (detailed history, clinical examination, investigation) of the trauma patient to find any other evidence of trauma. Specific clinical finding as per anatomical region during the secondary survey is shown in the table (**Table 9**: Secondary Survey). It is done after the primary survey (ABCDE) is completed. If additional trauma healthcare workers are available nearby, the secondary survey may be started along with the ongoing primary survey. It should not, however, interfere with the performance of the primary survey, which is the priority.

Table 8: Primary survey with resuscitation.

ABCDE steps	Assessment	Management
Airway	• Vocal response • Look for patency, facial trauma, secretions, neck injury, etc. • Confirmation of endotracheal tube if placed during prehospital care	• Basic airway maneuver • 100% oxygen
Breathing	• Inspection of the chest wall for contusions, penetrating trauma, symmetry, and adequacy of chest rise • Auscultation	• Intubation • Mechanical ventilation • Thoracostomy
Circulation	• Check central and peripheral pulses • Skin color • Temperature • Blood pressure and pulse rate • Focused assessment with sonography for trauma (FAST) in unstable patients	• Intravenous line • IV fluid and/or blood product administration • Pressure bandage in an open wound • Pelvic binder • Prepare for surgery
Disability	• Glassglow coma scale • Pupillary response • Sensory and motor function in all extremities	• Computed tomography (CT) head • Emergency surgery • Intracranial pressure monitoring
Exposure	• Expose the patient fully • Inspect for additional severe injuries e.g., penetrating back injury	Surgical intervention if needed

Any unstable patients, e.g., active thoracoabdominal bleeding, should be shifted directly to the operative room without completing the secondary survey. The examination can be completed once surgical hemostasis is achieved. Patients with suspected traumatic brain injury with a poor Glasgow coma scale should be sent for Computed Tomography (CT) of the head. They must be prepared for a surgical procedure if needed, such as intracranial hematoma evacuation.

LIFE-THREATENING THORACIC INJURIES

Tension Pneumothorax

Pneumothorax is a collection of air between the parietal and viscera pleurae. Tension pneumothorax develops due to air leaks through a "one-way valve" from the lung or the thoracic wall. Air gets collected into the pleural cavity without any escape, which leads to the collapse of the affected lung and mediastinum displacement to the opposite side [**Fig 27(a)**]. Severe mediastinum displacement causes decreased venous return and compression in the opposite lung. This is a life-threatening injury that needs immediate management. The most common cause of tension pneumothorax in trauma patients are penetrating/blunt chest trauma and fractured rib in which a parenchymal lung injury fails to seal.

The physical finding includes chest pain, tachypnea, tachycardia, hypotension, tracheal deviation away from the side of the injury, unilateral absence of breath sounds, elevated hemithorax without respiratory movement, hyper-resonance on the affected side, neck vein distention, cyanosis (late manifestation), etc. If the patient is hemodynamically stable and there is a high suspicion of

Table 9: Secondary survey.	
Anatomic region	Assessment
Head	• Lacerations over scalp/face • Fractures of skull/facial bone • Dental trauma • Evidence of basilar skull fractures (raccoon eyes and battle signs i.e. bruising behind the ears • Cerebrospinal fluid rhinorrhea/otorrhea
Neck	• Hematomas, lacerations, • Cervical spine tenderness • *Remove cervical collar and examined neck with manual in-line stabilization
Chest	• Chest wall excursion and breath sounds • Asymmetry, ecchymosis, open wounds, subcutaneous air
Abdomen	• Contusions over flank • Open wounds • Tenderness
Back	• Ecchymosis • Open wounds • Spinal tenderness • *For assessment of back: The patient is log-rolled with manual in-line stabilization.
Extremities	• Lacerations • Deformities or open fractures • Tenderness • Swelling • Diminished/no pulse.
Genitourinary	• Bruising or lacerations • Blood at the urethral meatus. • *Rectal examination: Unresponsive patients to evaluate for reflexes and tone
Central nervous system	• Pupillary response • Neurologic deficits • Loss of reflexes • Sensory and motor deficits

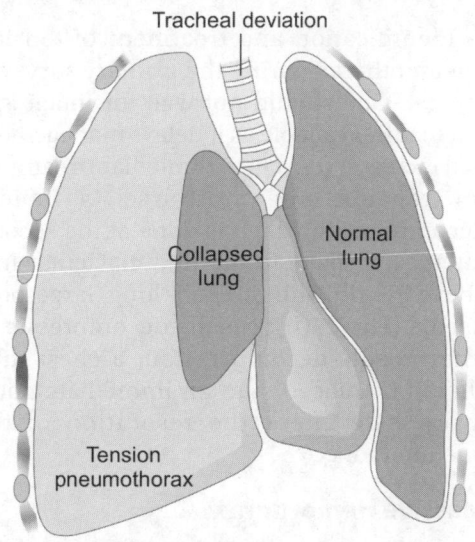

Fig. 27(a): Right side tension pneumothorax

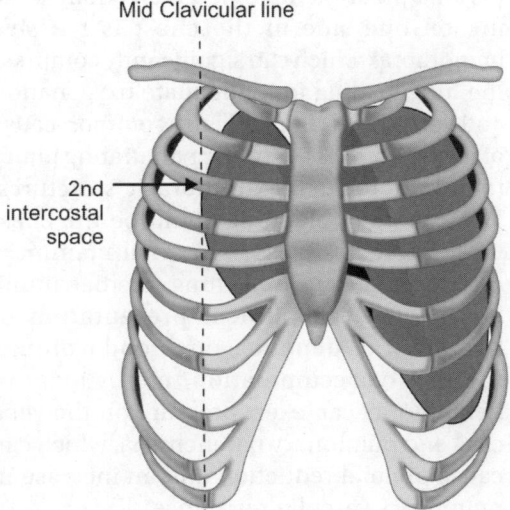

Fig. 27(b): Site for needle decompression.

pneumothorax, a radiological evaluation is done. The chest X-ray can show effacement of lung markings distally, a thin line representing the edge of the visceral pleura, ipsilateral lung collapse, mediastinum shift to the opposite side, subcutaneous emphysema, tracheal deviation to the opposite side, flattening of the hemidiaphragm on the ipsilateral side, etc.

Identification and treatment of tension pneumothorax during the primary survey is critical. One should not wait for imaging if not readily available as it delays management and increases mortality. Immediate treatment for tension pneumothorax is needle decompression which is done at the second intercostal space in the mid-clavicular line above the rib with the help long, large-bore needle [**Fig. 27(b)**: Needle decompression]. After needle decompression, a chest tube should be placed, and an immediate chest X-ray is to check the resolution of the pneumothorax.

Massive Hemothorax

Hemothorax is a blood collection in the pleural space (between the visceral and parietal pleura). The blood collection >1500 mL on one side of the chest is massive hemothorax which can significantly compress the lung leading to inadequate oxygenation and ventilation (**Fig. 28**). The common cause of hemothorax is a blunt or penetrating injury to intrathoracic or extrathoracic structures. The source of bleeding could be the chest wall, intercostal vessel, internal mammary arteries, major vessels, lung, mediastinum, heart, etc. The clinical presentation of hemothorax depends on blood volume, the rate of accumulation, etc. A massive hemothorax can exert pressure on the vena cava and pulmonary parenchyma, which can cause preload reduction and an increase in pulmonary vascular resistance.

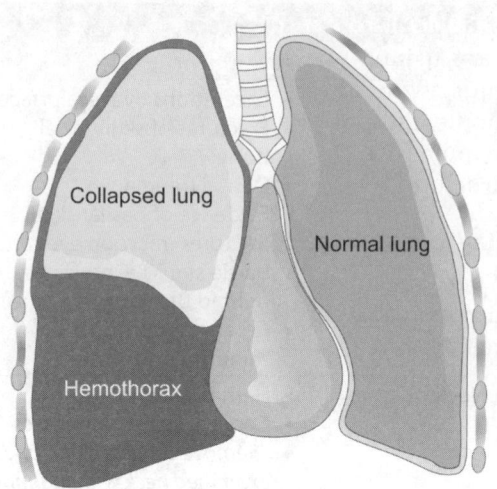

Fig. 28: Right side hemothorax.

Clinical findings of hemothorax are tachypnea, decreased or absent breath sounds, dull notes during percussion, asymmetrical chest wall, hypotension, etc. Physical findings of hemothorax may overlap with pneumothorax (**Table 10**). In massive hemothorax, the neck veins may be collapsed due to hypovolemia unless associated with tension pneumothorax.

Simultaneous resuscitation and decompression of the chest cavity is the primary goal of managing hemothorax. Secure wide bore intravenous lines and administer intravenous fluid to restore intravascular volume. Consider blood products as soon as possible. Place as a chest tube with the size of 28–32 French, usually at the fifth intercostal space and anterior to the midaxillary line. The patient needs

Table 10: Clinical signs of tension pneumothorax and massive hemothorax.

Clinical signs	Tension pneumothorax	Massive hemothorax
Neck veins	Full	Collapsed (unless associated with tension pneumothorax)
Trachea	Deviated to the opposite side	Midline
Chest movement	Minimal / No movement	Present
Percussion note	Hyper resonant	Dull
Auscultation	Decreased/Absent	Absent

thoracotomy if continues to bleed at the rate of ≥ 200 mL/hour, persistent need for blood transfusion, with a chest wall penetrating injury with anterior wounds medial to the nipple and posterior wounds medial to the scapula (possibility of injury to mediastinal structure).

Flail Chest

When a segment of the chest wall due to multiple rib fractures (i.e., ≥2 adjacent ribs fractured in ≥ 2 places) does not have bony continuity with the rest, known as a flail chest (**Fig. 29**). The flail segment moves paradoxically to the rest of the chest wall. This is usually associated with blunt trauma chest. This injury may be associated with significant pulmonary contusion, resulting in hypoxia. Impaired chest wall movement due to pain and pulmonary contusion can cause respiratory failure.

During the physical examination, abnormal respiratory motion and palpation of crepitus due to rib/cartilage fractures may suggest the diagnosis of flail chest. Visualization of abnormal chest movement may be difficult in muscular patients. A chest X-ray will show multiple rib fractures. Chest computerized tomogram is the better choice for investigation, which can also show other associated chest injuries.

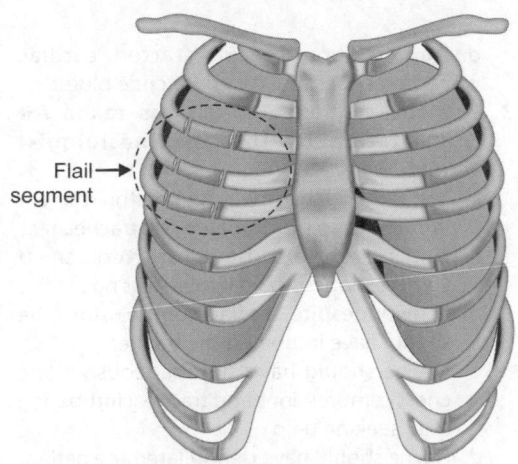

Fig. 29: Flail chest due to fractures of right-sided 3rd, 4th, and 5th ribs at two places.

The treatment of the flail chest includes oxygen therapy, adequate pain control, and surgical stabilization of the flail chest wall segment. The patients may need invasive mechanical ventilation if oxygen therapy and non-invasive ventilation. Intravenous fluid administration should be done cautiously, as it can compromise lung function. Surgical stabilization is done using metallic wires or mesh.

MULTIPLE CHOICE QUESTIONS

A patient in the medical ward has suddenly become unresponsive. The attendant calls the ward nurse. The nurse checks for the pulse on the patient's wrist, and she cannot palpate it. She shouts for help. The duty doctor comes to assess and says the patient has had a cardiac arrest. He calls for the anesthesiologist. The anesthesiologist comes after about 5 min and places an endotracheal tube, and then starts cardiopulmonary resuscitation. He delivered about 150 compressions every minute, all alone. Despite all efforts, the patient could not be revived.

1. **The nurse's method of recognizing cardiac arrest was wrong. What is the correct way to identify cardiac arrest?**
   a. To auscultate for the heartbeats with a stethoscope
   b. To look for pupillary signs
   c. To palpate the carotid artery
   d. All of the above

2. **Once the cardiac arrest was identified, the duty doctor called for the Anesthesiologist. Was this the correct way?**
   a. Yes. Anesthesiologists are resuscitation experts
   b. No, he should have called the cardiologist
   c. No, he should have activated code blue for the entire resuscitation team

d. No, he should have started cardiac compressions and called for code blue
3. **Was the sequence of actions taken for resuscitation by the anesthesiologist correct?**
   a. Yes, securing the airway for breathing is very important, so he intubated the trachea first
   b. No, he should have started chest compression first, and if there was no cardiac activity despite cardiac compressions, he should have intubated the trachea
   c. No, he should have simultaneously done chest compressions and tracheal intubation after seeking help
   d. No, he should have defibrillated the patient first
4. **Cardiopulmonary resuscitation is best given:**
   a. By chest compression with both hands with the heel of the hand in the left 4th- 5th intercostal space 5 cm lateral to the sternum
   b. By chest compression in the midline at the midpoint of the sternal length
   c. By chest compression at the lower end of the sternum
   d. By chest compression at the junction of the lower third of the sternum with the upper two-thirds
5. **Was the rate of chest compressions correct?**
   a. Yes, the higher the rate, the better the chance of success
   b. Yes, a high rate ensures higher cardiac output
   c. No, he should have compressed at a rate of 120/min for optimal cardiac output
   d. No, he should have compressed at a rate of 80/min
6. **The recommended depth of high-quality chest compressions during resuscitation is:**
   a. 3 cm
   b. 5 cm
   c. 7 cm
   d. 8 cm
7. **To administer a defibrillation shock with an automated external defibrillator (AED), the pads should be applied:**
   a. At the apex of the heart on the left side of the chest and below the clavicle on the right side in the mid-clavicular line
   b. At the apex of the heart on the left side of the chest and the other below the clavicle on the left side in the mid-clavicular line
   c. At the apex of the heart on the left side of the chest and the other on the sternum
   d. At the apex of the heart on the left side of the chest and the other on the right side in the mid-axillary line
8. **During cardiopulmonary resuscitation, an 1 mg bolus of adrenaline can be administered every:**
   a. 2 min
   b. 3–5 min
   c. 5–10 min
   d. 10 min
9. **In infant cardiopulmonary resuscitation:**
   a. The two-finger technique is used if there is a single rescuer
   b. The two-thumb technique is used if there are two rescuers
   c. The chest compression should be at least one-third of the anteroposterior diameter
   d. All of the above
10. **Triage is:**
    a. A Process of sequencing patients needing emergent, urgent, and less urgent care
    b. A process of prioritizing patients' treatment during mass-casualty or multiple casualties to ensure reasonable treatment for all patients with available resources
    c. A dynamic process in which the patient's priority may change if they either improve or worsen with interventions and time
    d. All of the above

Answers
1. c
2. d
3. b
4. d
5. c
6. b
7. a
8. b
9. d
10. d

22. Medicolegal Aspects and Investigation of Anesthetic Death

Mahima Singh, Sunil Singh

Learning Objectives

- Consent
- Understanding what is standard of care
- Importance of record-keeping and case notes
- Anesthesia-related mortality

INTRODUCTION

An anesthesiologist is never the primary consultant of the patient. Hence, anesthesia-related mortality is very difficult to explain, particularly in healthy individuals, since most activities are witnessed only by a handful of caregivers. Counseling, appropriate consent taking, high-quality medical recordkeeping, and knowledge of the legal nuances go a long way in ameliorating litigation. The anesthesia-associated death rate is negligible, yet it is not humane to equate a live individual to a number. It is crucial to understand the vital role orchestrated by autopsy and investigation into perioperative fatality in identifying the cause of death and its contribution to improving the quality of perioperative care.

"To err is human ...." In the practice of medicine, this may cause increased morbidity or even result in mortality. The error could be a consequence of inadequate knowledge and/or skill. Such a manifestation is perceived as an instance of "Malpractice" and is viewed through the lens of the Consumer Protection Act. The law of torts defines malpractice as negligence or incompetence on the part of a professional. The Merrian Webster dictionary defines malpractice as a dereliction of professional duty or failure to exercise an ordinary degree of professional skill or learning by one rendering professional services which result in injury, loss, or damage.

MEDICAL ETHICS

Details of medical ethics are described in Chapter 24.

CONSENT

An informed written consent has a legal connotation and characterizes its autonomous informed authorization. The consent document must address:

- *Disclosures*
  - Nature of the disease
  - Various treatment options are available (with their benefits and risks)
  - Prognostication with statistical data
  - Financial implications
- *Comprehension:* The information provided must be understood by the patient. It is

therefore important that the explanations and all discussions must happen in the language which the patient understands. Due caution must be used when handling compromised patients, viz deaf, dumb, mentally challenged, etc.

- *Absence of outside control:* It must be ensured that the consent is given voluntarily and with free will. There must be no external influence or pressure. Any acts of coercion or threat make the consent null and void. If the patient seeks any additional information, it must be provided.
- *Competence:* The person giving the consent has to be mentally sound, above 18 years of age, and not under the influence of any drug, alcohol, or anesthesia.
- *Actual consent:* The legal tenability of consent is only when it is in writing and signed by the consent giver in the presence of two independent witnesses. It must be for a specific purpose. If the purpose is to be revised or an addition made, the consent must be taken again. The anesthesiologist is personally responsible for taking the consent. The responsibility cannot be delegated to some other person.

Granting consent is the prerogative of the individual concerned or their surrogate. Respect for patient autonomy is at the core of the medical laws and ethics in vogue. The choice is placed in the hands of patients rather than physicians. Antihippocratic as it may seem, it forms the basis of patient-centered decision-making.

STANDARD OF CARE

Medical science is an ever-evolving and non-mathematical science, and hence it is prone to imperfections. These imperfections manifest because of multiple patient-centric variables and an ill-defined, empirical, and subjective definition of compromised service. To bridge the divide, various measurable objectives have been devised, namely, "Standard of Care," "Practice Protocols," "Guidelines," etc. This requires the use of a fair degree of skill sets, the acquisition of a reasonable knowledge base, and exercising an appropriate level of patient care. As elementary as it may seem, it is impossible to define and delineate specific standards of care for all forms and aspects of healthcare practices, situations, and contingencies. To cater to this phenomenon, the terminology of "reasonable and prudent physician" has been introduced. All this, however, involves prognostication of outcomes based on statistical values, which are, often confounding and difficult to comprehend, particularly since the individual is not a numeral.

The determinants of patient outcome comprise:
a. Physical limitations imposed by the primary pathology
b. Functional status of the other organ system systems
c. Treatment to be exhibited
d. nature and scope of the planned procedure
e. Availability of equipment and resources.

All these factors must be considered when applying the "standard of care" amidst the legal tenability and liability of the anesthesiologist.

RECORDKEEPING

The Professional Etiquette and Ethics Regulation of the Indian Medical Council has prescribed the duties and responsibilities of the physician regarding the maintenance, custody, and release of medical records. The Clinical Establishment (CE) Act and Rules (2012) also mandate the provisioning of electronic medical records for all patients. These records must adhere to the Electronic Health Record (EHR) Standards enunciated in the CE Act. All legal bodies and organizations give immense focus to recordkeeping and record preservation to attenuate the unreliability of memory over long periods during the arbitration.

On the patient's death, all medical records about the patient must be sealed and preserved. These are vital during investigating the cause of perioperative death because that is the only antemortem evidence available to corroborate post-mortem pathophysiology and other circumstantial evidence. Therefore, due diligence must be done to ensure documenting high-quality anesthesia records. Hence the rule, *If It Is Not Documented, It Was Not Done,* is coined.

CASE NOTES

The Indian Society of Anesthesiologists provides extensive guidelines for maintaining high-quality anesthesia records. These guidelines are based on the Latin proverb *Verba volant, Scripta manent*, i.e., spoken words fly away, and written words remain. The value of these records is realized during legal tangles. They illustrate the patient's clinical path and the standard of care provided. The anesthesia notes can be segregated into:

Preanesthetic Assessment

The preanesthetic assessment of the patient is performed to:
 i. Evaluate the general physical condition
 ii. Evaluate the functional status of organ systems
 iii. Evaluate the status of comorbid conditions
 iv. Evaluate the impact of preexisting drugs on anesthesia and surgery
 v. Evaluate for possible difficulties in the conduct of anesthesia, namely difficult airway, difficult spine, etc.

History

A detailed medical history of the current and past ailments coupled with a thorough clinical examination and diagnostics workup is vital to accomplish the first step towards ensuring patient safety. All of this helps to have an objective-based risk stratification using standardized grading systems, viz American Society of Anesthesiology (ASA), New York Heart Association (NYHA), Mallampatti Classification, Simplified Airway Risk Index (SARI), etc. It is important to remember that these scores do not provide a risk grading of perioperative morbidity or mortality. They help as alerts by prognosticating the likely occurrence of adverse events.

Identification of Anesthesia Risk

To date, no studies have been done to identify, preoperatively, the risk factors for anesthesia-related death. This is probably because of the rarity of anesthesia-related deaths. Rationality suggests that critically ill patients with multi-organ dysfunction shall have a higher incidence of anesthesia-related death than the healthier.

Anesthesia Notes

These depict the proceedings "behind closed doors" and must be documented in real-time or as close to it to prevent distortion due to time lag. The document must incorporate all events commencing from the preanesthesia room, through the conduct of anesthesia and surgery, till the patient's discharge from the Post Anesthesia Care Unit (PACU).

Monitoring

Pulse oximetry was introduced into clinical practice in 1980, and it is considered the watershed year for patient safety. The intraoperative use of capnography and pulse oximetry monitoring has helped reduce anesthesia-related mortality. Recording all patient monitored parameters, drugs administered along with their doses, and other interventions must happen in real-time/periodically. The minimum patient monitoring standards as advocated by the Indian Society of Anesthesiologists include all the vital parameters, viz temperature, pulse rate, blood pressure, respiratory rate, electrocardiogram, and oxygen saturation.

Continuous monitoring of inspired and expired concentrations of inhaled and exhaled gases and anesthetic agents with MAC levels when general anesthesia is administered. The amount of neuromuscular block must be monitored and documented, especially at the end of anesthesia, to exclude residual muscular paralysis.

Anesthesia Technique

The anesthetic technique and drugs used, the airway management strategy, type of patient monitoring, and compliance to Patient Safety Goals have to be indicated. The indication for invasive monitoring should be prescribed to demonstrate the critical nature of the event.

Anesthesia Record

The entire record must be available either as a manuscript or in digital form. HL7 standards system has made real-time safe and reliable patient recordkeeping a reality. The combination of HL7 compliant patient monitors and servo-based anesthesia delivery system, coupled with HL7 compliant drug injectors, allows for a real-time accurate record of the conduct of entire anesthesia.

Recovery

The monitoring done during the surgery must continue seamlessly into the PACU. The record of all monitored parameters, event occurrences, and medication administration details must be recorded with timelines. The criteria met by the patient before mobilization out from the PACU must be documented and signed by the anesthesiologist. In case the patient is shifted to a critical care bed, the reason for the same, along with the objective elements to be achieved during this phase, has to be documented, witnessed, and evidenced. The nurses' notes are equally vital and must also be perused to identify any early warning signs of an impending criticality. These notes, in combination with the clinicians' notes and other charts, help in documenting the whole clinical picture.

Other Charts

Various charts are maintained which record various other activities, viz Medication chart, Blood sugar chart, Vitals chart, Intake and Output chart, etc., which provide useful and timely information regarding the treatment activities and the condition of the patient.

MORTALITY RELATED TO ANESTHESIA

The first large-scale retrospective study to identify the mortality risk associated with anesthesia was done by Beecher and Todd. It involved ten teaching hospitals, covered 5,99,500 surgical patients, and extended over a period of 4 years from 1948 to 1952. This intensive exercise was pivotal to identifying anesthesia safety as a public health concern. It paved the way for the introduction of the concept and significance of the role of continued improvement in anesthesia safety. This led to better techniques, drugs, and enhanced training. The result is a decline in anesthesia-related mortality from 1/100 in 1940 through 1/10,000 in 1970 to 1/1,00,000 in the 1990s and early 2000s.

Lack of Data

The absence of monitoring through any established national surveillance data system, expansion in the horizon of the clinical application of anesthesia beyond therapeutics to encompass diagnostics, increase in ambulatory care surgical anesthesia, and the rarity of anesthesia-related deaths have all contributed to the woes of data analytics regarding exposure to anesthesia.

Defining Anesthesia Death

Anesthesia-related morbidity or mortality connotes death during the conduct of anesthesia. Anesthesia plays a vital role in comprehensive patient care requiring an invasive intervention. Being an independent specialty in clinical practice and having a common patient base with other surgical and nonsurgical specialties, the relationship is symbiotically targeted towards patient beneficence. Fatalities consequent to surgical procedures or anesthetic lapses are ill-defined.

Conventionally, deaths occurring within 24 hours of exposure to anesthetics and surgery are classified as unnatural deaths. These are required, by law, to be informed to the police, the statutory investigating body, for establishing the cause of death and accountability of any deficiency in service which is tantamount to malpractice, under section 39 of CrPC. Failure to do so may entail penal action under section 202 of the IPC.

Anesthesia deaths were earlier segregated based on clinical judgment into deaths primarily due to anesthesia and those in which anesthesia had a partial role. The International *Statistical Classification of Diseases and Related Health Problems* (ICD) is a standard classification system for recording and reporting diseases, injuries, and other health conditions. This system is used by many countries for the compilation of morbidity and mortality data. It is also a useful tool for disease-specific data analysis, outcome comparison, retrospective studies, health strategy development, and formulating projection trends.

Causes of Anesthesia Death

The combination of a loose definition for anesthesia-related mortality and its low incidence requires the denominator to be huge to facilitate meaningful conclusions. No available studies unequivocally identify specific preoperative anesthesia-related risk factors for morbidity or mortality. However, the most common causes of death linked to anesthesia are:

1. Circulatory failure
   a. Hypovolemia
   b. Anesthetic overdose
2. Hypoxia and hypoventilation
   a. Undetected esophageal intubation
   b. Failed intubation
   c. Failure to ventilate
   d. Gastric content aspiration
   e. Equipment malfunction
3. Drug reactions: Anaphylactic/anaphylactoid
4. Negligence
   a. Compromised vigilance
   b. Error in drug administration
   c. Inadequate maintenance of equipment and devices
      i. Defective vaporizer
      ii. Flowmeter assembly defects
      iii. Medical gas pipeline system malfunction.

The most vital prerequisite for identifying the cause of death is accurate, adequate, and high-quality documentation of all activities. Technology, based on HL7 standards, has now provided the capability of real-time recording of vital parameters, inspired and expired concentrations of volatile anesthetic agents, minimum alveolar concentration values, and the infusion rates of parenterally administered agents, viz, muscle relaxants, opioids, vasoactive and inotropic drugs, antiarrhythmic agents, etc.

Investigation of Death

First Actions

a. Report the occurrence to the hospital administration.
b. Seal the operation theatre. Ensure that nothing is removed or tampered with, including used syringes, ampoules, vials, parenteral fluid bottles, etc.
c. Do not allow the operating room to be cleaned.
d. The anesthesia machine must not be used till the investigation is completed.

e. The digital recording of the monitored parameters must be preserved till the completion of the investigation.
f. The case file must be completed promptly and sealed for handing over to the investigation team promptly.

Investigation

A pathologist must be the head of the investigation team and the following aspects must be considered:
a. *History*: It is important to do due diligence on the period preceding the present hospitalization.
b. *Indication and scope of surgery*: To determine the surgical risk to the patient
c. *Preanesthetic medication*: To identify medication errors
d. Injuries due to device malfunction/careless use and absence of adequate preventive measures
e. *Anesthetic agent*: Inadvertent mixing/leakage
f. Hypovolemia, hypotension and acidosis
g. Blood transfusion and transfusion reactions
h. Resuscitative measures.
i. *Equipment and qualified personnel*: A device is only as good as the operator behind it.

Autopsy

Autopsy findings are often useful to the defense of the anesthesiologist in malpractice suits. An autopsy is, unfortunately, an under-utilized investigation process in medical jurisprudence. An autopsy assists in deciphering the pathophysiology underlying anesthesia-related adverse events. There are no pathognomonic features of anesthesia-related fatalities. Hence the autopsy often does not reveal anything ominous. Pathological features associated with anoxia and cardiovascular collapse are the usual findings. The problem with the identification of the cause of death lies in the absence of any evidence for the sudden fall in blood pressure, irregularity of cardiac rhythm, or glottic spasm as the leading causes of fatality.

Surgical and anesthetic devices introduced into the patient should not be removed before autopsy. The endotracheal tube, if inserted for ventilating the patient, must not be removed, and its position must be checked by pre-autopsy radiography. All antemortem samples available are preserved for further studies by the investigation team.

Alveolar air must be sampled by pulmonary puncture underwater, blood should be collected under oil, and both lungs and brain must be preserved. Cerebrospinal fluid must be collected for chemical analysis if death results from neuraxial anesthesia. The gases used during anesthesia must also be sampled to evaluate the proportionate combination of the mixture before use. Approximately two grams of mesenteric fat, ten grams of skeletal muscle, and both kidneys must be subjected to toxicology analysis.

In suspected air embolism, the inferior vena cava must be thoroughly examined for the presence of air bubbles. To exclude the effects of post-mortem decay, the gas sample must be subjected to analysis by chromatography. A serological examination is mandatory to evaluate for possibilities of serological reactions. Exudates, blood, other body fluids, and tissue samples from the heart, liver, lung, and brain must be sent for histological examination.

MULTIPLE CHOICE QUESTIONS

OSCE

A 15-year-old boy was taken up for Laparoscopic Appendicectomy. The patient had no comorbidities. After induction of anesthesia, the anesthesiologist secured the airway with an endotracheal tube and verified the correct placement by chest lift. He did not use a capnometer to monitor end-tidal carbon dioxide as it was not available. The oxygen saturation of the patient started dipping after a few minutes, so his inspired oxygen concentration was increased. Despite this, the saturation fell further, and the patient had a cardiac arrest. Cardiopulmonary resuscitation was started by the surgeon. The Anesthesiologist checked the tube placement by laryngoscopy and found the endotracheal tube in the esophagus. He re-introduced the tube in the trachea. The patient could not be revived. The surgery was canceled, and patient was shifted to the ICU and placed on mechanical ventilation before he was declared dead.

1. Does this case qualify as Malpractice by the anesthesiologist?
    a. Yes, because the patient died during surgery
    b. Yes, because the anesthesiologist displayed negligence in not ensuring the correct placement of the endotracheal tube
    c. No, because it was an error of judgment, not a deliberate act
    d. No, because to err is human
2. The consent for anesthesia was only signed by the uncle of the patient. Is it valid?
    a. It is valid as in the case of minors, the consent has to be signed by a parent or a caretaker
    b. It is invalid as it should have been signed by one of the parents
    c. It is invalid as it should have been signed by the patient, a caretaker, and a witness as the patient was more than 12 years old
    d. It is invalid as it should have been signed by a witness too
3. The hospital is also liable in such a case because of:
    a. The surgery took place in it
    b. The anesthesiologist was a consultant employed by the hospital
    c. A capnometer, the standard of care, was unavailable for the case
    d. All of the above
4. Was it correct to shift the patient to the ICU and declare him dead there?
    a. Yes, otherwise, the body would need to be handed over to the police as it was an anesthetic death
    b. Yes, as the patient's relative could get violent
    c. No, the death should have been truthfully declared in the OT. Deaths occurring within 24 hours of exposure to anesthetic and surgery are classified as unnatural deaths, and police must be informed to establish the cause of death
    d. Yes, one should avoid being sued in a medicolegal case
5. The esophageal intubation was not recorded in the anesthesia chart, and all resuscitation measures taken were not recorded. Will this benefit the doctors?
    a. Yes, they can escape scrutiny by claiming no adverse event occurred in the OT
    b. No, their negligence will be compounded for not taking resuscitation measures as no record will be assumed as not done by the court
    c. Yes, no mention will help them to do a cover-up later
    d. It may or may not benefit the doctors

Answers
1. b 2. c 3. d 4. c 5. b

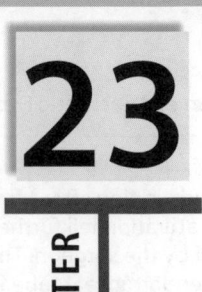

Career in Anesthesiology

Mukul Chandra Kapoor

Learning Objectives

- Evolution of modern anesthesiology
- Changed profile of anesthesiologists
- Extended role of anesthesiologists
- Advances in drugs and techniques
- Postgraduate training in anesthesiology
- Sub-specialization in anesthesiology
- Critical care physicians
- Increased demand for anesthesiologists
- Perioperative medicine
- Perioperative surgical home
- Safe surgery
- Pride of place in the medical profession

INTRODUCTION

AS1.4: Describe the prospects of anesthesiology as a career.

With the development of medicine, specialization has developed to cope with and facilitate growth in knowledge and standards of care and meet the aspirations and expectations that accompany these developments. Before the advent of anesthesia, there was hardly any advance in surgery, and operations were brief and limited to minor interventions. The advent of advanced anesthesia techniques and advanced perioperative care had a significant impact on the scale of surgery. Sophisticated surgery requires more skillful anesthetists, better physiological understanding, better equipment, and improved drugs. The surgeons took up complicated and challenging cases considered inoperable earlier with these available. This cycle has driven progress in surgery ever since and collaterally made significant contributions to advancing the specialty of anesthesia.

EVOLUTION OF MODERN ANESTHESIOLOGY

The standing of anesthesiologists as independent practitioners has improved. The need to ensure safe patient outcomes after surgery also enhanced the status of anesthesiologists. In 1948, anesthesiology was granted equal status with all British National Health Service specialties. By 1950, all of the elements of modern anesthesia were in place. Although very few drugs are still in use, their successors are improvements on the same theme. Modern anesthesia has achieved an impressive safety record thanks to the availability of better equipment and better protocols. Anesthesia workstations are commonplace across the country, and even tier 2/3 cities have modern anesthesia equipment and technology.

CHANGING PROFILE OF THE ANESTHESIOLOGIST

Anesthesiology has undergone remarkable changes over the past few decades. Anesthesiology was always considered a hospital-based specialty, always behind the curtain. Anesthesiologists were considered introverts, restricted to the confines of the operating room and under the command of surgeons. Anesthesiology has evolved into a mature specialty that today forms the backbone of any hospital and plays a pivotal role in almost all areas of hospital care. Anesthesiologists have progressed from technically competent assistant physicians to professional physicians with diverse knowledge and technical proficiency in multiple fields. Anesthesiologists have shed their introverted image and function as confident and skillful clinicians.

EXTENDED ROLE OF ANESTHESIOLOGISTS TODAY

The nonsurgical and noninterventional specialties may not appreciate an anesthesiologist's proficiency and role. However, anesthesiologists get all the kudos from surgical and nonsurgical interventional specialists. Apart from the established role of administration of anesthesia, anesthesiologists have majorly expanded into critical care, both as administrators and clinicians. Anesthesiologists run chronic pain clinics and perform ablation interventions. Anesthesiologists are the primary carers for labor analgesia. The awareness of and the demand for pain relief for labor has increased with the advanced methods of administering walking epidurals.

Anesthesiologists have taken advantage of some of these expanded roles and have gradually improved their profile. Anesthesiologists administer monitored anesthesia care to patients for endoscopy, bronchoscopy, magnetic resonance imaging scan, electroconvulsive therapy, radiotherapy, catheterization laboratory interventions, interventional radiology/neuroradiology procedures, and many such outpatient procedures. Anesthesiologists are also the primary members of the hospital resuscitation teams. Anesthesiologists are also responsible for emergent clinical management of various fluid, electrolyte, and metabolic disturbances.

ADVANCES IN DRUGS AND TECHNIQUES

The last few decades have seen remarkable improvements in anesthetic pharmacology with the development of several hypnotics, analgesics, and neuromuscular blocking agents. Tailored patient management with shorter-acting compounds and improved safety profiles has prevented injury from unwanted effects. In the current era, rapid onset and offset of a drug are prioritized to achieve enhanced recovery after surgery (ERAS). The available spectrum of drugs has hypnotics, opioids, muscle relaxants, and reversal agents of neuromuscular blockade, which nearly fall in the 'switch-on switch-off' category.

POSTGRADUATE TRAINING

Formal postgraduate training of medically qualified anesthesiologists began in 1935 with the Diploma in anaesthesia (DA) institution requiring one year's supervised clinical experience. With sophistication and complexity in the specialty, the training period for DA increased to 2 years. The essential qualification in anesthesiology now is Doctor of Medicine (MD) and Diplomate of the National Board (DNB). There is an increasing trend to have training as Doctorates in Medicine (DM) in anesthesiology subspecialties. Fellowships in certain niche areas are also in vogue. Competency-based training programs, introduced at the undergraduate level, are likely to be introduced at the postgraduate level.

SUBSPECIALIZATION IN ANESTHESIOLOGY

Anesthesiology is a specialty based on a state rather than a particular organ system and has an impressively diverse range of considerations to engage. In the last few decades, it has expanded to include multiple subspecialties (pediatric anesthesia, cardiothoracic anesthesia, obstetric anesthesia, transplant anesthesia, critical care, oncoanesthesia, and neuroanesthesia) that address specific clinical needs of patients undergoing surgical procedures. Anesthesiologists provide sedation, analgesia, and monitoring care to inpatients and outpatients. Other subspecialties evolving from the foundations in anesthesiology include pain medicine, palliative care, and sleep medicine. The skills of anesthesiologists have application outside the operating theatre. Other specialties seek anesthesiologists to perform trans-esophageal echocardiography and ultrasound-guided nerve interventions.

INCREASED DEMAND FOR ANESTHESIOLOGISTS

There is an expanding clinical demand for anesthesiologists. There is a significant deficiency in the smaller town and rural areas. The scope of practice had expanded from surgical suites and obstetric units to intensive care, pain clinics, preoperative evaluation centers, outpatient interventions, and other venues critical to the optimal care of surgical and medical patients. Anesthesiology is constantly facing the challenge of more and sicker patients. The aging population is expanding. Estimates say that those above 65 years will reach about 22% by 2050 (from about 17% in 2022). A corresponding increase of the 20–50% clinical anesthesia workload is expected. It will further accentuate the already deficient availability of qualified anesthesiologists. There has been a significant increase in the number of postgraduate trainees. However, despite these increased training positions, the shortage of trained anesthesiologists is expected to remain in the coming decades. The increased number of training positions has also increased the demand for eligible teachers.

CRITICAL CARE

Anaesthesiologists understand physiology and pharmacology and have resuscitation skills, and so are best suited to manage critical care units. Anesthesiologists have background knowledge of all medical conditions and surgical procedures and are trained to respond quickly. They have the requisite technical skills to treat the critically ill. They have an in-depth understanding of mechanical ventilation and hemodynamic management. They are experts in cardiopulmonary resuscitation. Their role in critical care is established and universally recognized. Their role during the COVID-19 epidemic has been lauded globally.

PERIOPERATIVE MEDICINE

Perioperative medicine encompasses the patient's care preoperatively, intraoperative, and postoperatively. Perioperative medicine involves surgeons, anesthesiologists, intensivists, and internal medicine consultants working in tandem. Anesthesiologists are being encouraged to take on the role of preoperative physicians. The specific knowledge needed includes risk assessment, risk reduction, management of operative complications, postoperative care, acquiring technical skills, and managing comorbid medical illness.

PERIOPERATIVE SURGICAL HOME

About a third of the costs related to perioperative care is attributable to hospital admission. Patient care is fragmented by multiple care transitions, with no ownership of a single provider in the perioperative period. Anesthesiologists, as perioperative physicians, can ensure seamless, coordinated care during transitions. Perioperative surgical home (PSH) has been proposed as a model to enhance surgical patient care. PSH is an extension of the perioperative medicine model. In this model, the anesthesiologist leads the perioperative care for surgical patients to improve outcomes. The PSH is a comprehensive pathway that includes the entire spectrum of care, from preoperative education and optimization processes to post-discharge and follow-up periods. The PSH is not intended to replace the surgeon's patient care responsibility but rather reduce his burden in perioperative care.

SAFE SURGERY

The advances in anesthesiology have dramatically reduced mortality rates from surgery by developing cutting-edge technologies, defining standards of care, and continuing education programs. The Anesthesia Patient Safety Foundation was founded to promote awareness and define protocols for managing critical incidents.

PRIDE OF PLACE IN THE MEDICAL PROFESSION

Anesthesiologists is increasingly gaining exposure to all aspects of clinical medicine, medical education, hospital-based utilization of resources, patient care, infection control, devising resuscitation programs, and leadership roles. They currently have an unprecedented representation among the country's medical university vice-chancellors, medical college deans, healthcare chief executive officers, chief operations officers of hospitals, advisory panels of the government, and other essential leadership positions.

ANESTHESIOLOGY AS A CAREER

Anesthesiology offers physicians unique opportunities. One can develop advanced expertise in pharmacology, manage the most vulnerable patients, work in acute care, emergencies, and pain palliation. A fresh anesthesiology postgraduate has the advantage of early settling down in clinical practice, unlike his counterparts in other specialties, who have a long learning curve.

The life of anesthesiologists is fast-paced, stressful, and intellectually demanding. However, the specialty is amenable to family life, with intense high-pressure workdays offset by ample personal time. Today, it is one of the better-paying medical specialties. It attracts outstanding talent as it offers reasonably high pay with an excellent work-life balance. Given this flexibility, anesthesiologists continue to practice well into their 70s. More and more women are entering the specialty considering the work-life balance.

MULTIPLE CHOICE QUESTION

1. Perioperative surgical home has been proposed as a model to enhance surgical patient care. In this:
   a. The surgical patient is managed in an entire surgery-based unit
   b. The patient is operated on for minor surgeries at his own home
   c. The anesthesiologist leads the perioperative care for surgical patients to improve outcomes
   d. The entire perioperative period is spent in a nursing home

Answers
1. c

CHAPTER 24

Ethics in Clinical Anesthesiology

Mukul Chandra Kapoor

Learning Objectives

- Principles of ethics
- Ethical responsibilities of anesthesiologists
- Ethical responsibilities of critical care Physicians
- International recommendations on ethics in anesthesia practice
- American society of anesthesiologists anesthesia-specific Ethics guideline

INTRODUCTION

The ethical principles described by Hippocrates have consistently guided the medical profession. The Hippocrates Oath focuses on benefiting the patient and providing the best care to him. These ethical principles have, over the years, been the guiding force for various medical councils, and all physicians take an oath to follow them. The principles are not laws but standards defining the moral behavior and conduct of the physician. Ethically, members of the medical profession are responsible primarily to the patient and secondarily to society, fellow professionals, and themselves.

Anesthesiologist John Bonica possibly shaped the future of medical ethics when he stated that pain was a "fundamental element of human suffering" and that pain relief is a fundamental human right. Anesthesiologists care for patients regardless of age, health, and illness. They administer life-sustaining technologies and procedures to support the patient.

ETHICS IN ANESTHESIA PRACTICE

AS1.3: Enumerate and describe the principle of ethics as it relates to anesthesiology.

The deplorable experimentation in the concentration camps during World War II and the beneficial advances in medical science have caused a rapid evolution in the ethical preservation of human rights. Ethics is a reflection of what is perceived as appropriate for society. It is based on the societal differentiation between right and wrong. The definition of ethics is, therefore, labile and is subject to the dynamics of the prevailing social, cultural, and economic vectors. The medical fraternity is severely regulated by ethical standards and statutory rules and regulations to benchmark ethical practice globally. The Indian Medical Council Act 1956 and the Professional Etiquette and Ethics Regulation 2002 govern and guide the specifics of the ethical practice of physicians in India.

Principle of Ethics

The treatise 'Principles of Biomedical Ethics' by Beauchamp and Childress is a magnificent discourse on the principles of ethics while analyzing alternative pathways. The four pillars of ethical practice are:
1. *Non-maleficence*: In essence, word, and spirit, the Hippocratic oath is an embodiment of non-maleficence. It promises a lifelong commitment to the tenet "Do no harm."
2. *Autonomy*: It respects the patient as an individual, capable of making learned decisions for themselves. It needs to be bereft of any form of external influence or coercion. This decision must be respected.
3. *Justice*: The provision of care has to be fair and without bias of race, religion, nationality, etc.
4. *Beneficence*: While non-maleficence involves the principle of *Do No Harm*, the principle of beneficence invokes the concept of *Do Good* to the patient in every situation.

Ethical Responsibilities of an Anesthesiologist

An anesthesiologist's prime responsibility is to ensure a legally valid and adequately explained informed consent for surgery or intervention. With the recognition of the autonomy of an aware and conscious patient in medical decision-making, it is essential to seek the patient's guidance and respect his/her decision within the constraints of the physician's own ethical belief. The patient has the right to refuse medical treatment, including life-sustaining therapy. The anesthesiologist should remember that there can be no informed consent without the opportunity for informed refusal.

Ethical Responsibilities of Critical Care Physicians

Critical care physicians face enduring questions of when to withdraw therapy, should they provide clinically nonindicated care, when to withdraw life support and when to declare an unconscious person dead. The biggest ethical dilemma faced by critical care physicians is to decide 'Do-not-resuscitate' (DNR) for non-salvageable patients. There is no legal support for a DNR order, but morally and ethically, the physician is bound to the wishes of the patient and his next of kin.

Major Ethical Issues

The major ethical issues faced by anesthesiologists are:
1. Patients' rights
2. Equity of resources
3. Patient confidentiality
4. Patient safety
5. Conflict of interests
6. Ethics of privatization
7. Informed consent: Ensure patient autonomy
8. Maintain sanctity of opposite sex
9. End of life
10. Healthcare team ethics
11. Nonmaleficence: '*do no harm*' to patients
12. Beneficence: physicians '*do good*' for the patient in every situation.

International Recommendations

The British Royal College of Anaesthetists signposted the general guidelines issued by the British Medical Association and the General Medical Council as the guiding principles. The Indian Society of Anesthesiologists has also issued some brief guidelines. Other national associations have issued guidelines covering consent.

The American Society of Anesthesiologists (ASA) recommends that its members adhere to the guidelines of the American Medical Association. Considering special issues faced by anesthesiologists, the ASA issued anesthesia-specific comprehensive ethics guidelines for its member anesthesiologists in 2013.

ASA ETHICAL GUIDELINE

(Excerpted from "Guidelines for the Ethical Practice of Anesthesiology, American Society of Anesthesiologists, 2020" of the American Society of Anesthesiologists. A copy of the full text can be obtained from ASA, 1061 American Lane Schaumburg, IL 60173-4973 or online at www.asahq.org")

There may be specific circumstances when elements of the following guidelines may not apply and wherein individualized decisions may be appropriate.

I. Anesthesiologists have ethical responsibilities to their patients.

1. The patient-physician relationship involves special obligations for the physician that include personal interaction with the patient, placing the patient's interests foremost, faithfully caring for the patient and being truthful.
2. Anesthesiologists respect the right of every patient to self-determination. Anesthesiologists should include patients, including minors, in medical decision-making that is appropriate to their developmental capacity and the medical issues involved. Anesthesiologists should not use their medical skills to restrain or coerce patients who have adequate decision-making capacity.
3. Anesthetized patients are particularly vulnerable, and anesthesiologists should strive to care for each patient's physical and psychological safety, comfort and dignity. Anesthesiologists should monitor themselves and their colleagues to protect the anesthetized patient from any disrespectful or abusive behavior.
4. Anesthesiologists should keep confidential patients' medical and personal information.
5. Anesthesiologists should provide preanesthetic evaluation and care and should personally provide or participate in the process of informed decision-making, especially regarding the choice of anesthetic technique.
6. Anesthesiologists should inform the patient if other physicians, physicians-in-training, or nonphysician providers are likely to participate in the patient's anesthesia care.
7. Anesthesiologists should be honest and forthcoming when describing their level of patient care involvement to their patient, the patient's family or surrogate, to hospitals, and the community. A description of such is an essential element of informed consent.
8. When working with nonphysician anesthesia providers or physicians-in-training in the provision of anesthesia care, anesthesiologists should remain personally and continuously available during the anesthetic; they should be able to directly participate in the most demanding aspects of the anesthetic care.
9. Anesthesiologists should provide for appropriate postanesthetic care for their patients.
10. Anesthesiologists should not participate in exploitive financial relationships.
11. Anesthesiologists share with all physicians the responsibility to provide care for patients irrespective of their ability to pay for their care. Anesthesiologists should provide such care with the same diligence and skill as for patients who do pay for their care.

II. Anesthesiologists have ethical responsibilities to medical colleagues.

1. Anesthesiologists should promote a cooperative and respectful relationship with their professional colleagues that facilitates quality medical care for patients. This responsibility respects the efforts and duties of other care providers including physicians, medical students, nurses, technicians and assistants.
2. Anesthesiologists should provide timely medical consultation when requested and should seek consultation when appropriate.
3. Anesthesiologists should cooperate with colleagues to improve the quality, effectiveness and efficiency of medical care.
4. Anesthesiologists should advise colleagues whose ability to practice medicine becomes temporarily or permanently impaired to appropriately modify or discontinue their practice. They should assist, to

the extent of their own abilities, with the re-education or rehabilitation of a colleague who is returning to practice.
5. Anesthesiologists should not take financial advantage of other physicians, nonphysician anesthesia providers or staff members. Verbal and written contracts should be honest and understandable, and should be respected.

III. Anesthesiologists have ethical responsibilities to the health care facilities in which they practice.
1. Anesthesiologists should serve on health care facility or specialty committees. This responsibility includes making good faith efforts to review the practice of colleagues and to help develop departmental or health care facility procedural guidelines for the benefit of the health care facility and all of its patients.
2. Anesthesiologists share with all medical staff members the responsibility to observe and report to appropriate authorities any potentially negligent practices or conditions which may present a hazard to patients or health care facility personnel.
3. Anesthesiologists personally handle many controlled and potentially dangerous substances and, therefore, have a special responsibility to keep these substances secure from illicit use. Anesthesiologists should work within their health care facility to develop and maintain an adequate monitoring system for controlled substances.

IV. Anesthesiologists have ethical responsibilities to themselves.
1. The achievement and maintenance of competence and skill in the specialty is the primary professional duty of all anesthesiologists. This responsibility does not end with completion of residency training or certification by the American Board of Anesthesiology.
2. The practice of quality anesthesia care requires that anesthesiologists maintain their physical and mental health and special sensory capabilities. If in doubt about their health, then anesthesiologists should seek medical evaluation and care. During this period of evaluation or treatment, anesthesiologists should modify or cease their practice.

V. Anesthesiologists have ethical responsibilities to their community and to society.
1. An anesthesiologist shall recognize a responsibility to participate in activities contributing to an improved community.
2. An anesthesiologist who serves as an expert witness in a judicial proceeding shall possess the qualifications and offer testimony in conformance with the ASA "Guidelines for Expert Witness Qualifications and Testimony."
3. An anesthesiologist shall not engage in misconduct in research and/or publication.
4. An anesthesiologist should take into account the environmental impact of their clinical management and decision-making.

Index

Page numbers followed by *b* refer to box, *f* refer to figure, and *t* refer to table

A
Abdomen 225
Accidental arterial injection 47
Acetaminophen 194
Acetylcholine 58, 61
Acid-base balance 112
Acidemia 216
Acidosis 206, 234
　metabolic 112
　respiratory 113
Activate emergency medical system 208*f*
Acupuncture 195
Acute coronary syndrome 206
Acute lung injury, transfusion-related 184
Acute respiratory distress syndrome 132
Acute transfusion reactions 184
Acute upper respiratory tract infection 16
Adenosine triphosphate 109
Advanced airway management 215
Advanced life support 210
Advanced monitoring 95, 134
Advanced trauma life support 223
Airway 11, 12, 22, 216, 221, 222, 224
　adjuncts 155
　assessment 31
　management 29, 40
　patency 29*f*
　protective reflexes 161
Aldrete recovery score, modified 126*t*
Alfentanil 142, 145
Alkalosis
　metabolic 113
　respiratory 113
Allay anxiety 166
Allodynia 187
Alpha 2-adrenergic receptors agonists 194
Ambulation 138
American Society of Anesthesiologists 38, 94, 147, 242
　classification 15
　features of 95*t*
　minimum monitoring standards 94
Amiodarone 215, 217
Amitrytiline 194
Anaerobic metabolism 117
Analgesia 20, 55, 145
　conscious 56
　postoperative 56
Analgesic
　drugs 155, 194*f*
　ladder 193*f*
　medications 193, 194*t*
　topical 195
Analyze rhythm 210*f*
Anesthesia 3, 42, 96*f*, 97*t*, 116, 145, 146, 160, 231, 232
　caudal 73, 74*f*
　combined spinal-epidural 67, 73
　continuous regional 84
　death 232
　　cause of 233
　delivery systems, development of 8
　dissociative 39, 148
　drug safety 200
　epidural 6, 67, 73, 156
　general 37, 78, 140, 153, 155
　global spread of 3
　induction of 56, 155
　infiltration 5
　inhalation 41
　intravenous 41
　　regional 6, 80, 82
　local 81*t*
　machine safety 200
　maintenance of 41, 56
　monitors, depth of 145
　nonoperating room 146, 147
　opioids free 42
　patient safety foundation 94
　practice 241
　record 232
　spinal 6, 67, 71, 153, 156
　technique 140, 232
　total intravenous 41, 140, 141, 155
Anesthesiology 238, 239
Anesthetic
　agents 234
　　development of 7
　　pharmacology of 44
　concerns 148
　death, investigation of 229
　management 163
　techniques 154
　　development of 5
Anterior spinal artery syndrome 76
Antibody screening 181
Anticipation 218
Antidepressants 194, 195
Antiepileptics 194
Anxiolysis 20
Apfel scoring system 155*t*
Arachnoiditis 76
Arterial blood
　gas 132
　pressure control 108
Arterial oxygen saturation 118
Artificial implants 202
Arytenoid cartilage 25
Asepsis 167
Aspiration, pulmonary 173
Assisted ventilation modes 131
Asthma 16
Atherosclerosis 108
Atracurium 63, 145
Atropine 64
Automated drug delivery systems, types of 143
Automated external defibrillator 206, 209, 209*f*
Autopsy 234
Autoregulation 117
Axillary approach 88
Axillary block 85, 86

B
Baclofen 195
Bag and mask ventilation 213*f*
Balanced anesthesia 7, 37
　triad 38
Basic anesthesia monitoring 95*t*
Basic cardiopulmonary life support 206, 206*f*, 207*f*
Benzocaine 82

Index

Benzodiazepines 194
Bicarbonate 81
Bier's block 82
Biopsy, collection of 203
Bio-psycho-social therapy 195
Bispectral index 41
Blood 18, 178
   components 178
     preparation 181
     quality of 183
     shelf-life of 183t
     uses of 182
   count 15
   disorders 180
   grouping 180
   management 178
   pressure 94, 96f, 114, 132
     invasive 100
     monitoring 100
   production, quality control of 182
   products 180
     transfusion 178, 179
     types of 179
   supply 23, 105, 119
   transfusion 178, 184, 234
     importance of 179
     reactions 184
Bloodstream infection, central line-associated 136, 137
Body temperature 95, 113
Bone 29f
   marrow 179
Botulinum toxin 195
Bowel care 127
Boyle's machine 8, 8f
Brachial block 88, 88f, 89f
Brachial plexus 84, 85t
   block 84, 85t, 86, 87f
     distribution of 84f
     organization of 84f
Bradycardia 75
Brain 105, 117, 189
   metabolism 117
Breathing 126, 213f, 216, 222, 224
   normal 208
Bronchi 28
Bronchioles 28
Bupivacaine 76, 80, 83

C

Cannabinoids 194
Cannulation 168
Capnography, phases of 104, 104f
Capsaicin 195
Carbamazepine 194
Carbon dioxide
   carriage 110
   partial pressure of 118
Carbon monoxide poisoning 112
Cardiac arrest 76, 216t
   cause of 205, 206t, 215
Cardiac disease 108
Cardiac function 161
Cardiac output 102, 118, 160, 179
   monitoring methods 102
Cardiopulmonary life support 205
Cardiovascular function 108
Cardiovascular system 13, 16, 74, 160
   protection 119
Carotid pulse 208
Cauda equina syndrome 76
Centers for Disease Control and Prevention 223
Central nervous system 18, 44, 54, 161, 225
   disease 108
   protection 116
Central neuraxial blockade 67, 74t, 76t
   complications of 76
   contraindications of 73
   indications of 73
   physiological effects of 74
   principle of 73
   types of 71
Central pain inhibiting mechanisms 190, 191
Central venous cannulation 170t
Central venous catheter 171
   insertion, complications of 172b
   measurement of 101
   placement, techniques of 169
Central venous pressure 102
   monitoring 101
Cerebral
   blood flow 116
   metabolic rate 117
   oxygenation 105, 118
Cerebrospinal fluid 72, 118
Cerebrovascular accident 17
Cervical spine, manual in-line stabilization of 221
Chemical linkage 79t
Chest 225
   compression 20f, 208, 209f, 213, 214f, 216, 217f, 218
   depth of 216
   ventilation ratio 217
   X-ray 15
Chin lift 213f

Chlorprocaine 80, 83
Cholinesterase inhibitor 64, 64t
   drugs 64t
Chronic obstructive pulmonary disease 11, 16
Circulation 95, 125, 126, 216, 222, 224
Cis-atracurium 63
Citrate-phosphate-dextrose-adenine 182
Clonidine 194
Coagulopathy, prevention of 119
Cocaine 5
Colloids 174
   classification of 174
Combat blood infections 179
Combitube 34f
Comprehensive cardiopulmonary life support 205, 210, 212f
Computer assistance 143
Computer assisted continuous infusion 146
Conduction block 5
Consciousness 126
Continuous noninvasive arterial pressure 100
Continuous positive airway pressure 132
Cord management 218
Coronary arterial disease 17
COVID-19 epidemic 238
Crash cart 126
Credé maneuver 127
Cricoid cartilage 24
Cryoprecipitate 179
Crystalloids 173
   classification of 173
Cuneiform cartilages 25

D

Daily spontaneous
   awakening trial 133
   breathing trial 133
Daycare anesthesia 151
   goals of 153
   mode of 153
   principle of 152
Daycare surgery 151
Death, investigation of 233
Deep sedation 158
Deep venous thrombosis 127, 138, 200
   prophylaxis 127, 164
Defibrillation 221
   early 209, 214
Dehydration 172
Dental surgery 153

Index

Depolarizing neuromuscular blocking agents 61, 62
Desflurane 52
Dexamethasone 155
Dexmedetomidine 49, 158
   dose of 49*t*
Dextrans 174
Diastolic dysfunction 134
Dibucaine 80
Diclofenac 194, 195
Disseminated intravascular coagulation 179
Dissociative drugs 148
Dobutamine 135
Dopamine 135
Dorsal root ganglion 189
Dorsolateral pontine tegmentum 190
Doxepin 195
Droperidol 155
Drugs 221
   administration of 44-46, 48-56, 215
   therapy 217
Duke activity status index 14, 16*t*
Duloxetine 194
Dyspnea 76

E
Early anesthesia delivery systems 8
Echocardiography, intraoperative 106
Edrophonium 64
Electrical therapy 217
Electrocardiogram 132, 145
   artifacts 98
   display modes 97
   monitoring 96
      benefits of 98
Electrocardiographic leads 96*f*
Electrocautery burns 202
Electrode placement 97
Electroencephalogram 145
Electrolytes 15
   balance 18, 206
Electronic health record 230
Embolism 206
Endocrine system 13, 18, 75, 162
Endotracheal intubation 30-32
Endotracheal tube 32, 32*f*, 40
End-tidal carbon dioxide 94, 114
   monitoring 103
Enhanced recovery after surgery 42, 173
Enteral nutrition 137
Enzyme acetylcholinesterase 59
Epiglottis 25

Epinephrine 135, 215, 217
Etomidate 45, 142
   induction dose of 46*t*
Extended-spectrum beta-lactamase inhibitors 137
Extravascular lung water index 136
Extremities 225
Eye protection 121

F
Face mask 29*f*
   design 29
   parts 29
Factors influencing cerebral oxygen
   consumption 118
   delivery 118
Femoral vein 169, 171
   cannulation of 171*f*
Fentanyl 55, 142, 145, 158, 194
Fetal hemoglobin 112
Fever 127
Flail chest 227, 227*f*
Fluid
   gelatins, modified 174
   intake, preoperative 173
   responsiveness 102
   status monitoring 102
   therapy 166, 172
      preoperative 174
Focused airway examination 12
Fresh frozen plasma 183

G
Gabapentin 194
Gamma-amino butyric acid 44, 50
Gantacurium 63
Gastric
   motility 20
   secretions 20
Gastrointestinal system 75
Gastrointestinal tract 121
Gelatins 174
Gelofusine 174
Genitourinary system 75
Global end-systolic volume 136
Glottis, laryngoscopic view of 25*f*
Glucose 15, 117, 206
Glycemic control 128, 199
Glycopyrollate 64
Good postoperative pain relief 154
Graft-versus-host disease, transfusion-associated 184
Granisetron 155
Guillain-Barre syndrome 62
Gynecology 153

H
H ions 206
Haldane effect 110
Hartmann's solution 175
Head 225
   tilt 213*f*
Hearing loss, transient 76
Heart
   functions 134
   protection of 119
   rate 96*f*, 113, 132
Hemodynamic management and vasoactive drug therapy 133
Hemoglobin
   level 118, 179
   oxygen
      absorption spectrum of 99*f*
      binding kinetics 111
      dissociation curve 111, 111*f*, 112*t*
   role of 110
Hemorrhage control 221
Hemothorax
   massive 226, 226*t*
   right side 226*f*
Hepatic system 14, 161
High-frequency jet ventilation 146
High-quality cardiopulmonary resuscitation 208, 211
Holding face mask 30
   CE technique of 30*f*
Horner's syndrome 76
Hydrogen ion 216
Hydroxy-ethyl starch 174
Hyperalgesia 187
Hyperglycemia 206
Hyperkalemia 206, 216
Hypertension 108
Hypertonic solutions 174
Hypoglycemia 206, 216
Hypokalemia 206, 216
Hypotension 96, 234
Hypothermia 206, 216
   prevention 220
Hypotonic solutions 174
Hypovolemia 172, 206, 216, 234
   preoperative 172
Hypoxemia 133
Hypoxia 206, 216

I
Iatrogenic patient injury 198
Ibuprofen 194
Indian Resuscitation Council 205, 206*f*, 207*f*, 211*f*, 212*f*
Indian Society of Anaesthesiologists 94

Indomethacin 194
Infections
  control 136, 200
  prevention of 136
  treatment of 136
Infraclavicular block, anatomical landmark of 88*f*
Inhalation agents 49, 155
Inhalation anesthetics 163
In-hospital cardiac arrest, pediatric chain of survival for 216*f*
Intensive care unit 129
  function of 129
  structure of 129
Intermittent positive-pressure ventilation 41
Internal jugular vein 169, 171
  cannulation of 170*f*
Interscalene block 84
  anatomical landmarks of 87*f*
Intra-arterial cannula 101*f*
Intracranial pressure 11, 74
Intravenous cannulae 168*t*
Intravenous fluids 173, 175*t*
Intravenous induction 39
Intravenous infusion set, components of 167*f*
Intubation 31, 31*f*
Invasive arterial monitoring 134
Ischemic attack, transient 17
Isoflurane 51
Isotonic solutions 173

J
Jaw thrust 213*f*

K
Ketamine 47, 142, 145, 149, 158
  dose of 47*t*
Kidney 18
  disease 108
  protection 120
Knee surgery, combination blocks for 90

L
Laryngeal mask airway 32, 33*f*
  uses of 33
Laryngeal nerve palsy, types of 27*f*
Laryngoscope 32*f*
  blades 40*f*
Laryngoscopy 31, 31*f*, 32
Laryngospasm 27
Larynx 24, 24*f*
  bone of 26
  muscles of 26
  nerve supply of 27

Laughing gas frolic party 2*f*
Left ventricular ejection fraction 146
Levobupivacaine 76, 80, 83
Life-threatening thoracic injuries 224
Ligaments 29*f*
Lignocaine 76, 80, 83, 215, 217
Limb protection 121
Liver 18
  function 15
  protection 121
Local anesthesia 81*t*
  discovery of 4
Local anesthetics 5, 6, 76, 79, 80, 81*t*, 189, 195
  agents
    classification of 79*t*, 80*t*
    comparative pharmacology of 80*t*
    clinical uses of 83*t*
Lower airway, anatomy of 28
Lumbar
  plexus nerve distribution 89
  puncture 6
Lung
  changes 161
  injury
    self-inflicted 131
    ventilator-induced 131, 132
  protective ventilation 41, 120, 132

M
Macintosh blade 32*f*
Major vessels, protection of 119
Mallampati classification, modified 12, 13*f*
Manual in-line stabilization 221, 221*f*
Marey's law 75
Mask holding C-E technique 213*f*
McGill pain 192
Mean arterial pressure 117, 118, 134, 176
Mechanical ventilation 41, 131
Meninges 68, 68*f*
Mental care 125
Mepivacaine 76, 80
Methemoglobinemia 82, 112
Methohexital 142, 145
Metoclopramide 155
Midazolam 48, 142, 145, 158
  dose of 48*t*
Minimal alveolar concentration 41
Minimum monitoring standards 94
Mivacurium 145
Modern anesthesia workstation 9*f*

Monitored anesthesia care 153, 156, 164
Morphine 53, 194
Mouth to mask ventilation 209*f*
Mucosal gland secretions 20
Muscles 26, 29*f*
  relaxants 7, 40, 145, 155
Musculoskeletal system 162
Myelitis 76
Myocardial infarction 17

N
Nasal cavity, lateral wall of 23*f*
Nasopharyngeal airway 214*f*
Nausea 76, 125
Neck 225
Needle stick injury 202
Neostigmine 64
Nerve
  blocks 195
  distribution of 85*t*
  localization techniques 82
  locators 83
  pathway 79*f*
N-ethylmaleimide-sensitive factor attachment protein receptors 60
Neural tissue toxicity 82
Neurologic system 11, 13
Neuromuscular blockade 61, 63, 64*f*, 133
  antagonism of 63
  reversal of 42
Neuromuscular junction 58
  structure of 59*f*
Neuromuscular monitoring 105
Neuromuscular transmission 58, 60
  physiology of 60*f*
Neurosurgery 118, 153
New York Heart Association 231
  classification 16, 17*t*
Nitric oxide 117
Nitrous oxide 1, 4, 49
N-methyl-D-aspartate 47, 50, 51, 190
Nondepolarizing neuromuscular blocking agents 61, 63, 63*t*
Noninvasive blood pressure 100, 134
  limitations of 100
  working principle of 100
Nonmalignant pain 187
  types of 188*t*
Non-steroidal anti-inflammatory drugs 20, 42, 154, 164, 194
Norepinephrine 135
Nortryptiline 194

Nose 22
Nosocomial infections 136
Numeric analog scale 191*f*
Numeric rating scale 191
Nursing care 138
Nutrition 128, 137

O

Obstructive sleep apnea 153
Ondansetron 155
Open tracheostomy 34
Ophthalmology 153
Opioids 39, 53, 81, 194, 195
    analgesia 193
Oral care 138
Organ
    protection 116
    systems, preoperative assessment of 13
Oropharyngeal airway 33*f*, 214*f*
Orthopedics 153
Otolaryngorhinology 153
Out-of-hospital cardiac arrest, pediatric chain of survival for 216*f*
Oxygen
    carriage 109, 110
    cascade 109, 110
    cerebral metabolic rate of 117
    content 110
    saturation 96*f*, 114, 126
        derivation of 98
    transport of 109
Oxygenation 95, 125
Oxy-poly-gelatins 174

P

Packed red blood cells 183
Pain 118, 186
    assessment 191
    central sensitization of 190
    chronic 186, 187
    inhibitory mechanisms 190
    malignant 187
    management 124, 164, 192
        methods of 193
    mediators 190, 190*f*
    pathways 186, 188, 191*f*
    physiology of 79
    processing 188
    relief, interventions for 195
Pancuronium 63
Parenteral nutrition 137
Peak-end-expiratory pressure 131
Pediatric
    advanced cardiac life support 219*f*
    basic life support 218*f*
    cardiopulmonary resuscitation 215
    surgery 153
Percutaneous central venous access 166
Peripheral intravenous access 166
Peripheral nerve
    block 80, 82, 153, 156
    locators 83*f*
    protection of 118
Peripheral nervous system 80
Peripheral pain inhibiting mechanisms 190
Peripheral vein, cannulation of 169*f*
Peripheral venous access 166
    devices 166
Pharmacodynamics 79
Pharmacokinetics 44-47, 49-56
    models 142*t*
    principles 141
Pharmacology 44, 162
Pharynx 23, 24*f*
Physostigmine 64
Plasma 179, 182
    normal 175
Plasmagel 174
Plasmalyte 175
Platelets 179, 182
Pneumomediastinum 132
Pneumonia, ventilator-associated 132, 136
Pneumothorax 132, 216
Poisons 206
Positive end-expiratory pressure 41, 102
Positive-pressure ventilation 218
Post-anesthesia
    care unit 43, 123
    sedation and respiratory depression, minimal risk of 154
Post-operative care unit
    protocols 124
    recovery assessment 125
Postoperative cognitive dysfunction 125, 165
Postoperative nausea and vomiting 42, 125, 146, 155, 157
    minimal risk of 154
Postoperative pain management 156
Post-resuscitation care 215
Preanesthetic assessment plan 11*t*, 231
Precardiac arrest condition, management of 211
Pregabalin 194
Pregnancy test 15
Premedication 19, 20*t*, 38
    purposes of 20
Preoperative airway examination, components of 12*t*
Preoperative drug therapy 18
Preoperative intravenous fluid therapy, goals of 172
Preoxygenation 39
Preprocedural medications 147
Pressure
    controlled ventilation 41
    support ventilation 132
    transducer
        system 101*f*
        working principle of 101
Prilocaine 80, 82, 83
Procaine 80
Procedural sedation, drugs used for 158
Prophylaxis, stress-related 138
Propofol 44, 45*t*, 142, 145, 158
Pulmonary artery catheter 102
Pulmonary vascular resistance 134
Pulse 213*f*
    oximeter plethysmograph 96*f*
    oximetry 98
        limitations of 99
    plethysmograph 99, 99*f*
        normal 99*f*
Puncture 71
Pyridostigmine 64

R

Radiculitis 76
Radiological procedure 157
Raised intracranial pressure 206
Rapid sequence induction 40
Red blood cells 178, 179, 182
Regional anesthesia 7, 78, 84*t*, 140, 153, 156, 163
    potential complications of 84
    techniques 82*t*
Rehabilitation 165
Remifentanil 56, 142, 145
Renal system 14, 161
Residual neuromuscular blockade 64
Respiratory gas monitoring 105
Respiratory system 16, 75, 161
    protection 119
Respiratory tract, optimization of 17
Respiratory waveform 96*f*
Resuscitation 174, 205, 220*f*, 224*t*
    cardiopulmonary 205, 217
    ensure safe place for 211
    equipment 126*t*

Revised cardiac risk index 15, 16t
Ringer's lactate 175
Rocuronium 63
Ropivacaine 76, 80, 83
Rostral ventral medulla 190

S
Sacral
   canal 70f
   hiatus 74f
Sacrum 70, 70f
Safe surgery 239
Safe transfusion 183
Salivary gland 20
Scene safety 206, 208f
Schimmelbusch mask 8, 8f
Scoline 62
Sedation 138, 145
   levels of 157
   moderate 158
Seldinger's technique 169f
Sevoflurane 51
Shock 133
   electric 210f
Shoulder, position of 209f
Skeletal muscles 58
Society for Ambulatory Anesthesia 151
Sodium
   pentothal 7
   thiopental 46
Spinal cord 67, 68f, 69f, 188
   anatomy 67
   cross-section of 189f
   protection 118
   stimulation 195
Spinal nerves 68f, 69
Spirometry 105
Spontaneous breathing trial 132
Steroid 81
Stimulation techniques 195
Subarachnoid hemorrhage 206
Subclavian vein 169, 170f, 171
Succinyl choline 62
Succinylated fluid gelatins 174
Succinylcholine 145
Sufentanil 142, 145
Sugammadex 64
Supraclavicular block 85-87
   anatomical landmark of 87f
Surgeries, cardiac 118
Surgical hand hygiene technique 201f
Suxamethonium 62
Swan Ganz catheter 102

Synaptic cleft 59
Synchronized intermittent mandatory ventilation 132
Synchronized mandatory minute ventilation 133
Systemic vascular resistance 134
Systolic dysfunction 134

T
Tamponade 206, 216
Target controlled infusion system 143
Temperature 114, 206
   homeostasis 75
   management 124
   monitoring 103
   safety 202
Tension pneumothorax 206, 216, 224, 226
   clinical signs of 226t
   right side 225f
Therapeutic hypothermia 103
Thermodilution cardiac output 102
Thiopentone 142, 145
Thoracic compliance 161
Three-compartment pharmacokinetic model 141f
Three-electrode system modifications 98t
Thrombophlebitis prevention 169
Thrombosis 216
   pulmonary 206
Thyroid cartilage 25
Total intravenous anesthesia 144b, 145
   advantages of 146
   conduct of 142
   disadvantages of 146
   indications of 141, 141b
Toxins 206, 216
Trachea 28
Tracheal extubation 42
Tracheal protection 120
Tracheostomy 34
   percutaneous 34, 35f
Transcutaneous cerebral oximetry 118
Transcutaneous electrical nerve stimulation 195
Trauma
   care 221
   victim, triage of 222
Triage color coding 223t

Tricyclic antidepressants 195
Triple airway maneuver 30, 30f
Triptans 194
Tuberculosis 11
Tubocurarine 63
Two thumb technique 217f
Typical crash cart 126t

U
Upper airway
   anatomy of 22
   cervical fascia of 29f
   obstruction 28
Upper extremity, peripheral nerves of 89
Upper limb, veins of 168f
Urea-cross-linked gelatins 174
Urinalysis 15
Urinary care 127
Urinary retention 76
Urinary tract infection, catheter-associated 127, 136
Urology 153

V
Vascular access 220
Vascular surgeries 118, 153
Vasoactive drug therapy 134
Vasoconstrictors 81
Vasopressin 135
Vecuronium 63, 145
Venlafaxine 194
Ventilation 95
Ventilator function 133
Vertebral column 69f, 70
   cross-section of 69f
Visual analog scale 124, 191, 192f
Vocal cord 26
   palsy 27
   position of 26f, 27f
Volatile anesthetic, effect of 117
Volume controlled ventilation 41
Vomiting 76, 125

W
Weaning off ventilator 133
White blood cells 179
Wong-Baker face pain rating scale 192, 192f
Wound care 126

Z
Ziconotide 195